PEDIATRIC HEMATOLOGY & ONCOLOGY

PEDIATRIC HEMATOLOGY & ONCOLOGY

SECRETS

MICHAEL WEINER, MD
Hettinger Professor Emeritus of Pediatrics, Columbia University Irving Medical Center, New York, NY

DARRELL J. YAMASHIRO, MD, PhD
Professor of Pediatrics, Pathology & Cell Biology, Pediatrics, Columbia University Irving Medical Center, New York, NY

PRAKASH SATWANI, MD
Professor, Pediatrics, Columbia University Irving Medical Center, New York, NY

MONICA BHATIA, MD
Associate Professor, Pediatrics, Columbia University Irving Medical Center, New York, NY

CINDY NEUNERT, MD, MSCS
Associate Professor, Pediatrics, Columbia University Irving Medical Center, New York, NY

ELSEVIER

Elsevier
1600 John F. Kennedy Blvd.
Ste 1800
Philadelphia, PA 19103-2899

PEDIATRIC HEMATOLOGY & ONCOLOGY SECRETS   ISBN: 978-0-323-81047-0
Copyright © 2024 by Elsevier, Inc. All rights reserved.

Notice

Practitioners and researchers must always rely on their own experience and knowledge in evaluating and using any information, methods, compounds, or experiments described herein. Because of rapid advances in the medical sciences, in particular, independent verification of diagnoses and drug dosages should be made. To the fullest extent of the law, no responsibility is assumed by Elsevier, authors, editors, or contributors for any injury and/or damage to persons or property as a matter of products liability, negligence or otherwise, or from any use or operation of any methods, products, instructions, or ideas contained in the material herein.

Previous edition copyrighted 2002.

Content Strategist: Marybeth Thiel
Content Development Specialist: Casey Potter
Project Manager: Julie Taylor
Design Direction: Bridget Hoette

Printed in India

Last digit is the print number: 9 8 7 6 5 4 3 2

Working together
to grow libraries in
developing countries

www.elsevier.com • www.bookaid.org

CONTRIBUTORS

Maha Al-Ghafry, MD
Transfusion Medicine Fellow
Columbia University Irving Medical Center
New York, NY

Charlotte Alme, MD
Pediatric Bone Marrow Transplant Attending
Oslo University Hospital
Oslo, Norway

Bachir Alobeid, MD
Professor of Pathology and Cell Biology
Pathology and Cell Biology
Columbia University Irving Medical Center
New York, NY

Staci D. Arnold, MD, MBA, MPH
Associate Professor
Pediatrics
Aflac Cancer and Blood Disorders Center at Children's
    Healthcare of Atlanta, Emory University, Atlanta, GA

Megan Askew, MD
Hope and Heroes Fellow
Division of Pediatric Hematology, Oncology,
    and Stem Cell Transplantation
Columbia University Irving Medical Center
New York, NY

Melissa P. Beauchemin, PhD, RN, CPNP
Postdoctoral Research Fellow
Epidemiology
Columbia University Irving Medical Center
New York, NY

Monica Bhatia, MD
Associate Professor
Pediatrics
Columbia University Irving Medical Center
New York, NY

Michelle Bombacie, MS, LAc, LMT
Program Manager
Integrative Therapies
Division of Pediatric Hematology, Oncology,
    and Stem Cell Transplantation
Columbia University Irving Medical Center
New York, NY

Mary Ann Bonilla, MD
Assistant Professor of Pediatrics
Rowan University School of Osteopathic Medicine
Stratford, NJ
Attending Physician
Pediatric, Hematology/Oncology
St. Joseph's Children's Hospital
Paterson, NJ

Gary M. Brittenham, MD
James A. Wolff Professor of Pediatrics and Professor of
    Medicine
Pediatrics
Columbia University Irving Medical Center
New York, NY

Larisa Broglie, MD, MS
Assistant Professor
Pediatrics
Medical College of Wisconsin
Milwaukee, WI

Jing Chen, MD
Division of Pediatric Oncology
Hackensack University Medical Center
Hackensack, NJ

Eileen Connolly, MD, PhD
Assistant Professor of Radiation Oncology
New York Presbyterian/Columbia University Medical
    Center
Department of Radiation Oncology
Columbia University Irving Medical Center
New York, NY

Caitlin Constantino, MA Ed
Educational Liaison
Department of Pediatrics
Division of Hematology, Oncology & Stem Cell
    Transplantation
Columbia University Medical Center
New York, NY

Laurie Davis, MD, PhD
Assistant Professor
Division of Pediatric Hematology, Oncology,
    & Stem Cell Transplantation
Children's Hospital of San Antonio
Baylor College of Medicine
San Antonio, TX

Larisa Debelenko, MD, PhD
Associate Professor
Pathology and Cell Biology
Columbia University Irving Medical Center
New York, NY

Filemon S. Dela Cruz, MD
Assistant Attending
Department of Pediatrics
Memorial Sloan Kettering Cancer
    Center/MSK Kids
New York, NY

Nader Kim El-Mallawany, MD
Assistant Professor
Texas Children's Cancer & Hematology Centers
Baylor College of Medicine
Houston, TX

Katie Ender, MDMD, MD
Assistant Professor
Pediatric Anemia and Red Blood Cell Hematology
Pediatric Coagulation Disorder Hematology
Pediatric Platelet Disorder Hematology
Columbia University Irving Medical Center
New York, NY

Erica M. Fallon, MD
Assistant Professor of Surgery
Division of Pediatric Surgery
Morgan Stanley Children's Hospital of
    NY-Presbyterian
Columbia University Irving Medical Center
New York, NY

Marc D. Foca, MD
Associate Professor of Pediatrics
Columbia University
New York, NY
Department of Pediatrics
Albert Einstein College of Medicine
Children's Hospital at Montefiore
Bronx, NY

Matthew Gallitto, MD
Resident Physician
Department of Radiation Oncology
Columbia University Irving Medical Center
New York, NY

Bradley Gampel, MD, MS
Chief Fellow
Division of Pediatric Hematology, Oncology,
    and Stem Cell Transplantation
Columbia University Irving Medical Center
New York, NY

Robyn D. Gartrell, MD, MS
Assistant Professor of Pediatrics
Division of Pediatric Hematology, Oncology,
    and Stem Cell Transplantation
Department of Pediatrics
Columbia University Irving Medical Center
New York, NY

James Garvin, Jr, MD, PhD
Professor of Pediatrics
Pediatrics
Columbia University Irving Medical Center
New York, NY

David Gass, MD, MS
Assistant Professor of Pediatrics
Wake Forest School of Medicine
Atrium Health Levine Children's Cancer and Blood
    Disorders
Charlotte, NC

Gabriella E. George, Psy.M.
Doctoral Candidate, School Psychology
Graduate School of Applied and
    Professional Psychology
Rutgers the State University
Rutgers University
New Jersey, NJ

Julia Glade Bender, MD
Vice Chair
Clinical Research
Department of Pediatrics
Memorial Sloan Kettering Cancer Center
New York, NY

Chana L. Glasser, MD
Associate Professor of Pediatrics
Pediatric Hematology/Oncology
NYU Langone Hospital — Long Island
Mineola, NY

Rudi-Ann Graham, MD, BSc
Clinical Fellow
Division of Pediatric Hematology, Oncology,
    and Stem Cell Transplantation
Columbia University Irving Medical Center
New York, NY

Linda Granowetter, MD
Professor of Pediatrics (retired)
Pediatrics
NYU Grossman School of Medicine
New York, NY

Nancy S. Green, MD
Professor
Pediatrics
Columbia University Irving Medical Center
New York, NY

Nitya Gulati, MBBS
Department of Pediatrics
Section of Hematology/Oncology
Baylor College of Medicine
Texas Children's Cancer & Hematology Centers
Houston, TX

Nobuko Hijiya, MD
Department of Pediatrics
Columbia University Irving Medical Center
New York, NY

Jess Hochberg, MD
Assistant Professor Pediatrics
Director Hematologic Malignancy Program
Children and Adolescent Cancer and Blood Diseases
Center Maria
Fareri Children's Hospital New York Medical
College
Valhalla, NY

Lenat Joffe, MD, MS
Division of Pediatric Hematology, Oncology,
and Stem Cell Transplantation
Columbia University Irving Medical Center
New York, NY

Angela V. Kadenhe-Chiweshe, MD
Assistant Professor of Surgery
Weill Cornell Medical College
New York, NY

Justine M. Kahn, MD, MS
Assistant Professor of Pediatrics
Department of Pediatrics
Division of Pediatric Hematology, Oncology,
and Stem Cell Transplantation
Columbia University Irving Medical Center
New York, NY

Shipra Kaicker
Associate Professor of Pediatrics
Division of Pediatric Hematology/Oncology
Weill Cornell Medical College
New York, NY

Dominder Kaur, MD
Assistant Professor
Pediatrics
Columbia University Irving Medical Center
New York, NY

Kara M. Kelly, MD
Waldemar J. Kaminski Endowed Chair of Pediatrics
Pediatric Oncology
Roswell Park Cancer Institute
Division Chief, Pediatric Hematology/Oncology and
Research Professor
Pediatrics
University at Buffalo School of Medicine and
Biomedical Sciences
Buffalo, NY

Michael D. Kinnaman, MD
Instructor
Department of Pediatrics
Memorial Sloan Kettering Cancer Center/MSK Kids
New York, NY

Manpreet Kochhar
Attending Physician, Pediatric Hematology-Oncology
Hasbro Children's Hospital
Assistant Professor, Department of Pediatrics
The Warren Alpert Medical School of Brown University
Providence, RI

Jennifer Krajewski, MD
Attending Physician
Pediatric Transplantation and Cellular
Therapy
Hackensack University Medical Center
Assistant Professor
Pediatrics
Hackensack Meridian School of Medicine
Hackensack, NJ

Justin L. Kurtz, MD
Clinical Laboratory Director
Children's National Hospital
Washington, DC

Elena J. Ladas, PhD, RD
Sid and Helaine Lerner Associate Professor for Global
Integrative Medicine
Division of Pediatric Hematology, Oncology,
and Stem Cell, Transplantation
Department of Pediatrics in Epidemiology and in the
Institute of Human Nutrition
Columbia University Irving Medical Center
New York, NY

Jennifer Levine, MD, MSW
Associate Professor of Clinical Pediatrics
Department of Pediatrics
Division of Hematology-Oncology
Weill Cornell Medicine
New York, NY

Margaret T. Lee, MD, MS
Division of Pediatric Hematology, Oncology,
and Stem Cell Transplantation
Columbia University Irving Medical Center
New York, NY

Kristin Lieb, MD
Assistant Attending
Pediatric Oncology
Memorial Sloan Kettering Cancer Center
New York, NY

Chinwe Madubata, MD, MSCI
Clinical Residency Fellow
Department of Pathology and Cell Biology
Columbia University Irving Medical Center
New York, NY

Mahesh M. Mansukhani, MD
Professor of Pathology and Cell Biology
Director, Laboratory of Personalized Genomic
  Medicine
Columbia University Irving Medical Center
New York, NY

Lianna J. Marks, MD
Clinical Assistant Professor
Pediatrics
Stanford University School of Medicine
Palo Alto, CA

Catherine McGuinn, MD
Assistant Professor
Pediatrics
Weill Cornell Medicine
New York, NY

Jill S. Menell, MD
Assistant Professor of Pediatrics
Rowan University School of Osteopathic
  Medicine
Stratford, NJ
Chief, Pediatric Hematology/Oncology
St. Joseph's Children's Hospital
Paterson, NJ

Regina Myers, MD
Instructor of Pediatrics
Division of Oncology and Cancer,
  Immunotherapy Program
Children's Hospital of Philadelphia
Philadelphia, PA
Department of Pediatrics
University of Pennsylvania School of Medicine
Philadelphia, PA

Hanna E. Minns
Research Technician
Division of Pediatric Hematology/Oncology
Department of Pediatrics
Columbia University Irving Medical Center
New York, NY

Hanna Moisander Joyce, MD, MSc
Assistant Attending
Department of Pediatrics
Division of Hematology, Oncology,
  and Stem Cell Transplantation
Columbia University Irving Medical Center
New York, NY

Cindy Neunert
Associate Professor
Pediatrics
Columbia University Irving Medical Center
New York, NY

Jennifer Oberg, EdD, MA
Assistant Professor of Pediatrics
Division of Pediatric Hematology, Oncology,
  and Stem Cell Transplantation
Columbia University Irving Medical Center
New York, NY

Manuela Orjuela, MD, ScM
Assistant Professor
Pediatrics (Oncology)
Columbia University Irving Medical Center
New York, NY

Andrew Myles Parrott, MD, PhD
Pathology & Cell Biology
Columbia University Irving Medical Center
New York, NY

Jovana Pavisic, MD, MA
Assistant Professor of Pediatrics
Division of Pediatric Hematology, Oncology,
  and Stem Cell Transplantation
Columbia University Irving Medical Center
New York, NY

Lia N. Phillips, MD, MPH
Clinical Fellow
Division of Pediatric Hematology, Oncology,
  and Stem Cell Transplantation
Columbia University Irving Medical Center
New York, NY

Evelyn M. Ramirez, PhD
Clinical Postdoctoral Fellow
Division of Child and Adolescent Psychiatry, Psychiatry
Columbia University Irving Medical Center
New York, NY

Angela Ricci, MD
Assistant Professor of Pediatrics
Section of Pediatric Hematology/Oncology
Dartmouth-Hitchcock Medical Center
Lebanon, NH

Jaclyn D. Rosenzweig, MD
Pediatric Hematology/Oncology Fellow
Department of Pediatrics
Memorial Sloan Kettering Cancer Center
New York, NY

Prakash Satwani, MD
Professor of Pediatrics
Director, Cellular Therapy Program
Director, Hope and Heroes Fellowship Program
Division of Pediatric Hematology, Oncology,
  and Stem Cell Transplantation
Columbia University Irving Medical Center
New York, NY

Andrew M. Silverman, MD
Pediatric Hematology and Oncology
Department of Pediatrics
K. Hovnanian Children's Hospital
Jersey Shore University Medical Center
Hackensack Meridian Health
Neptune City, NJ

Dara M. Steinberg, PhD
Assistant Professor of Medical Psychology
Department of Pediatrics
Division of Hematology, Oncology,
   and Stem Cell Transplantation
Department of Psychiatry
Division of Child and Adolescent Psychiatry
Columbia University Irving Medical Center
New York, NY

Sujit Sheth, MD
Professor
Pediatrics
Weill Cornell Medicine
New York, NY

Maria Luisa Sulis, MD, MS
Member, Attending Physician
Pediatrics
Memorial Sloan Kettering Cancer Center
New York, NY

Luca Szalontay, MD
Assistant Professor of Pediatrics
Division of Pediatric Hematology, Oncology,
   and Stem Cell Transplantation
Department of Pediatrics
Columbia University Irving Medical Center
New York, NY

Amy Tang, MD
Assistant Professor
Pediatrics
Children's Healthcare of Atlanta, Emory University
Atlanta, GA

Meghan F. Tomb, PhD
Assistant Professor of Medical Psychology
Division of Child and Adolescent Psychiatry
Psychiatry
Columbia University Irving Medical Center
New York, NY

Joyce Varkey, DO
Assistant Professor
Department of Pediatrics, Section of Hematology-Oncology
Baylor College of Medicine
Houston, TX

Andrea Webster Carrion, MD
Fellow in Pediatric Neuro-Oncology at The Children's
   Hospital of Philadelphia
Philadelphia, PA

Michael Weiner, MD
Hettinger Professor Emeritus of Pediatrics
Columbia University Irving Medical Center
New York, NY

Stuart P. Weisberg, MD, PhD
Assistant Professor of Pathology and Cell Biology
Department of Pathology and Cell Biology
Columbia University Irving Medical Center
New York, NY

Cheng-Chia Wu, MD, PhD
Tenure Track Assistant Professor
   of Radiation Oncology
New York-Presbyterian/Columbia University Medical
   Center
Department of Radiation Oncology
Columbia University Irving Medical Center
New York, NY

Darrell J. Yamashiro, MD, PhD
Professor of Pediatrics, Pathology & Cell Biology
Pediatrics
Columbia University Irving Medical Center
New York, NY

Stergios Zacharoulis, MD
Division of Pediatric Hematology, Oncology,
   and Stem Cell Transplantation
Pediatrics
Columbia University Irving Medical Center
New York, NY

PREFACE

Pediatric Hematology/Oncology Secrets, Second Edition, is a textbook targeted to physicians in training, practitioners, and other health professionals engaged in the diagnosis and care of children with blood disorders, cancer, and immune deficiencies. This book contains a comprehensive set of questions and answers to a variety of childhood disorders, including hemoglobinopathies, hemolytic anemias, coagulation disorders, marrow failure syndromes, and immune dysregulation, and also addresses stem cell transplant, cellular therapies, and gene replacement therapy. This multidisciplinary and comprehensive review of pediatric hematology-oncology provides the reader with an easy-to-read format and suggested reading lists with current "secrets" to the diagnosis and management of children with these specific disorders.

We trust that this book will be a valuable resource and will provide secrets that will enable our colleagues to enhance the care of children and adolescents afflicted with cancer and blood disorders.

ACKNOWLEDGMENTS

We wish to acknowledge the protean contributions of physicians and healthcare providers engaged in the care of children and adolescents with cancer and blood diseases.

Michael Weiner, MD
Darrell J. Yamashiro, MD, PhD
Prakash Satwani, MD
Monica Bhatia, MD
Cindy Neunert, MD

To our patients, their families, and the entire staff at the Herbert Irving Child and Adolescent Oncology Center.

CONTENTS

III ONCOLOGIC DISEASES

IV   STEM CELL AND CELLULAR THERAPIES

TOP 100 SECRETS

HEMATOLOGY

1. The prothrombin time (PT) represents the extrinsic clotting system. Prolongation of just the PT is an indication of low factor VII levels. This can be because of congenital factor VII deficiency, vitamin K deficiency, liver disease, or disseminated intravascular coagulopathy (DIC). The activated partial thromboplastin time (aPTT) represents the intrinsic pathway. Prolongation of just the aPTT is because of deficiencies in factors XII, XI, IX, and/or VIII. These deficiencies may be congenital or because of the acquired conditions previously listed. Prolongation of both the PT and aPTT is usually because of a deficiency in more than one factor (liver disease, vitamin K deficiency, or DIC) or a common pathway factor (factor X, V, II, and fibrinogen). Factor XIII deficiency is the only factor deficiency that will have a normal PT and aPTT.

2. The coagulation system is immature in the neonatal phase, with many of the coagulation proteins being reduced at birth. In the procoagulant system, the contact factors (high-molecular-weight kininogen, prekallikrein, factors XII and XI) and the vitamin K–dependent factors (II, VII, IX, and X) are reduced to about 30% to 50% of the adult range in the term newborn infant and even more reduced in a preterm infant. For this reason, coagulation studies in neonates need to be compared with age-appropriate normal values.

3. The incidence of deep vein thrombosis (DVT) in children is reported to be 0.07 to 0.14 per 10,000, and although incidence may be rising, DVTs in children are much less frequent than in adults. There is a bimodal distribution, with neonates/infants and teenagers being at highest risk. In the majority of the cases (>95%), thromboses are secondary to other risk factors (i.e., central venous catheters and any underlying medical conditions). Therefore most children with a DVT do not need testing for thrombophilia unless they have a family history of thrombosis or recurrent DVTs.

4. Hemorrhagic anemia is the most common cause of anemia in the full term newborn infant. Antepartum fetomaternal hemorrhage (FMH) occurs in approximately 75% of pregnancies. The risk is increased with pre-eclampsia, the need for instrumentation, and cesarean delivery. Massive FMH is defined as more than 20% blood loss from the fetoplacental circulation. Fetomaternal hemorrhage can be quantified either by staining the blood film of the mother for the proportion of fetal cells (the Kleihauer Betke test) or by flow cytometry.

5. Sickle cell disease (SCD) is an autosomal recessive inherited blood disorder caused by mutation in the ß-globin gene. Hemoglobin (Hb) S (an abnormal hemoglobin) polymerizes under deoxygenated conditions, leading to formation of distorted "sickle-shaped" erythrocytes. It is prevalent in individuals of African, Middle Eastern, Southern European, and Indian ethnicity. Globally, an estimated 300,000 babies are born with the disease annually, with 80% in Africa.

6. Functional asplenia develops in almost all individuals with HbSS or HbSß^0-thalassemia by age 3 to 5 years, making them susceptible to infections caused by *Streptococcus pneumoniae, Haemophilus influenzae,* and other encapsulated organisms. To decrease risk of sepsis, penicillin prophylaxis is started at 1 to 2 months of age or as soon as diagnosis is made for patients with Hb SS and HbSß^0-thalassemia. Penicillin prophylaxis can be discontinued at age 5 years unless the patient has a history of splenectomy or previous invasive pneumococcal infection.

7. Hydroxyurea is the most widely used medication for SCD. The primary function is fetal hemoglobin (HbF) induction, which retards erythrocyte sickling. Hydroxyurea use reduces vaso-occlusive events, hospitalizations, acute chest syndrome, and the need for red cell transfusions. Its use has also been shown to have protective effects against silent organ damage in kidneys, spleen, lungs, brain, and more.

8. Hemolytic disorders of the red blood cell (RBC) can originate either inside the RBC (intrinsic) or outside of the RBC (extrinsic). Hemolysis can be classified as either intravascular or extravascular. Intravascular hemolysis occurs, as its name suggests, within the blood vessels and is complement or shear mediated. Extravascular hemolysis occurs in the reticuloendothelial system (spleen or liver) as a result of macrophage digestion of RBC.

9. Two common intrinsic red cell disorders include hereditary spherocytosis (HS) and G6PD deficiency. HS is caused by deficiency of RBC membrane proteins of spectrin, ankyrin, and band 3. HS is the most common RBC membrane disorder. Although it is most commonly inherited in autosomal dominant fashion, HS can also be the result of autosomal recessive inheritance. G6PD deficiency is the most common enzymopathy. Normal G6PD functions to protect RBC from oxidative damage. With G6PD deficiency, RBCs are susceptible to damage from oxidative insults, leading to RBC destruction, intravascular hemolysis, and anemia. It is inherited as an X-linked disorder.

10. Intravascular and extravascular hemolysis can be differentiated by labs. Intravascular hemolysis typically causes more profound elevation of lactate dehydrogenase (LDH) and reduction of haptoglobin, as well as hemoglobinemia and hemoglobinuria. Extravascular hemolysis typically leads to more modest changes in LDH and haptoglobin. Overall, extravascular hemolysis is more common in pediatrics.

11. Normal Hb is a heterodimer of two globins produced as a result of expression of genes from the α-globin gene cluster on chromosome 16 and two globins produced as a result of expression of genes from the β-globin gene cluster on chromosome 11. Thalassemia refers to a group of congenital disorders of globin synthesis in which there is decreased or absent production of one of the two subunits of hemoglobin. Thus, it is a quantitative hemoglobinopathy.

12. The clinical severity of α-thalassemia depends on the number of genes affected. When a single α-globin gene is abnormal, this is α-thalassemia silent carrier state (α-/$\alpha\alpha$), which is typically associated with a normal complete blood count (CBC). When two genes are abnormal, this is α-thalassemia trait, which is associated with mild microcytic anemia. The two deleted genes can be inherited in a cis formation with both deletions on the same gene (–/$\alpha\alpha$), more common in Southeast Asia, or a trans formation with one deletion on each gene (α-/α-), more common in Africa. When three genes are abnormal (α -/–), the result is HbH disease, which is associated with a moderate symptomatic microcytic anemia. Finally, when all four genes are nonfunctional (–/–), no α-globin is produced, resulting in the absence of HbF in the second trimester of pregnancy, with resulting severe anemia and hydrops fetalis, termed α-thalassemia major.

13. Beta thalassemia severity also varies based on the genotype. At one end of the spectrum of severity is (β0/β0) thalassemia or β-thalassemia major. With the inability to make any normal HbA, these individuals are transfusion dependent from early infancy. Individuals with less severe genotypes (β+/β+, β0/β+), in which some functional β-globin is produced, have an intermediate phenotype (β-thalassemia intermedia) with variable severity of anemia and transfusion requirements, depending on the mutations. Lastly, there is β-thalassemia trait (β/β0 or β/β +), or minor, where individuals have an asymptomatic mild microcytic anemia and no other complications.

14. Globally, iron deficiency is by far the most common cause of nutritional anemia in infants, children, and adolescents. Deficiencies of vitamin B12 (cobalamin) and folate are much less common but account for most other nutritional anemia.

15. A full CBC and serum ferritin are optimal for screening for iron deficiency, with or without anemia. Universal screening for iron deficiency, with or without anemia, is suggested at 9 to 12 months of age, again at 15 to 18 months of age, and lastly for females at about age 14 for those who are at least one-year post-menarche and for males during their peak growth period. Additional screening should be considered for those with heightened risk of iron deficiency, such as low iron diets, blood donation, and females with increased menstrual losses.

16. Benign ethnic neutropenia can occur commonly in individuals of African, Caribbean, Middle Eastern, and West Indian descent. Most patients have an absolute neutrophil count (ANC) between 1000 and 1500 cells/μL. The diagnosis is confirmed by demonstrating a stable platelet count at least 2 weeks apart. No treatment is needed.

17. Autoimmune neutropenia of childhood is generally a benign disorder. Affected individuals are often found incidentally with a routine blood count or when diagnosed with a minor infection. Despite ANCs of less than 500 cells/μl, 80% to 90% of patients do not have severe infectious complications. The median age at diagnosis is 8 months with a range of 3 to 30 months. The disease is self-limited, often resolving by 4 years of age.

18. Immune thrombocytopenic purpura (ITP) in children is most often acute and self-limited. The decision to treat is based on the severity of bleeding symptoms (past or present), lifestyle and activity of the patient, and other comorbidities that may increase the risk of bleeding. The platelet count alone should not be used as a reason to treat in a child with no or mild bleeding, and many of these children can be managed with observation alone.

19. Neonatal alloimmune thrombocytopenia (NAIT) is caused by alloantibodies produced and transferred by the mother against a specific fetal platelet antigen that the baby inherited from the father and that is absent in the mother. The most common platelet antigen involved is the human platelet antigen (HPA)-1a. It is recommended that infants with NAIT be transfused to maintain a platelet count greater than 30×10^9/L in the absence of bleeding, and higher based on clinical bleeding symptoms. Transfusion with matched platelets is preferred; however, if giving random donor platelets, intravenous immunoglobulin (IVIG) can also be given.

20. Thrombocytosis is defined as platelet count above the upper limit of normal value ($> 450 \times 10^9$/L). This can be further classified as either essential (primary) or reactive (secondary) thrombocytosis. Reactive thrombocytosis is the most common cause of an elevated platelet count in children. The treatment involves treating the underlying condition.

21. Screening for causes of constitutional marrow failure is indicated for patients with aplastic anemia.

22. In children with severe aplastic anemia, if a human leukocyte antigen (HLA)–matched related donor is available, the treatment of choice is hematopoietic stem cell transplant (HCT). If no such donor is available, patients can be treated with immunosuppressive therapy (antithymocyte globulin [ATG] and cyclosporine). If immunotherapy fails, matched unrelated donor transplant is a suitable option.

23. Almost all systemic conditions can result in some degree of derangement of hematologic system. Conditions associated with inflammation can cause an increase in platelets, which are an acute phase reactant, as well as anemia. In other cases, particular organ dysfunction, such as liver and kidney disease, can disrupt production and regulation of blood cells and factors. Lastly, some conditions can result in impairment of blood cell function.

24. Anemia of chronic disease is common in any condition, acute or chronic, that results in inflammation. The primary cause is disruption in iron metabolism caused by inflammation because of increased increase hepcidin. The anemia is usually normochromic and normocytic; it is occasionally hypochromic and microcytic.

25. Anemia of chronic disease and iron deficiency anemia can both result in microcytic anemia. In anemia of chronic disease, plasma iron, total iron binding capacity, and transferrin saturation are usually diminished, whereas the ferritin can be normal or increased. This is the main difference when compared with iron deficiency, which will have low ferritin.

ONCOLOGY

26. National Cancer Institute SEER (Surveillance, Epidemiology, and End Results) data indicate the incidence of cancer from birth through 14 years of age is 14 cases per 100,000 per year. For patients between 15 and 19 years, the incidence approaches 20 cases per 100,000 per year. Thus, in the United States, there are approximately 15,000 to 16,000 new cases of cancer per year diagnosed in children and teenagers.

27. Survival rates for children and adolescents have improved dramatically in the last half century. In the 1960s, the overall survival rate for all diagnoses was less than 30%; in the 21st century, 5-year survival outcome exceeds 80%. Survival data are comparable for children 0 to 14 years and for teenagers who are 15 to 19 years of age.

28. The difference between traditional chemotherapy and targeted therapy is that the former is commonly cytotoxic and cannot discriminate between cancer and normal cells, whereas targeted therapies differentiate cancer cells from normal cells either by recognizing a specific cell surface marker (monoclonal antibody or antibody drug conjugate) or blocking a growth pathway upon which the cancer cell is uniquely dependent.

29. The application of precision oncology is emerging within pediatric oncology as we shift from directing the diagnosis, classification, and management of tumors from the site of tumor origin alone to incorporating individual tumor information at the gene, protein, and environment level to provide targeted therapy that is less toxic and more effective for the patient.

30. Immunotherapy is a form of cancer therapy that uses the innate or adaptive immune system of a patient to eradicate malignant cells.

31. Monoclonal antibodies are proteins developed in vitro by the adaptive immune system that directly target malignant cells, deliver cytotoxic molecules to malignant cells, or retarget cellular immune activation against malignant cells.

32. Compared with adult cancers, pediatric cancers are much rarer, are more often induced by inherited or sporadic errors in development rather than environmental exposures, and are typically of mesenchymal rather than epithelial origin.

33. Comprehensive tumor sequencing is indicated to characterize patients diagnosed with high-risk malignancies, outlier phenotypes, rare cancers lacking standard therapies, cancer predisposition syndromes, and relapsed/refractory disease to inform patient care.

34. The WAGR (Wilms tumor, aniridia, genitourinary defects, and mental retardation) and Beckwith-Wiedemann syndromes (BWS) are both associated with a predisposition to the development of Wilms tumor, and both are associated with developmental abnormalities, as well as with germline abnormalities involving gene loci on chromosome 11.

35. Compared with White children, Black and Hispanic children experience lower survival from many cancers, including leukemias, lymphomas, central nervous system (CNS) tumors, and extracranial solid tumors.

36. The tumor lysis syndrome is defined by hyperuricemia, hyperkalemia, hyperphosphatemia, hypocalcemia, and an increasing serum creatinine that results from massive release of intracellular contents into the systemic circulation secondary to the initiation of cytotoxic therapy and may cause renal failure, cardiac arrhythmias, seizures, or sudden death.

37. The cytokine release syndrome describes a spectrum of reactions seen after administration of targeted therapies, such as chimeric antigen receptor (CAR) T-cell and bispecific T-cell engaging antibodies, that cause activation of the immune system, resulting in symptoms of a flu-like illness and sepsis to vasodilatory shock, acute respiratory distress syndrome, multi-organ failure, and DIC.

38. Typical infectious complications in children with cancer include bacterial sepsis, systemic or organ specific infections caused by either primary or reactivated viruses, respiratory viruses, and invasive fungal.

39. Empiric antibiotic coverage for patients with febrile neutropenia should be based on the local hospital antibiogram and offer combined coverage for *Pseudomonas*, related gram-negative organisms, typical gram-positive organisms such as *Staphylococcus aureus*, and *Streptococcus viridans*.

40. Hodgkin lymphoma (HL) is composed of two distinct disease entities: classical HL (cHL) and nodular lymphocyte predominant HL. The four subtypes of cHL include nodular sclerosis, mixed cellularity, lymphocyte depleted, and lymphocyte rich.

41. High hyperdiploidy, or more than 50 chromosomes, which is present in 30% of childhood B-cell acute lymphoblastic leukemia (B-ALL), is associated with mutations in the Ras pathway, chromatin modifiers such as CREBBP, and favorable outcomes; on the other hand, low hypodiploidy, involving 31 to 39 chromosomes, and near haploidy, involving 24 to 30 chromosomes, which present in up to 2% of children, are characterized by IKZF2 deletion, near-universal TP53 mutations, and Ras pathway mutations and deletions of IKZF3, respectively, are associated with unfavorable outcomes.

42. Post-transplant lymphoproliferative disorders (PTLDs), often driven by the oncogenic Epstein-Barr virus (EBV), are a major complication of solid organ and allogeneic HCT (alloHCT) that develop as a consequence of immunosuppression.

43. DNA is the preferred target for mutation testing and for chimerism analysis, whereas RNA is the preferred target for detecting gene fusions and performing gene expression analysis.

44. With childhood cancer survival rates exceeding 80%, survivorship clinics provide screening, intervention, health education, anticipatory guidance, and promotion of healthy lifestyles and facilitate the transition for adolescents and young adults from a pediatric to an adult healthcare system, steps that are all critical to long-term health.

45. Patients with cancer often seek the use of complementary and integrative health therapies, which include nonmainstream practices such as natural products, mind-body practices, and whole-system approaches like traditional Chinese medicine (TCM), Ayurvedic medicine, homeopathy, and naturopathy, to help manage the side effects associated with cancer therapy, to augment the efficacy of conventional therapy, or to provide support for coping with the diagnosis of cancer.

46. Palliative care is an interdisciplinary collaborative approach to improve the quality of life of children with life-threatening, profound acute and chronic conditions and their families, inclusive of physical, emotional, social, and spiritual elements.

47. Long-term neurocognitive effects are most common in children diagnosed with brain tumors, ALL, non-Hodgkin lymphoma (NHL), or tumors of the eye, ear, or face when the disease or its required treatment directly involves the CNS.

48. Globally, more than 85% of the greater than 400,000 children and adolescents who develop cancer each year live in low- and middle-income countries where the estimated survival is less than 30%, contrasting starkly with the 80% survival achieved for the approximately 45,000 children diagnosed with cancer in high-income countries. Although innumerable factors contribute to this unacceptable disparity in survival, the relationship between poverty and poor survival is inseparable.

49. Although sporadic Burkitt lymphoma (BL) is the most common pediatric lymphoma in the world, endemic BL is the most common overall childhood cancer in equatorial sub-Saharan Africa, and it shares geographic overlap with the incidence of malaria and chronic antigenic stimulation from plasmodium falciparum, which is thought to play a role in the malignant transformation of this germinal center mature B-cell lymphoma.

50. Tumor tissue samples obtained in the operating room should be placed in sterile saline, not formalin, and immediately collected by the pathologist for transport to the laboratory. Fixatives, contamination, and tissue decay compromise the retrieval of tissue for biological evaluation.

ONCOLOGIC DISEASES

51. There is an increased risk for development of ALL in individuals with Down syndrome, Schwachman syndrome, Bloom syndrome, and ataxia-telangiectasia.

52. The outcomes for children with ALL have improved dramatically over the last several decades because of refinements in risk stratification, improved diagnostics and high-level minimal residual disease (MRD) detection, and novel targeted therapies, with overall survival from 94% to 97%.

53. Acute myeloid leukemia (AML) accounts for about 25% of pediatric leukemia and has a bimodal distribution, with a higher incidence in both children younger than 2 years of age and adolescents 15 to 20 years old.

54. Length of first remission is the most important prognostic factor for AML patients who relapse, with approximately 80% of patients who relapse more than 12 months from diagnosis achieving a second complete remission compared with 50% of patients who relapse less than 12 months from diagnosis.

55. The Philadelphia chromosome—or t(9;22)(q34.1;q11.2) resulting in a *BCR-ABL1* fusion gene—is the hallmark of 90% to 95% of chronic myeloid leukemia (CML) cases.

56. Embryonal rhabdomyosarcoma is more common in younger children (<8 years) with primary tumors in the head and neck or genitourinary regions.

57. Alveolar rhabdomyosarcoma tends to occur in older patients (adolescents and young adults), presenting with extremity tumors, and tends to be clinically more aggressive with metastatic disease and a worse prognosis.

58. The most common malignant bone tumors in children, adolescents, and young adults are osteosarcoma (56%) and Ewing sarcoma (34%).

59. The most common chromosomal translocation in Ewing sarcoma (85%) is the t(11; 22) (q24; q12), which leads to the expression of the EWSR1-FLI1 transcription factor.

60. Neuroblastoma can originate from any site in the sympathetic nervous system, with the primary site being the adrenal gland occurring more frequently in children older than 1 year (40%) than in infants (25%), whereas cervical and thoracic tumors occur more frequently in infants (33%) than older children (15%).

61. Metastatic neuroblastoma classically presents with proptosis and periorbital ecchymoses, as well as bone pain, pancytopenia, irritability, limp, or refusal to walk.

62. In infants and toddlers, the most common malignant liver tumor is hepatoblastoma and is characterized by an asymptomatic abdominal mass and an elevated alpha fetoprotein (AFP).

63. More than two-thirds of pediatric hepatocellular carcinomas (HCCs) occur during the second decade of life with HCC divided into classic or adult type HCC and fibrolamellar HCC.
64. Children with sporadic aniridia, WAGR syndrome, hemihypertrophy, and BWS are at increased risk for developing Wilms tumor and should have routine screening with an abdominal ultrasound until the age of 7 years.
65. B symptoms describe the extent of systemic or constitutional symptoms that accompany a diagnosis of HL, with patients presenting with unintentional weight loss, drenching night sweats, or unexplained fevers.
66. Salvage regimens and second-line treatment for HL is extraordinarily effective, and thus overall survival rates at 5 years approach 98% for the majority of pediatric and adolescent patients.
67. There are unique geographic distinctions in the epidemiology of childhood NHL; endemic BL is the most common overall childhood cancer in equatorial regions of sub-Saharan Africa, whereas East Asia and Central and South America have a higher incidence of rare EBV-associated T and natural killer (NK)–cell lymphomas and lymphoproliferative disorders.
68. Upfront treatment considerations in pediatric NHL include the following general concepts: multiagent chemotherapy achieves high cure rates without the need for surgical resection or radiation therapy; and intrathecal chemotherapy is incorporated in most treatment regimens, even for CNS-negative patients.
69. Supratentorial tumors (tumors of the cerebral hemispheres, basal ganglia, thalamus, and hypothalamus) can show signs of increased intracranial pressure, such as early morning headache or headache that goes away after vomiting; focal deficits, such as memory loss, weakness, visual changes, hearing problems, speech problems, and deterioration of school performance; and seizures.
70. Infratentorial tumors (tumors of the cerebellum and brainstem) can block cerebrospinal fluid (CSF) outflow, leading to headache and vomiting; they can also become apparent with localizing signs such as cranial nerve palsies or ataxia (loss of balance and trouble walking).
71. Diffuse intrinsic pontine glioma carries the worst prognosis of any childhood brain tumor, being nearly uniformly fatal within 18 to 24 months, with radiation therapy providing only temporary relief of symptoms.
72. EBV infection in patients with compromised T-cell immunity after transplantation because of immunosuppression can lead to the development of PTLD.
73. Children with bilateral retinoblastoma usually have RB1 mutations in their germline, whereas only 15% of children with unilateral disease have germline mutations.
74. The most frequent endocrinopathy in Langerhans cell histiocytosis (LCH) is diabetes insipidus (DI), which may occur before, concurrently, or subsequent to the development of the disease in other sites, especially with bone lesions of the skull.
75. A high index of suspicion is required for diagnosing hemophagocytic lymphohistiocytosis (HLH); children with unexplained fever of more than 5 days duration should have a serum ferritin checked, with ferritin levels of more than 3000 ng/mL raising suspicion for HLH and levels greater than 10,000 ng/mL strongly associated with HLH.

STEM CELL AND CELLULAR THERAPIES

76. Autologous HCT (autoHCT) uses a patient's own hematopoietic cells and is used for malignant conditions such as lymphomas, CNS tumors, and solid tumors. The goal of an autoHCT is restore the body's ability to make normal blood cells after high-dose chemotherapy or radiation. Such intensive treatments usually destroy cancer cells better than standard treatments, but these high-dose treatments are toxic and also destroy the blood-producing stem cells in the bone marrow.
77. Stem cells for autoHCT are collected during recovery from initial conventional dose chemotherapy with filgrastim. Leukapheresis is initiated when the peripheral blood CD34$^+$ count is 20 million per liter. Harvest yields can be improved by the addition of plerixafor, a CXCL4 antagonist, to filgrastim. This may be seen in heavily pretreated patients. In those with inadequate peripheral blood stem cell (PBSC) collections, bone marrow harvest may be considered.
78. AlloHCT uses donor hematopoietic cells to provide a graft versus malignancy effect, replace a missing gene or enzyme in the hematopoietic/immune system, or replete a failed bone marrow. This type of transplant can be used in both malignant and nonmalignant conditions. AlloHCT was first performed in 1956 in a patient with leukemia; however, this was quickly applied to nonmalignant disorders only a decade later in a patient with severe combined immunodeficiency.
79. When performing alloHCT, donor sources include sibling donors and alternate donors. Alternate donors can then be subdivided into mismatched family donors or unrelated donors. Stem cell sources include bone marrow, peripheral blood, and umbilical cord blood.
80. HLA typing has had a tremendous impact on alloHCT outcomes. HLA genes are part of the major histocompatibility complex, responsible for alloreactivity because of minor and major HLA mismatch between patient and donor. HLA genes are located on chromosome 6, and HLA antigens are divided into two groups: Class I- HLA-A, HLA-B, and HLA-C and Class II- HLA-DP, HLA-DQ, and HLA-DRBI. When considering donors for alloHCT, HLA matching between the donor and recipient is the most important consideration. Other factors to take into account include donor age, sex, parity, cytomegalovirus status, and ABO blood group.

81. The majority of patients receive chemotherapy and some receive total body irradiation (TBI) therapy before infusion of hematopoietic cells. The purpose of the conditioning regimen is to partially or completely eliminate the bone marrow and immune system. In patients with malignant diseases, it is also used to minimize disease burden so that the donor immune system has a better chance to eliminate MRD. Myeloablative conditioning (MAC) regimens are used to maximize disease control and facilitate engraftment; however, their use is often limited by toxicity. Reduced intensity conditioning regimens use less chemotherapy and radiation myeloablative ones. The goal is to decrease the transplant related complications, toxicity, and mortality. Nevertheless, there is a higher risk of rejection with this approach.

82. Acute graft versus host disease (aGVHD) occurs when donor T cells recognize recipient antigens as foreign and is usually within the first 100 days after alloHCT. The organ systems usually involved in aGVHD are skin, gastrointestinal tract, or hepatobiliary. The single most important factor associated with the development of aGVHD is the degree of HLA mismatch between the donor and the recipient. T-cell depletion using serotherapy or graft processing have resulted in lower rates (approximately 20%–40%).

83. Chronic graft versus host disease (cGVHD) is more common in adults than children but can have a significant impact on quality of life. The biggest risk factor for the development of cGVHD is a history of aGVHD and PBSC transplantation. It is caused by an impaired immune tolerance between both alloreactive and autoreactive donor-derived T and B cells, resulting in chronic inflammation and scarring. Symptoms usually develop 3 to 24 months after alloHCT and can involve nearly all organ systems. Those with mild cGVHD tend to have better outcomes than those with more severe disease.

84. Most patients with ALL do not requires allogeneic transplant. Patients with high risk for relapse, however, are considered for allogeneic transplant. Patients who are unable to achieve a morphologic remission (<5% bone marrow blasts) after induction chemotherapy or who have persistent MRD should be referred for consideration of allogeneic transplant in first complete remission. For patients that relapse after therapy, early relapses are at higher risk of subsequent relapses and death and should be considered for allogeneic transplant in second remission. Patients who relapse less than 18 months from initial diagnosis were noted to have an extremely poor outcome with only 21% overall survival (OS) with chemotherapy alone. Patients who suffer a third relapse in ALL should also be considered if able to achieve remission.

85. Survival among children with AML remains suboptimal. Nevertheless, incremental progress in survival after alloHCT has occurred over the last 3 decades. Relapsed AML is the most common indication for alloHCT. In the current era, 40% of newly diagnosed AML pediatric patients receive it because of a high risk of relapse. After alloHCT, the 5-year AML-free survival in the current era is approximately 60%. Mortality because of transplant-related toxicities and relapse of AML post-alloHCT are the main cause of treatment failure.

86. Among leukemia patients undergoing alloHCT, the MRD is one of the most important prognostic indicators of relapse post-alloHCT. MRD is measured by flow cytometry and next-generation sequencing (NGS). The sensitivity of leukemia detection in flow cytometry is 1 leukemia cell among 10,000 normal cells and NGS is 1 leukemia cell among 1 million normal cells. Within reasonable limits, every effort should be made to achieve MRD negative status by flow cytometry before alloHCT because positive MRD increases the risk of relapse by 30% to 40%.

87. Two potentially serious complications after alloHCT or autoHCT include veno-occlusive disease of the liver (VOD) and transplant-associated thrombotic microangiopathy (TA-TMA). VOD, also known as sinusoidal obstructive syndrome (SOS), occurs from small microthrombi that form in the sinusoids of the liver. The obstructive microthrombi lead to liver dysfunction and manifest as hepatomegaly, right upper quadrant pain, ascites leading to weight gain, and cholestatic liver disease. TA-TMA is another complication after transplantation that occurs secondary to systemic endothelial damage. It can present as a limited finding or can have multisystem involvement. Organs typically involved with TA-TMA include the kidney, the intestines, the liver, and the lungs.

88. The use of CAR-T cells offer patients who are ineligible for alloHCT an opportunity for remission. CAR-T cells are a powerful form of adoptive cell therapy. In their native state, T cells do not express antigens targeted to bind to malignant cells. In CAR-T therapy, T cells are harvested from a patient and then genetically engineered using a viral vector (most commonly a lentiviral or retroviral vector) to produce proteins on their surface that can directly bind to the malignant cells. Binding of CAR-T cells with malignant cells leads to activation and proliferation of CAR-T cells, which results in the killing of malignant cells.

89. Antigens that can be targeted by CAR-T cells in pediatric malignancies include the following: for B-ALL, CD19 and CD22; for T-cell ALL, CD7 and C5; for AML, CD33 and CD123; for NHL, CD19; and for neuroblastoma, GD2. The most well-studied CARs to date target CD19. In 2017, the US Food and Drug Administration Agency (FDA) approved tisagenlecleucel, a CD19-directed CAR-T cell therapy in patients up to 25 years of age who have B-ALL that is either: (1) refractory, or (2) in second or greater relapse.

90. The major unique toxicities of CAR-T cells include cytokine release syndrome (CRS) and immune effector cell–associated neurotoxicity (ICANS). The activation and proliferation of CAR-T cells results in the release of various inflammatory cytokines. One of the key cytokines driving toxicity is interleukin-6 (IL-6), which is predominantly released by macrophages. The cornerstone of severe CRS management is administration of tocilizumab, an IL-6 receptor antibody, that has led to rapid reversal of CRS in many cases. Other common toxicities include cytopenias, infection, hypogammaglobulinemia, and other organ toxicity.

91. For nonmalignant transplants, conditioning regimens have historically been myeloablative. Nevertheless, this approach is associated with numerous short-term and long-term complications, such as aGVHD and cGVHD,

infections, infertility, and organ damage. Full-donor chimerism levels are usually associated with success in the malignant setting but in the nonmalignant setting, mixed-donor chimerism levels can be curative. Lowering the intensity of conditioning regimens has been used in an attempt to decrease complications but can also be associated with higher rates of graft failure and rejection.

92. HCT can be curative for patients with inherited bone marrow failure syndromes. These include those with Fanconi anemia (FA), Kostmann syndrome, Diamond Blackfan syndrome, and Dyskeratosis congenita. For those with FA, special caution must be taken with regards to conditioning regimens. Because FA is an inherited DNA repair disorder, patients are particularly sensitive to chemotherapy and radiation therapy and cannot tolerate standard doses of chemotherapy and radiation therapy.

93. Acquired aplastic anemia (AA) is the result of an immune-mediated destruction of hematopoietic stem cells. The modified Camitta criteria is used to assess severity. To diagnose severe AA (SAA), there must be two of the following: hemoglobin concentration less than 100 g/L, platelet count less than 50×10^9/L, and neutrophil count less than 0.5×10^9/L. A bone marrow biopsy is mandatory and will confirm an empty marrow; it should also exclude MDS, leukemia, or marrow metastasis from solid tumors. Cytogenetics and/or fluorescence in situ hybridization (FISH) analysis should also be sent to determine any chromosomal abnormalities.

94. The standard of care for those with newly diagnosed SAA is a bone marrow transplant if a full-sibling match is available with event-free survival rates of approximately 90%. For those lacking a sibling donor, immunosuppressive therapy (IST) is given consisting of equine ATG and cyclosporine, with hematological recovery in 50% to 70% of patients and excellent long-term survival among responders.

95. In patients with severe combined immunodeficiency (SCID), early transplantation is crucial with those less than 3.5 months of age at the time of transplant having excellent outcomes. Having an active infection was found to be significantly higher in those greater than 3.5 months and contributed to the lower success rates.

96. Curative options for patients with SCD include alloHCT and gene therapy. Those receiving sibling HCT have event-free survival rates of more than 90%. Gene therapy is currently only being offered through clinical trials.

97. Among SCD patients undergoing alloHCT, patients are more at risk for neurologic complications, such as posterior reversible encephalopathy syndrome, seizures, and hemorrhage during and after bone marrow transplant.

98. In patients with thalassemia receiving regularly scheduled monthly transfusions, control of iron overload and prevention of iron-related tissue damage is crucial for successful transplantation and for decreasing transplant-related complications such as VOD/SOS.

99. Gene therapies using gene addition and gene editing approaches are currently being studied as curative options in those with SCD and thalassemia. Gene therapy for hemoglobinopathies consists of the autologous transplantation of hematopoietic stem and progenitor cells (HSPCs) transduced with a viral vector (i.e., lentivirus) encoding a modified β-globin gene, which results in the production of an antisickling hemoglobin. Gene editing technologies such as CRISPR/Cas9 are currently being investigated that use endonucleases and guide RNA to manipulate the target gene. This system is able to repair, insert, and delete genes to either modify the expression of β-globin genes or promote the expression of HbF.

100. Gene therapy carries a risk of secondary malignancy and infertility because engraftment of genetically modified HSPCs primarily depends on the use of a busulfan-based conditioning regimen. Although newer lentiviral viral vectors have improved safety profiles, there is the potential for insertional mutagenesis/oncogenesis. This can result in the insertion of viral promoters upstream of a pro-oncogene or within a regulatory gene resulting in aberrant expression of cell cycle regulatory proteins, which can lead to cellular dysfunction, myelodysplasia, or the development of malignancy, such as leukemia or lymphoma.

HEMATOLOGY

I

COAGULATION OVERVIEW

Dominder Kaur, MD and Catherine McGuinn, MD

NORMAL HEMOSTASIS

1. **Describe normal hemostasis.**
   Hemostasis is the physiological process of cessation or prevention of bleeding from a site of vascular injury involving the interplay of three important participants: the blood vessel, the platelets, and the coagulation system.
   When a blood vessel is damaged, the following events occur:
   - Vasoconstriction
   - Platelet adhesion and aggregation mediated by von Willebrand factor (VWF) and fibrinogen forming a platelet plug
   - Exposure of collagen and tissue factor from the damaged endothelium causing initiation of coagulation by the activation of factor VII (FVII) and subsequent activation of a series of clotting factors leading to the formation of fibrin thrombus
   - Regulation of extension of the thrombus by the natural anticoagulants
   - Activation of the fibrinolytic system causing lysis of the thrombus
   - Remodeling and healing of the injury site after control of bleeding

2. **What are the differences between primary and secondary hemostasis?**
   Primary hemostasis is defined as platelet-mediated activity at the site of injury, with four involved phases, namely vasoconstriction, platelet adhesion, platelet activation, and platelet aggregation. The result is the formation of a platelet plug where bleeding was occurring from.
   Secondary hemostasis involves activation of the proteolytic coagulation cascade, involving contribution from various coagulation factors, and results in the formation of a stable fibrin thrombus.

3. **What is cell-based hemostasis?**
   The traditional waterfall model of coagulation describes it as a series of proteolytic processes, with coagulation factors being proenzymes leading to activation of downstream enzymes. We now understand that in vivo, a number of these processes take place simultaneously. The hemostatic pathway is triggered by vessel wall injury, with a number of these proteolytic and activation steps occurring on the cell surface. This led to the development of "cellular model of hemostasis," which describes various phases: initiation, amplification, propagation, and stabilization.
   The extrinsic pathway is triggered in vivo in response to trauma, whereas the intrinsic pathway plays a role in the continued formation of fibrin by supporting and increasing thrombin generation. *Initiation*, or start of the extrinsic pathway, happens with vessel wall injury, with release of tissue factor from cells in the vascular bed. It comes in contact with and activates factor VII and forms a complex in the presence of calcium ions. This *factor VIIa–tissue factor complex* then converts factor X to Xa (thrombin spark), as well as IX to IXa.
   Factor Xa binds to factor Va in the presence of calcium and phospholipid, forming the *prothrombinase complex,* which rapidly converts prothrombin to thrombin. Thrombin generated from this phase activates factors V and VIII, playing a cofactor role in prothrombinase complex and leading to *amplification* of other factors. Factor Xa is formed by a series of enzymatic conversion of factor XII, factor XI, prekallikrein, high-molecular-weight kininogen, and factor IX. The activated factor IX, along with factor VIIIa as a cofactor in the presence of calcium and phospholipid, then forms the *ten-ase complex*, which converts factor X to Xa (*propagation phase*). Thrombin generated from these pathways (thrombin burst) is a key effector enzyme that finally converts fibrinogen to fibrin. It also causes feedback amplification of coagulation by activation of factors V, VIII, XI, and XIII. Fibrin is then covalently crosslinked by factor XIIIa during the *stabilization* phase to form a stabilized thrombus (Figure 1.1).

4. **Discuss the regulation of blood coagulation by the natural inhibitors and anticoagulants.**
   Blood coagulation is regulated by several natural anticoagulants that limit and localize thrombus formation at the site of injury. Endothelial cells act as inhibitors by being physical barriers between platelets and the matrix proteins, cofactors, and substrates, preventing their activation and binding.
   At each level of the hemostatic pathway, there are processes of either enzyme inhibition or cofactor modulation to keep thrombosis in check. The tissue factor pathway inhibitor (TFPI) inactivates the factor VIIa–tissue factor complex. Antithrombin inactivates thrombin and other serine proteases (XIIa, XIa, Xa, and IXa). Its action is enhanced in the presence of heparin or heparan sulfate in the vessel wall. The protein C system inactivates factors Va and VIIIa. This is initiated by thrombin, which binds to thrombomodulin (an endothelial cell membrane protein) and forms activated protein C (APC). APC acts most efficiently in the presence of its cofactor protein S, which exists in the plasma as either a free protein or bound to the complement component C4b–binding protein. (See next question for fibrinolytic modulators.)

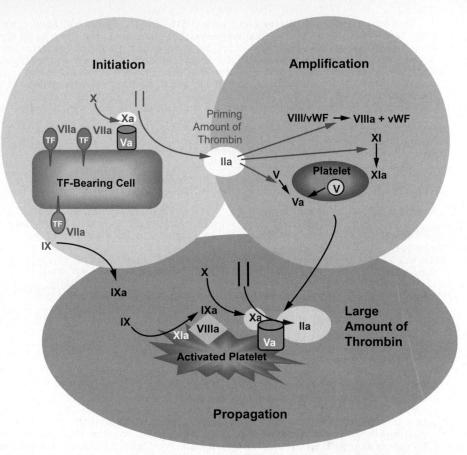

Figure 1.1 Cell-based model of hemostasis. (Adapted from Hoffman M, Monroe DM. Reversing targeted oral anticoagulants. *Hematology Am Soc Hematol Educ Program.* 2014;2014[1]:518–523.)

5. **Describe the fibrinolytic system.**

   The fibrinolytic system (Figure 1.2) is responsible for lysis of fibrin cross-linking in the thrombus. It is composed of plasminogen and its activators and inhibitors. Plasminogen is converted to plasmin through activation by tissue plasminogen activator (tPA), which is synthesized and released from vascular endothelium, or by urokinase plasminogen activator (uPA), which is produced in the kidney.

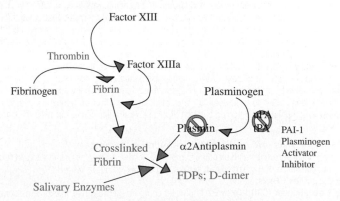

Figure 1.2 Overview of the fibrinolytic system.

The fibrinolytic process is regulated by specific protease inhibitors: (1) PAI-1 (plasminogen activator inhibitor), which inhibits the plasminogen activators (tPA and urokinase), and (2) α2-antiplasmin, which inhibits plasmin. Plasmin acts on both fibrinogen and fibrin, forming the fibrinogen degradation products (FDPs). Crosslinked fibrin lysed by plasmin leads to the production of fragments such as D-dimer and soluble fibrin monomers. Thrombin activatable fibrinolysis inhibitor (TAFI) is a fibrinolysis regulator. TAFI, activated by the thrombin-thrombomodulin complex, cleaves plasminogen and tPA binding sites from fibrin fragments. This prevents action of plasminogen and tPA on fibrin, inhibiting fibrinolysis.

Evaluation of the fibrinolytic system can be done by individual assays of these aforementioned components. A whole blood evaluation is also possible via thromboelastography (TEG) or rotational thromboelastometry (ROTEM).

6. **Where are the coagulation proteins synthesized and stored?**
Most of the coagulation proteins are synthesized in the liver, with some exceptions:

Cells/Site	Role/Activity	Respective Factors and Coagulation Proteins
1. Liver Hepatocytes	Production of coagulation proteins	Fibrinogen, prothrombin, factors V (80%), VII, IX, X, XI, XII, XIII, protein C & S, and antithrombin
2. Liver Sinusoidal Endothelial Cells	Production and storage	Factor VIII and von Willebrand factor (VWF)
3. Vessel Wall Endothelial Cells	Production of VWF and tissue factor pathway inhibitor (TFPI) Storage of other proteins listed	VIII, VWF, tissue plasminogen activator (tPA), thrombomodulin, TFPI, and urokinase
4. Platelets	Production of one factor Storage of the other factors and proteins	Factor V (rest 20%) [also calcium ions] Storage of fibrinogen, factors V, VIII, XI, XIII, platelet factor 4

7. **Which are the vitamin K–dependent factors and proteins?**
Vitamin K is a fat-soluble compound that occurs naturally in the diet (fruits and vegetables) and is synthesized by the bacterial flora in the gut. Vitamin K is important for the synthesis of the procoagulant factors II, VII, IX, and X and the anticoagulants proteins C and S. Vitamin K promotes the post-translational modification of specific glutamic acid residues to γ-carboxyglutamic acid, which is essential in their calcium binding to negatively charged phospholipid surfaces.

Deficiency states can be seen in malnutrition or starvation, prolonged antibiotic therapy and warfarin ingestion, and conditions that cause fat malabsorption, such as biliary obstruction, pancreatic insufficiency, short-bowel syndrome, cystic fibrosis, and diarrhea.

8. **Which clotting factors are "acute phase reactants"?**
Factor VIII, fibrinogen, and VWF are often elevated during infection and the inflammatory processes. In such scenarios, they can lead to shortening of the activated partial thromboplastin time (aPTT).

9. **How would you approach a patient with concern for a bleeding disorder?**
Obtaining a good and reliable history is important in making an accurate diagnosis of a bleeding disorder. The type of bleeding (e.g., skin, mucous membrane, joint or deep muscle bleeds), its severity, and the duration of symptoms guide us for further evaluations. Because reporting and interpreting bleeding symptoms is subjective, bleeding assessment tools (BATs) can be helpful to standardize this process. BATs are questionnaires that guide the review of bleeding symptoms in a comprehensive and systematic manner. The Pediatric Bleeding Questionnaire (PBQ) and the BAT standardized per the International Society of Thrombosis & Haemostasis (ISTH-BAT) are two such tools that include review of pediatric symptoms.

A careful family history must also be obtained because many common bleeding disorders are familial or inherited (e.g., von Willebrand's disease [VWD], hemophilias). Acquired causes must also be sought, such as intake of drugs that are known to affect hemostasis (e.g., aspirin, warfarin, certain anticonvulsants and antibiotics), as well as medical conditions known to be associated with bleeding (e.g., liver or kidney disease, lupus and other autoimmune disorders). Further screening and hematological evaluation can be carried out based on the information from this history.

10. **What laboratory tests are used for the screening of hemostasis?**
In patients presenting with concerning bleeding symptoms, positive history (personal or that of family), and a positive bleeding score, evaluation of the hemostatic system can be carried out as follows:
Screening Coagulation Tests
• **Complete blood count (CBC):** To evaluate platelet count (and ensure reasonable hematocrit) as part of initial screening tests

- **Prothrombin time (PT):** To measure the "extrinsic pathway"
- **aPTT:** To measure the "intrinsic pathway"; together, the PT and aPTT also assess the common pathway

Additional Coagulation Tests

- **Mixing studies:** Carried out by mixing patient plasma with normal plasma to assess if PT or aPTT prolongation is because of factor deficiency or an inhibitor (see detail in question 11)
- **Thrombin time (TT):** Measures the quality and amount of fibrinogen and the rate of conversion of fibrinogen to fibrin. It is the time required for plasma to clot after the addition of thrombin. It is prolonged in hypofibrinogenemia and dysfibrinogenemia and by substances that interfere with the thrombin-induced fibrinogen conversion to fibrin, such as heparin and FDPs. Can be sent when suspicion is high for a fibrinogen-related issue or when common pathway testing is abnormal.
- **Fibrinogen activity:** Fibrinogen deficiency does not prolong the other commonly used screening tests (PT, aPTT, TT) until the level is well below the normal (<100 mg/dL).
- **Platelet function assay:** Screening test for platelet dysfunctions and primary hemostatic pathway (i.e., can also screen for VWD). More specific platelet function evaluation can be done via platelet aggregometry.
- **Specific coagulation factor assays:** Based on the aforementioned screening tests, to assess for qualitative or quantitative factor deficiencies.

11. **What is a "mixing study"?**

A mixing study is a method to differentiate innate or acquired factor deficiency from the presence of an inhibitor in the patient plasma. A mixing study is typically carried out if either of the screening coagulation tests—the PT or aPTT—is noted to be prolonged to identify direction of further evaluation.

Normal plasma is added to the patient's plasma (in equal volume), and the PT/aPTT assays are performed. If the PT/aPTT of the mixture corrects or becomes normal, factor deficiency is present. If the PT/aPTT remains prolonged, however, this indicates the presence of an inhibitor (lupus anticoagulant, heparin/other anticoagulant, or a specific-factor inhibitor, more commonly II, VIII, IX, or XI). There is also a warming process and a delayed assessment (incubation) in the mixing study to look for heat labile and time/temperature-dependent delayed-binding inhibitors; this additional testing should be undertaken especially if the patient has a negative mixing study but normal factor levels and clinical symptoms of bleeding consistent with an acquired factor deficiency.

Some conditions can additionally interfere with this test, leading to nonspecific normalization or prolongation of PT/aPTT after mixing; these include D-dimer/other FDPs and elevated C-reactive protein.

12. **What are some of the artifacts in sample collection and processing of coagulation testing that affect interpretation of the tests?**

A properly collected and processed sample is crucial in the interpretation of coagulation tests. Some of the causes of errors include:

- **Traumatic and repeated punctures and slow blood flow**: This can contaminate the sample with procoagulant materials in the tissue juice (tissue factor or thrombin), causing shortening of the aPTT and positive D-dimer or FDPs.
- **High hematocrit:** This leads to a reduced plasma concentration in proportion to the measured citrate anticoagulant in the tubes, thereby causing extra citrate to bind calcium and thus prolong the clotting time. Similarly, if the hematocrit is too low, some shortening of clotting times can be erroneously noted.
- **Incomplete filling of the collection tube ("short" draw):** If the amount of blood drawn is reduced in proportion to the citrate anticoagulant, the excess citrate depletes the calcium in the plasma and leads to prolongation of PT/aPTT.
- **Heparin contamination:** This may occur when specimens are drawn from arterial or venous catheters flushed with heparin. To obtain an accurate coagulation test, 3 to 5 mLs of blood must be discarded before collecting the sample to get rid of the heparin.

13. **Are there any screening tests for the natural inhibitors or anticoagulants?**

Specific tests for measuring the activity and concentration of some inhibitors exist (e.g., antithrombin, PAI-1, α2-antiplasmin, protein C, and protein S tests are available). Many other natural anticoagulants cannot be measured though, making it difficult to assess their reduction. Also, reduced amounts of these natural anticoagulants or inhibitors do not cause "shortening" of the PT or aPTT.

NEONATAL AND DEVELOPMENTAL HEMOSTASIS

14. **How is the coagulation system in neonates different from that in the adults? Does gestational age affect the coagulation system?**

The coagulation system is immature in the neonatal phase, with many of the coagulation proteins being reduced at birth. In the procoagulant system, the contact factors (high-molecular-weight kininogen, prekallikrein, and factors XII and XI) and the vitamin K–dependent factors (II, VII, IX, and X) are reduced to about 30% to 50% of the adult range in the term newborn infant and are even more reduced in a preterm infant.

On the other hand, factors V and VIII and fibrinogen are present in the normal adult level range, even in the premature neonate. Newborns also have increased VWF, which has an altered multimeric structure with increased high-molecular-weight forms producing increased reactivity with ristocetin. The coagulation inhibitors (antithrombin, protein C, and protein S) are also reduced to less than or equal to 50% of normal. In the fibrinolytic system, plasminogen, tPA, and α2-antiplasmin show decreased plasma concentrations, and there is reduced plasmin generation and overall fibrinolytic activity, whereas there is modest elevation of α2-macroglobulin and PAI-1.

Moreover, there are a few clotting factors in the neonate that exhibit unique structural and functional differences from the adult proteins. For instance, "fetal" fibrinogen has increased sialic acid content associated with a prolonged TT and reptilase time. The functional significance of this is unknown. Table 1.1 shows various factor levels at different gestational ages in infants.

15. **When do these coagulation proteins reach the adult values?**
The procoagulant proteins gradually increase postnatally and reach the adult values by about 6 months of age. Nevertheless, although the values fall within the adult normal range, the mean levels remain reduced throughout infancy when compared with the mean levels of adults. The inhibitors also increase during the first 3 to 6 months of life, except for proteins C and S, which remain lower for a few additional months.

16. **Describe how this difference in the coagulation system between newborns and adults can affect the commonly used coagulation screening tests.**
The reduced level of most of the coagulation proteins is reflected as prolongation of the coagulation screening tests. The PT is minimally prolonged in the normal term infant, whereas the aPTT is markedly prolonged because of the reduced levels of the contact factors disproportionately affecting the aPTT. In the premature infant, these test results are even more prolonged and results for these tests must be interpreted based on established reference range for neonates according to their gestational and postnatal age and in consideration of the interlaboratory variation in relation to the adult normal range for that laboratory.

17. **How do bleeding disorders present in the neonate?**
Hemorrhage in the neonatal period can be occult or overt. Bleeding is typically from sites of access or injury, such as prolonged bleeding from heelstick or venipuncture sites and large hematomas at sites of arterial puncture. Babies can present with blood in urine or stool. Specific bleeding sites related to some factor deficiencies can also occur (e.g., umbilical cord stump site bleeding with factor XIII deficiency) as well as increased risk of intracranial hemorrhage (severe deficiency). Neonates, especially preterm babies, have friable and thin vessel walls and go through circulatory pressure readjustments, making them prone to intracranial hemorrhages. Birth trauma–related risk of intracranial hemorrhage is also high in other congenital bleeding disorders like hemophilias and type 3 VWD. Neonates can also present with bleeding from the scalp, large cephalohematomas, and bleeding after circumcision. Hemarthrosis and deep muscle bleeding are rather unusual because babies do not bear weight in their large joints (which leads to the increased risk of bleeding at these sites).

17a. **A two-day-old, healthy full-term male infant developed bleeding after circumcision. What laboratory evaluation is indicated in this patient?**
In a healthy full-term infant who presents with bleeding manifestation, severe thrombocytopenia from immune causes, congenital or inherited factor deficiencies, and vitamin K deficiency should be considered. Initial screening tests include a platelet count and coagulation studies including PT, aPTT, and specific factor levels if there is concern based on family history.

17b. **The laboratory work-up reveals an isolated prolongation of aPTT of 95 seconds. What are the possible diagnoses?**
Factor VIII (hemophilia A) and factor IX (hemophilia B) are the two most common congenital factor deficiencies that can cause isolated prolongation of the aPTT. These are both x-linked recessive and more commonly occur in males with severe disease having factor levels less than 1. Factor XI deficiency can also present with a prolonged aPTT. It is an autosomal recessive condition. An additional consideration should be a type 3 VWD with low FVIII level and absent VWF activity.

17c. **How would you treat this patient to control the bleeding?**
Replacement therapy with the appropriate factor concentrate is indicated to control the bleeding. Nevertheless, when the diagnosis of a specific factor deficiency is pending, fresh frozen plasma (FFP), which contains all the clotting factors, is the blood product of choice. Cryoprecipitate contains factor VIII, VWF, fibrinogen, and FXIII and can be used if work-up/history has led to suspicion of one of these four deficiencies, but it does not contain factors IX or XI.

18. **A 5-day-old full-term female infant presents with prolonged bleeding from the umbilical cord site. Initial laboratory evaluation showed normal platelet count and normal results for coagulation studies (PT, aPTT, fibrinogen). What further work-up is needed, and what could be the diagnosis?**
The coagulation screening tests do not include factor XIII; therefore, if this is suspected, a specific assay must be performed. Homozygous deficiency of this factor classically presents with delayed umbilical cord bleeding.

Table 1.1 Coagulation Factors, Antithrombin, and D-Dimer Separated for Every Week of Gestational Age (Median and Range)

GA (WEEKS)	FIBRINOGEN (MGDL⁻¹)	F II (%)	F V (%)	F VII (%)	F VIII (%)	F X (%)	ANTITHROMBIN (UML⁻¹)	D-DIMER (MGDL⁻¹)
23 (n=26)	114 (1–430)	20 (12–42)	55 (25–156)	18 (5–54)	64 (20–195)	29 (14–76)	0.26 (0.14–0.45)	1.8 (0.1–10)
24 (n=24)	136 (54–547)	28 (13–51)	56 (24–171)	23 (4–59)	93 (13–168)	31 (17–62)	0.28 (0.03–0.54)	1.8 (0.3–11.2)
25 (n=22)	93 (20–446)	27 (10–55)	57 (13–111)	28 (5–47)	72 (29–174)	33 (10–79)	0.27 (0.14–0.37)	2.6 (0.7–61.4)
26 (n=39)	128 (42–526)	34 (13–55)	66 (20–132)	28 (6–76)	86 (26–174)	44 (18–102)	0.30 (0.08–0.44)	1.1 (0.3–10)
27 (n=21)	103 (26–318)	28 (14–62)	62 (3–122)	32 (9–69)	107 (29–173)	39 (13–82)	0.27 (0.03–0.54)	1.1 (0.2–40)
30–36a (n=137)	243 (150–373)	45 (20–77)	88 (41–144)	67 (21–113)	111 (50–213)	41 (11–71)	0.38 (0.14–0.62)	NA
Newborn (n=72)	283 (160–390)	48 (26–70)	72 (34–108)	66 (28–104)	100 (50–180)	40 (12–69)	0.63 (0.51–0.75)	NA

F II, Coagulation factor II; *F V*, coagulation factor F V; *F VII*, coagulation factor VII; *F VIII*, coagulation factor VIII; *F X*, coagulation factor X; *NA*, not applicable.
(From Poralla C, Traut C, Hertfelder H-J, Oldenburg J, Bartmann P, Heep A. The coagulation system of extremely preterm infants: Influence of perinatal risk factors on coagulation. *J Perinatol*. 2012;32[11]:869–873; and M Andrew, B Paes, R Milner, M Johnston, L Mitchell, DM Tollefsen, V Castle, P Powers; Development of the human coagulation system in the healthy premature infant. Blood 1988; 72 (5): 1651–1657.)

The urea solubility test is a useful screening test for homozygous deficiency but only detects levels in the less than 5% range. For milder deficiencies or confirmation, a factor XIII activity can be performed.

19. **What are the three forms of hemorrhagic disease of the newborn (HDN) secondary to vitamin K deficiency?**

Hemorrhagic disease of the newborn, which can present with various hemorrhagic manifestations, such as gastrointestinal, postcircumcisional, umbilical, or intracranial bleeding, occurs in three forms:

- **Early:** The early form occurs within the first 24 hours after birth and is because of maternal ingestion of medications that pass through the placental circulation and affect the neonatal production of vitamin K. These drugs include warfarin, carbamazepine, barbiturates, phenytoin, rifampin, isoniazid, and certain cephalosporins.
- **Classic:** The classic form manifests between days 2 and 7 of life and is caused by inadequate intake of vitamin K seen in breastfed babies with marginal intake of breast milk. Commercial infant formulas contain higher amounts of vitamin K compared with breast milk. The classic form of HDN is prevented by the routine practice of prophylactic administration of vitamin K at birth.
- **Late:** The late form of HDN presents 2 weeks to 6 months after birth because of inadequate intake (low vitamin K content in breast milk) or inadequate absorption in hepatobiliary disease. This form occurs more frequently in males and has a high incidence of intracranial bleeding. Intramuscular injection of vitamin K at birth provides improved protection against late-onset HDN compared with oral vitamin K.

20. **Why are neonates and young infants prone to thrombosis? Name some of the predisposing issues.**

Within the pediatric age group, the peak incidence of thrombotic disorders occurs in neonates and infants younger than 1 year. Although the immature coagulation system in the newborn is "physiological," the balance is perturbed in favor of thrombin formation rather than inhibition, especially in sick infants (those needing neonatal/cardiac intensive care, surgeries, having gastrointestinal issues or infections). The majority of neonatal thromboses occur in association with indwelling vascular catheters. In vitro studies on thrombin regulation in neonates and cord blood indicate that their blood exhibits a deficiency of thrombin inhibition and reduced plasmin generation. Other associated conditions include polycythemia, hypoxia, infection, maternal diabetes, and maternal lupus anticoagulant. Neonatal thromboses most frequently involve the large major vessels, such as the inferior vena cava, renal veins, aorta, and middle cerebral artery.

21. **Describe the treatment for thromboses in the neonate.**

The optimal treatment for neonatal thrombosis depends on the location, extent of vessel occlusion, and symptoms. Treatment options include anticoagulation with unfractionated heparin or low-molecular-weight heparin (LMWH), surgical thrombectomy, or thrombolytic therapy with tPA. Current approaches include 7 days of anticoagulation with heparinoids for arterial thromboses, followed by reassessment and extension of treatment as needed and tolerated. For venous thromboses, 6 to 12 weeks of anticoagulation with LMWH is typical, and shorter or longer courses can be considered based on resolution of thrombosis and ability to administer medication. Oral anticoagulation with warfarin can be challenging in a neonate, and options with direct oral anticoagulants (DOACS) are being studied. Interventions like thrombectomy and thrombolysis are reserved for life/limb-threatening situations and are dependent on available local expertise. Thrombolytic therapy is used typically for large arterial or venous thrombi, where surgical intervention is not feasible, and limited intracardiac thrombi in patients where no contraindications to use of thrombolytic agents exist.

22. **Why is it difficult to treat neonates with heparin?**

Newborns require higher doses of heparin compared with older children and adults for anticoagulation. Heparin works by accelerating the inactivation of thrombin and other activated clotting factors by antithrombin, which is physiologically reduced in the neonate. Furthermore, heparin has a faster clearance in the newborn because of an increased volume of distribution. Heparinoids also require parenteral administration and monitoring, which is difficult because of smaller vessels and difficult access issues in neonates.

DISORDERS OF COAGULATION

23. **Can hemophilia A and B be clinically distinguished?**

No. Hemophilia A and B cannot be clinically distinguished and present as similar pathologies. Hemophilia A, deficiency of factor VIII, and hemophilia B, deficiency of factor IX, are X-linked bleeding disorders. There are an estimated 25 in 100,000 live male births with hemophilia A and, less commonly, 5 in 100,000 live male births of hemophilia B.

Although there is some suggestion that the bleeding phenotype may be less severe for patients with hemophilia B on a population basis, on an individual basis, laboratory testing is needed to differentiate these diagnoses. The screening coagulation testing for both hemophilia A and B patients will show a prolonged PTT because factor VIII and factor IX are both in the intrinsic factor pathway; the best way to make a clear diagnosis would be factor-specific assays for factor VIII and factor IX activity.

Another clinical entity that can be difficult to distinguish from hemophilia is type 3 or type 2N VWD (discussed later in question 35), and this should be included in the differential diagnosis.

24. **Classify hemophilia A and B according to the degree of severity.**

The factor activity level correlates with clinical severity of disease:

Factor level less than 1%: Severe hemophilia

Factor level greater than 1% and less than 5%: Moderate hemophilia
Factor level greater than 5% and less than 40%: Mild hemophilia

25. **Does a negative family history exclude the diagnosis of hemophilia?**
No, hemophilia is a X-linked recessive disorder, and although there may often (~70% of the time) be a significant maternal family history, in the other 30% of patients it is a newly recognized mutation in the family. In these families, it can be a spontaneous mutation in the child newly diagnosed with hemophilia or, in some cases, the genetic mutation occurred in the mother and is now identified upon diagnosis of the child with hemophilia.

26. **Are there female patients with hemophilia (PWH)?**
Females can have hemophilia, but it is rare. There is an X-linked recessive pattern of inheritance. It is typically males who have hemophilia A/B. Females can present, however, with low factor levels and bleeding symptoms in the setting of Turner syndrome (one X chromosome), skewed X-inactivation, or two affected X chromosomes (maternal heterozygous carrier and paternal hemophilia, or an additional de novo mutation). Additionally, there are some females who are carriers for hemophilia with low factor levels and bleeding symptoms that can be classified as mild hemophilia patients.

27. **What types of bleeding can be encountered in patients with hemophilia?**

Life/Limb-Threatening Bleeds	*Moderate/Minor Bleeds*
• Head (intracranial)	• Joints
• Spinal cord	• Epistaxis
• Neck (airway)	• Mouth
• Iliopsoas muscle	• Cutaneous/Soft tissue
• Limb compartment syndrome	• Superficial lacerations
• Gastrointestinal hemorrhage	
• Ocular hemorrhage	
• Intra-abdominal hemorrhage	
• Fractures/Dislocations	
• Deep lacerations	
• Uncontrolled hemorrhage	

Hematuria: Bed rest/hydration. Avoid antifibrinolytics and factor concentrate balancing risk of obstructive uropathy.

28. **What are inhibitors, and how are they diagnosed?**
Inhibitors are neutralizing alloantibodies towards factor VIII/IX, typically developed in the setting of replacement therapy, making it ineffective to provide hemostasis. They can be classified as:
Low titer inhibitor: Titer measures less than 5.0 BU
High titer Inhibitor: Titer measures greater than 5.0 BU
    Features of inhibitors in hemophilia A and B are outlined in the table below:
Diagnosis (any of the below):
• Routine laboratory surveillance
• Lack of appropriate response to FVIII/FIX concentrate to control bleeding
• Diagnosed when decreased measured recovery of factor level
• Shortened half-life compared with expected

Inhibitors	Hemophilia A	Hemophilia B
Incidence	Severe: High (~30%)	Severe: Low (2%–10%)
	Mild/Moderate:13% with >100	
	exposure days (ED) or high-risk mutations	Mild/Moderate: Not seen
Risk Factors	Family history	Family history

29. **List the principle of bleeding treatment with replacement therapy for hemophilia.**
Treatment Principles:
• Bleeding must be treated promptly while waiting on diagnostic testing. Factor first!
• Dosing of factor replacement therapy is guided by volume of distribution, half-life, and hemostatic requirement of type of bleeding.

Factor replacement for hemophilia A: 1 international unit/kg ➔ ↑ FVIII Level 2% (Half-life ~12 hours)
[a]Factor replacement for hemophilia B: 1 international unit/kg ➔ ↑ FIX Level 1%[a] (Half-life ~24 hours)

[a]Typically increase dose by 1.2 to 1.4 for recombinant product.

- Monitor for inhibitor development during initial 20 exposures, which may present with allergic-type hypersensitivity reactions, including anaphylaxis, in a healthcare setting. Increased risk in severe FIX patients with large deletional mutation.

Treatment of Specific Hemorrhages

Hemorrhage	Hemophilia A	Hemophilia B	Duration	Comments
Central nervous system (CNS) bleeding	Initial 80%–100% Maintenance 50%	Initial 60%–80% Maintenance 30%	7 days 8–21 days	21 days for CNS
Airway Gastrointestinal (GI) bleeding				14 days for other sites of major bleeding
Iliopsoas muscle Muscle compartment with neurovascular injury	Initial 80%–100% Maintenance 30%–60%	Initial 60%–80% Maintenance 30%–60%	2 days until asymptomatic 3–14 days	May require reimaging to help guide planning and consider dosing with physiotherapy
Hemarthrosis Muscular bleeding (no neurovascular injury)	40%–60%	40%–60%	1–4 days	Consider duration of treatment based on response. May decrease to half initial dose during subsequent infusions
Deep laceration	50%	50%	5–7 days	
Renal	50%	40%	3–5 days	
Ophthalmology	100%	100%		Obtain ophthalmology consultation
Mouth Simple dental extractions	40%	20%–30%		Increased dose if molar or wisdom tooth extraction Benefit from anti-fibrinolytic therapy
Epistaxis	None	None		Local control: Pressure Topical agents Anti-fibrinolytics If conservative measures fail, 30%–40%

(Adapted from Di Paola J, Montgomery RR, Gill JC, Rood V. Hemophilia and von Willebrand disease. In Orkin SH, Nathan DG, Ginsburg D, Look AT, Fisher DE, Lux SE (eds). *Nathan and Oski's Hematology and Oncology of Infancy and Childhood.* 8th ed. Elsevier, 2015:1031; and Srivastava A, Brewer AK, Mauser-Bunschoten EP, et al. Guidelines for the management of hemophilia. *Haemophilia.* 2013;19[1]:e1–e47.)

30. **What type of hemophilia replacement products are available for treatment or prevention of bleeding?**
    Factor replacement products can be classified based on their half-lives or their production source:
    - **Standard half-life products:**
      - Can be plasma or recombinant factor concentrates
      - Plasma derived and may contain FIX or FVIII (+/- VWF), manufactured with antiviral after collection from healthy donors
      - Doses based on half-life of FVIII (~12 hours) or FIX (~24 hours)

- **Typical prophylaxis schedule:**
  - **Hemophilia A:** Every other day or 3 times per week
  - **Hemophilia B:** Twice per week
- **Extended half-life (EHL):**
  - Created by fusion to Fc part of IgG1 or albumin or PEGylation to prolong time between infusions
  - Typically, FVIII has an approximately 1.5-fold increase in half-life; FIX has a fivefold to sixfold increase in half-life
  - FVIII is less impressive than FIX EHL and likely limited by its VWF interaction (see question 34)
- **Nonfactor therapy:**
  - **Emicizumab:** Humanized bispecific antibody (approved 2017/2018) subcutaneous therapy for prevention of bleeding in hemophilia A patients with and without inhibitor
  - Mild hemophilia A patients can benefit from desmopressin (DDAVP) therapy (see question 37 for details on use of DDAVP in hemostatic therapy)

31. **What is a target joint?**

    Target joints are those joints where there are three or more spontaneous bleeds that occur in a 6-month period. These joints are more prone to rebleeding and are at risk for chronic damage and progression to hemophilic arthropathy.

32. **What is nonfactor therapy?**

    A new approach for managing bleeding disorders not based on replacement but rather on providing hemostasis by either inhibiting anticoagulant pathways (with drugs like fitusiran and concizumab) or by promoting coagulation (i.e., emicizumab) has been developed. Emicizumab is a humanized monoclonal bispecific antibody anti-FIXa/FX that functions as a mimetic of the FVIIa cofactor to form the ten-ase complex. Because it has no structural homology with FVIII, it is effective in the presence of inhibitory allo-antibodies. It has several advantages and disadvantages as therapy, which are outlined in the table below.

Advantages	Challenges

• Hemophilia A patients with and without an inhibitor can have prevention of bleeding
• Steady state, no peaks and troughs
• Infrequent infusions
• Weekly to monthly schedule
• Subcutaneous administration
  • No venous access
  • No central venous access device (CVAD)
  • May permit earlier initiation of prophylaxis
• Quality of life improvement
• No risk of FVIII inhibitor development
• Potential use for patients allergic to FVIII
	• Cannot be used to treat acute bleeding events
	• Safety signal with aPCC (FEIBA®) for thrombosis and thrombotic microangiopathic events.
	• No peak hemostatic levels, may provide less protection for active patients
	• Limited data for managing surgical procedures and breakthrough bleeding
	• Lack of exposures to FVIII
	• Anti-drug antibodies (<5%)
	• Limited hemostatic monitoring
	• No monitoring of level
	• No using standard PTT based assay for monitoring factor levels or inhibitors. Need chromogenic bovine based assays.

MANAGEMENT OF INHIBITOR PATIENT

33. **What are treatment options for PWH with inhibitors?**

    Hemophilia patients with inhibitors have an increased risk of morbidity and mortality and are medically complex with a high risk of bleeding.

    It is therefore recommended that they receive care in collaboration with the local hemophilia treatment center (HTC). Principles of management in inhibitor eradication, bypassing agents and nonfactor therapy, are as follows:

	Bleeding Management	Prevention of Bleeding	Inhibitor Eradication
Hemophilia A	**Bypassing Agents** **rFVIIa** • 90 mcg/kg every 2–3 hours • 270 mcg/kg • *Recombinant* • *Small volumes* • *Thrombosis risk* **APCC** • 50–100 IU/kg every 6–12 hours • Max 200 IU/kg/day	**Bypassing Agents** rFVIIa • Daily dose • Incomplete protection from bleeding based on short half-life • Thrombosis risk **APCC** • 85 IU/kg 2–3 times per week • Incomplete protection from bleeding based on short half-life	**Immune Tolerance Induction (ITI)** • Regular infusion of FVIII • Goal to allow body to be accustomed to FVIII replacement and stop making neutralizing antibodies (i.e., tolerized) • Allow for FVIII replacement to be effective treatment for bleeding

- Plasma derived
- Contains FIX/FVIII for re-exposure risk
- Large volume
- Thrombosis risk
- Risk of thrombotic microangiopathy (TMA) combined with emicizumab

Porcine rFVIII
- 200 unit/kg
- *Monitor for anti-porcine FVIII inhibitor*

High-Dose FVIII
- Low titer inhibitor <5.0 BU
- Twofold to threefold increased dose
- *Monitor for anamnestic response with rapid rise in inhibitor titer*

DDAVP
- Mild hemophilia patients
- Low titer inhibitor <5.0 BU with kinetics supporting incomplete inactivation of endogenous FVIII
- Minor bleeding

Hemophilia B **Bypassing Agents**
- rFVIIa > FEIBA given risk of anaphylaxis with exposure to FIX containing product

- Thrombosis risk

Nonfactor Therapy
Emicizumab
Dosing:[a]
1.5 mg/kg every week
3 mg/kg every 2 weeks
6 mg/kg every 4 weeks
- Steady state improved protection from bleeding
- Extended dosing interval
- Subcutaneous dosing
- Does **not** treat acute bleeding
- *Unable to monitor inhibitor level or FVIII levels with conventional testing (Bovine-based reagents are needed for accurate results)*

Bypassing Agent
- rFVIIa as earlier

ITI successful tolerization ~70%
ITI Protocols
Bonn Protocol
FVIII 100–150 IU/kg twice per day
Dutch "Low-Dose" Protocol
25 IU/kg every other day
International ITI Study
High-dose: FVIII 200 IU/kg daily
Low-dose: FVIII 50 IU/kg 3 times per week
Alternative Regimen
FVIII 100 IU/kg daily
Additional Considerations:
- Pd-FVIII/VWF concentrate
- Role of EHL FVIII in ITI
- Immunosuppression
Evolving role of ITI therapy, dosing, timing, and duration in the setting of new nonfactor therapies.

ITI *less* successful (~30%)
Immunosuppression often may be needed for inhibitor eradication:
- Rituximab
- Steroids
- MMF
- Cyclosporin
- IVIG

Challenges:
- Allergic reaction with re-exposure to FIX therapy
- Nephrotic syndrome may develop with ITI
- Lack of evidence to support decision making

---

[a]Emicizumab loading dose 3 mg/kg subcutaneous weekly for 4 weeks, then maintenance dosing as above.
APCC, Activated prothrombinase concentrate complex; *DDAVP*, desmopressin; *EHL*, extended half-life; *FEIBA*, factor eight inhibitor bypassing activity; *IVIG*, intravenous immunoglobulin; *MMF*, mycophenolate-mofetil; *pd-FVIII*, plasma-derived factor VIII; *rFVIIa*, recombinant factor VIIa; *VWF*, von Willebrand factor.

34. Name the two functions or physiological roles of VWF.
    The VWF protein acts through two main functions. First, it is the carrier protein for factor VIII, protecting it from rapid proteolysis in its activated form by activated protein C.
    Second, it promotes hemostasis by mediating platelet adhesion to damaged vascular sub-endothelial matrix (e.g., collagen) and furthers platelet aggregation by being present at the site of vessel injury. The adhesive activity of VWF depends on the size of its multimers, with larger multimers being the most hemostatic. When there is exposure of the subendothelium and modified flow dynamics with a vascular injury, a conformal change occurs in the VWF protein. As a result, the higher molecular weight multimers interact with collagen and platelet receptors with eventual regulatory participation from FVIII as well in thrombus generation.

35. **Describe the classifications of VWD.**
    VWD is broadly classified into three types:
    Type 1: Partial quantitative deficiency of VWF
    Type 2: Qualitative deficiency
    Type 3: Complete deficiency

Type 1	Decreased synthesis	Most common	80%	Autosomal dominant
Type 1C	Increased clearance	↑ VWFpp compared with VWF:Ag		Autosomal dominant
Type 2A	Defects in multimer formation or cleavage site	Loss of HMWM	10%–20%	Autosomal dominant
Type 2B	↑ affinity for platelet binding (Gain of function)	Loss of HMWN Low-dose RIPA	5%	Autosomal dominant
Type 2N	Mutation in binding site for FVIII	Low FVIII because of rapid clearance without VWF protection	Uncommon	Autosomal recessive
Type 2M	Loss of function VWF binding platelets	Normal multimers	<5%	Autosomal dominant
Type 3	Absent VWF	Phenotype overlaps with hemophilia A FVIII % <10%	Rare (1:million)	Autosomal recessive
Low VWF	VWF:Ag 30–50 IU/dL VWF Activity 30–50 IU/dL	Risk factor for bleeding		

HMWM, High molecular weight multimers; *RIPA,* ristocetin-induced platelet aggregations; *VWF,* von Willebrand factor; *VWF:Ag,* von Willebrand factor antigen; *VWFpp,* von Willebrand factor propeptide.

VWD types 1 and 3 are quantitative defects, whereas type 2 VWD is because of qualitative defect of the VWF protein. Type 1 VWD accounts for about 75% of all VWD cases and severity of symptoms in type 1 VWD typically co-relates with degree of deficiency of the factor. Type 2 VWD has four clinical subtypes (2A, 2B, 2M, and 2N) caused by qualitative defects in the VWF protein. Bleeding in types 2A, 2B, and 2M cannot be differentiated from type 1 or among themselves.

36. **What are the clinical manifestations of VWD?**
    VWD is typically a primary hemostatic pathway defect, and patients present with skin and mucosal lining–related bleeding. Symptoms can include epistaxis, easy and frequent bruising, gum and oral bleeding (prolonged bleeding after tooth extractions, from biting cheek or lips, frequent mouth bleeding from flossing/brushing), gut bleeding with angiodysplasia, and/or menorrhagia. The presentation can vary based on the severity and type of disease.
    VWD 2N is named after "Normandy" where the first individuals with this subtype were identified; they were noted to have decreased FVIII because of VWF defects of FVIII binding. The presentation is very similar to hemophilia A, and often these patients can initially be misdiagnosed as having hemophilia. As opposed to type 1 and other subtypes of type 2 VWD, there can be spontaneous bleeding into joints and muscles and large hematoma formation with minor trauma. The family history is helpful in those scenarios because type 2 N is inherited in an autosomal recessive fashion and can occur in females.

37. **How does DDAVP work for the treatment of VWD?**
    DDAVP (1-Desamino-8-D-Arginine-Vasopressin; desmopressin) is a synthetic derivative of antidiuretic hormone vasopressin acting at the V2 receptor. It acts by promoting release of stored FVIII and VWF from endothelial Wiebel-Palade bodies, thereby increasing circulating plasma levels of both. There have to be decent stored volumes of these factors for DDAVP to be an effective therapeutic option, limiting its use in severe hemophilia and type 3 VWD and in surgical or major trauma (e.g., motor vehicular accident), where high increment in circulating levels of factors may be needed. This increase is factor levels is typically transient, lasting 4 to 6 hours, peaking at about an hour since dose. Not everyone responds to DDAVP, so a trial beforehand (i.e., in a nonbleeding patient and in a nonsurgical setting) is advised to document magnitude and duration of response.

38. **What is hemophilia C (factor XI deficiency)?**
    Factor XI deficiency (also known as hemophilia C) is a rare disease (incidence 1 in 1 million) found predominantly and much more commonly in Ashkenazi Jews (1 in 8 heterozygous to 1 in 190 homozygous). Individuals with severe factor XI deficiency are primarily at risk for excessive bleeding after surgery and injury, particularly when trauma involves tissues rich in fibrinolytic activity. This is typically a mild bleeding disorder with patients presenting with easy bruising, epistaxis, and menorrhagia but no joint or deep muscle bleeds.

There is a poor correlation between factor XI level and bleeding in patients with factor XI deficiency. In some people with severe FXI deficiency (e.g., levels <20 IU/dL), there is no excessive bleeding, whereas other individuals with levels only moderately below the normal range bleed after surgery.

Diagnosis can be made after identifying isolated prolongation of aPTT, followed by specific factor after excluding other factor deficiencies. Need for replacement therapy with plasma infusions is rare, usually only indicated for high-risk surgical procedures like neurosurgical, cardiac, urologic and ear, and nose and throat procedures. Mucous membrane and dental bleeding usually respond well to adjunctive treatment with antifibrinolytic agents like epsilon aminocaproic acid or tranexamic acid.

39. **Name a few acquired causes of combined PT/aPTT prolongation.**
    After excluding artefactual reasons for combined PT and aPTT prolongation (heparin contamination, inadequate filling of the testing tubes, low hematocrit), the following causes can be considered:
    1. **Vitamin K deficiency** (factors II, VII, IX, and X) or true deficiency of one of the factors of the common pathway (fibrinogen, factors II, V and X): Vitamin K deficiency can cause isolated PT prolongation in the initial stages, because among vitamin K–dependent factors, factor VII has the shortest half-life (4–6 hours). It is, therefore, easily depleted in both vitamin K deficiency (and liver disease) compared with the other factors, resulting in isolated prolongation of the PT.
    2. **Liver disease:** All clotting factors will be low except the acute phase reactants factor VIII (and VWF) and fibrinogen, which are elevated or normal until the late or severe stage of hepatic injury.
    3. **Consumptive coagulopathy or disseminated intravascular coagulation (DIC):** Except in the early or mild stage, all coagulation factors can be diminished.
    4. **Recent use of an anticoagulant:** Warfarin toxicity would present similar to vitamin K deficiency as previously mentioned.

40. **What is disseminated intravascular coagulation?**
    Disseminated intravascular coagulation (DIC) or intravascular coagulation and fibrinolysis (ICF) is an acquired disorder of hemostatic dysregulation wherein widespread fibrin formation occurs with resultant thrombosis of small and mid-size vessels, compromising blood supply to organs. This sets off a consumptive coagulopathy in return, leading to acquired decrease in platelets and coagulation proteins, with subsequent increased risk of bleeding.
    DIC is always a secondary event typically in the setting of a systemic infection (commonly bacterial), trauma, malignancy, or giant hemangiomas. Diagnosis can be made based on lab findings of prolonged PT and aPTT, low fibrinogen, low platelet count, and elevated FDPs (D-dimers or soluble fibrin monomer concentration) in the correct clinical setting.

41. **Define thrombophilia.**
    The term "thrombophilia" or "hypercoagulable states" refers to a group of inherited or acquired abnormalities that predispose to thromboembolism. Thrombophilic states could be congenital or acquired. The common congenital thrombophilias including factor V Leiden and PG20210 mutations; deficiencies of protein C, protein S, and antithrombin; and elevated levels of FVIII, homocysteine, and lip (a). Incidence of these conditions range from very common (5% of population for Factor V Leiden heterozygosity) up to 6.5% to rare (1 in 2000–5000 for antithrombin deficiency).
    Factor V Leiden is a point mutation leading to replacement of arginine by glycine at position 506 (R506Q) in the factor V protein, making it resistant to degradation by activated protein C. Protein C and S are both responsible for proteolytic degradation of factor Va and VIIIa, and their respective deficiencies lead to unregulated prothrombotic predisposition from these activated factors. PG20210 variant is a guanine to adenine transition at nucleotide 20210 in the prothrombin protein, leading to higher plasma prothrombin levels. Increased risk of VTE in children with these conditions ranges from twofold to threefold for FV Leiden heterozygosity and PG20210 to approximately 10-fold for antithrombin deficiency.
    There can also be anatomic thrombophilic states (i.e., anatomic conditions that predispose one to thromboses), such as May-Thurner syndrome (when the left iliac vein is compressed by the right iliac artery) or Paget-Schroetter syndrome (compression of the subclavian vein at the thoracic outlet). Pregnancy and immobilization because of fractures/surgeries also can lead to such acquired thrombophilic states.
    Acquired thrombophilia also includes antiphospholipid syndrome (APS). APS is characterized by recurrent venous or arterial thrombosis and/or fetal loss because of immune dysregulation–related antibodies (most commonly because of systemic lupus erythematosus) that are directed against membrane anionic phospholipids (i.e., anticardiolipin [aCL] antibody, antiphosphatidylserine) or their associated plasma proteins, predominantly beta-2 glycoprotein, or evidence of a circulating anticoagulant.

42. **Discuss the presentation of thrombosis in children.**
    Incidence of deep vein thrombosis (DVT) in children is reported to be 0.07 to 0.14 per 10,000, and although incidence may be rising, DVTs in children are much less frequent than in adults. There is a bimodal distribution to pediatric thromboses, with neonates/infants and teenagers being at highest risk. In the majority of cases (>95%), thromboses are secondary to other risk factors, such as central venous catheters, and other underlying medical conditions, including prematurity, congenital heart disease, cancer, surgery, and systemic lupus erythematosus.

Thromboembolic events can be arterial or venous. Arterial thrombosis usually is related to catheters, such as umbilical artery catheterization in neonates, and cardiac catheterization through the femoral artery but can also occur spontaneously, as in ischemic stroke.

Venous thrombi could be in the deep veins of the extremities or other sites like pulmonary veins, inferior vena cava, renal vein, right atrium, portal vein, and cerebral sinus. Extremity DVTs present with redness/discoloration, pain, and swelling of the affected limb. For other DVTs, symptoms can vary according to affected site (e.g., hematuria with renal vein thrombosis, headaches, nausea, vision changes with cerebral or ophthalmic thromboses).

BIBLIOGRAPHY

1. Andrew M, David M, Adams M, et al. Venous thromboembolic complications (VTE) in children: first analyses of the Canadian Registry of VTE. *Blood.* 1994;83(5):1251–1257.
2. Blanchette VS, Key NS, Ljung LR, et al. Definitions in hemophilia: communication from the SSC of the ISTH. *J Thromb Haemost.* 2014;12 (11):1935–1939.
3. Franchini M, Mannucci PM. Haemophilia B is clinically less severe than haemophilia A: further evidence. *Blood Transfus.* 2018;16(2): 121–122.
4. Franchini M, Santoro C, Coppola A. Inhibitor incidence in previously untreated patients with severe haemophilia B: a systematic literature review. *Thromb Haemost.* 2016;116(1):201–203.
5. Gouw SC, van der Bom JG, Marijke van den Berg H. Treatment-related risk factors of inhibitor development in previously untreated patients with hemophilia A: the CANAL cohort study. *Blood.* 2007;109(11):4648–4654.
6. Male C, Andersson NG, Rafowicz A, et al. Inhibitor incidence in an unselected cohort of previously untreated patients with severe haemophilia B: a PedNet study. *Haematologica.* 2021;106(1):123–129.
7. Martensson A, Letelier A, Hallden C, Ljung R. Mutation analysis of Swedish haemophilia B families - high frequency of unique mutations. *Haemophilia.* 2016;22(3):440–445.
8. Miller CH, Benson J, Ellingsen D, et al. F8 and F9 mutations in US haemophilia patients: correlation with history of inhibitor and race/ethnicity. *Haemophilia.* 2012;18(3):375–382.
9. Peyvandi F, Mannucci PM, Garagiola I, et al. A randomized trial of factor VIII and neutralizing antibodies in hemophilia A. *N Engl J Med.* 2016;374(21):2054–2064.
10. Schwaab R, Brackmann HH, Meyer C, et al. Haemophilia A: mutation type determines risk of inhibitor formation. *Thromb Haemost.* 1995;74(6):1402–1406.
11. Srivastava A, Brewer AK, Mauser-Bunschoten EP, et al. Guidelines for the management of hemophilia. *Haemophilia.* 2013;19(1):e1–47.
12. van Ommen CH, Heijboer H, Büller HR, Hirasing RA, Heijmans HS, Peters M. Venous thromboembolism in childhood: a prospective two-year registry in The Netherlands. *J Pediatr.* 2001;139(5):676–681.
13. Young G, Albisetti M, Bonduel M, et al. Impact of inherited thrombophilia on venous thromboembolism in children: a systematic review and meta-analysis of observational studies. *Circulation.* 2008;118(13):1373–1382.

CHAPTER 2

DEVELOPMENTAL ERYTHROPOIESIS

Rudi-Ann Graham, MD and Nancy S. Green, MD

1. **Define fetal erythropoiesis.**

   In the fetus, erythropoiesis begins at approximately the fourth gestational week and is primarily formed in the extravascular yolk sac. By the fifth gestational week, erythropoiesis begins within the liver. Only in the last gestational trimester does erythropoiesis (and myelopoiesis) take place in the bone marrow. Simultaneously, major changes occur in the structure of hemoglobin (Hb). Initially, embryonic Hbs are expressed. Subsequently these are replaced by fetal Hb (HbF), and then ultimately, predominately by adult Hb.

   The first globin chains to be produced are the epsilon (ϵ) chains, similar in structure to the beta (β) chains. The ϵ chains (similar to later β globins) initially form symmetrical tetramers (ϵ^4). Next, other embryonic Hbs develop: The zeta (ζ) chains (similar to the later alpha [α]-globin) pair with the ϵ chains form the tetramer $\zeta^2\epsilon^2$. These primitive Hbs are called Gower-1.

   Gradually the α chain develops. Initially, it pairs with the ϵ chain and forms the complex $\alpha^2\epsilon^2$, the Gower-2 hemoglobin. Subsequently the gamma (γ) chains appear (γA and γG). These globin chains initially pair with the ζ chain to form the tetramer $\zeta^2\gamma^2$ (Hb Portland). Later, HbF ($= \alpha^2\gamma^2$) is formed.

   In the third trimester, the adult β chain appears, at which point adult-type Hb (HbA $= \alpha^2\beta^2$) begins to replace the HbF. At birth, approximately 40% to 60% of the Hb is HbA. Normally HbF continues to decline after birth and reaches the very low (1%–2%) adult level by 4 to 5 months of age.

2. **Describe erythropoiesis at birth.**

   At birth, the Hb level is remarkably high (15–18 g/dL) and the red cells are extremely large (120–130 μ^3). As the erythropoiesis progressively turns to mostly HbA, the red cells decrease in size to less than 80 μ^3 and the Hb concentration drops to 11 to 12 g/dL. This low concentration persists throughout childhood until puberty, when Hb concentration starts to rise toward the adult level.

DISORDERS OF HEMOGLOBIN IN THE NEONATAL PERIOD

3. **How does occult blood loss before delivery occur?**

   Hemorrhagic anemia is the most common cause of anemia in the full-term newborn infant. Antepartum fetomaternal hemorrhage (FMH) occurs in approximately 75% of pregnancies. The risk is increased with preeclampsia, the need for instrumentation, and cesarian delivery. The severity of FMH is related to the volume of blood lost in relation to the overall fetal blood volume and whether the event is acute or chronic. Massive FMH is defined as more than 20% blood loss from the fetoplacental circulation. Clinically significant bleeding will therefore vary by gestational age. Infrequently (less than <1% of cases) bleeding is substantial enough to result in fetal anemia. In severe cases nonimmune hydrops fetalis may result. FMH can be quantified either by staining the blood film of the mother for the proportion of fetal cells (the Kleihauer Betke test) or by flow cytometry; the latter is less labor-intensive.

   In the antepartum period, loss of fetal red blood cells (RBCs) can also occur with reduced placental integrity (abruptio placentae, placenta previa, or traumatic amniocentesis), anomalies of the umbilical cord or placental vessels (vasa previa, umbilical cord hematoma), or with twin-twin transfusion. Twin-twin transfusion syndrome (TTTS) may occur in monozygotic twins who share a placenta or placental vessels. Although uncommon, TTTS can result in one anemic and one polycythemic newborn. The anemic donor twin is at risk for congestive heart failure (CHF), whereas the recipient plethoric twin may develop signs of hyperviscosity syndrome.

4. **Discuss hemoglobinopathies and thalassemias at birth.**

   Most β-chain hemoglobinopathies are not clinically obvious at birth because HbF synthesis persists and thus may obscure the symptoms associated with β hemoglobinopathies (e.g., reduced production with β thalassemia). This is true for many types of β hemoglobinopathies (e.g. sickle cell disease) and with β thalassemias. An exception is when there are large deletions within the β-globin gene cluster that result in loss of both γ-globin genes and the delta (δ) and β-globin genes. In the homozygous state, this γ-δ-β-thalassemia is incompatible with life, whereas heterozygotes manifest a transient but moderate to severe microcytic anemia in the newborn. Infants born with homozygous β thalassemia major, β^0/β^0 thalassemia (discussed in full in Chapter 5, Thalassemia), although clinically normal at birth, will have almost exclusively HbF (or "F") on newborn screen because of an inability to produce HbA.

   Nevertheless, defects of the α chains can be clinically apparent in the neonatal period. Humans normally have four α genes, which are all coexpressed in the newborn period. Newborns with α-thalassemia trait (deletion of one or two of the four α genes) may have mild to moderate microcytosis and have low amounts of Hb Barts, a γ Hb tetramer (γ^4), on newborn screening. Newborns with Hb H (HbH) disease (deletion of three of the four α genes) have higher concentrations of Hb Barts, a γ Hb tetramer generally at levels of 20% to 40% at birth. In babies with HbH disease, some HbH (β^4) is found at birth and rises postnatally as Hb switches from being predominantly fetal to adult. These babies present with moderately to severe anemia, hemolysis, and jaundice. They need to be monitored for possible kernicterus because of excess hemolysis of these unstable abnormal Hbs, especially if affected babies are premature.

Hydrops fetalis occurs in fetuses that are homozygous for α-thalassemia (absence of α genes). As soon as embryonic erythropoiesis abates, these fetuses become profoundly anemic in utero because the absence of α chains precludes the synthesis of any hetero-tetramer of Hb. This condition leads to fetal CHF and generalized edema. When unrecognized, this syndrome is fatal in utero (hydrops fetalis). Nevertheless, if a diagnosis is made sufficiently early in utero, the pregnancy can continue with repeated intrauterine RBC transfusions. The newborn will need chronic RBC transfusions or a hematopoietic stem cell ("bone marrow") transplantation to reduce or eliminate chronic RBC transfusions.

Cases in which α thalassemia trait (1 or 2 α-globin gene absence) is not clinically evident at birth may be initially discovered with positive results from a routine newborn screen by the presence of Hb Barts. Many of these children have some microcytosis at birth (mean corpuscular volume [MCV] less than 100 fL in a full-term baby.) The diagnosis of α thalassemia is best confirmed by molecular globin gene testing, which can be performed by routine commercial laboratories. When molecular analysis is not available, the diagnosis can be made by the presence of elevated amounts of Hb Barts when performed during the newborn period. Later, Hb Barts will not be found once the baby has switched to HbH. Because HbH is an unstable Hb, it will not be present in sufficient amounts in children with α thalassemia trait and therefore is not a useful marker on Hb electrophoresis.

5. Describe other disorders of hemoglobin.
Many Hb variants have been described. Those that result in a reduction of the red cell life span and/or hemolysis are of clinical significance. Other than in α or β thalassemia (when α or β Hb synthesis is decreased or absent), in most hemoglobinopathies, the synthesis of Hb is normal, but the Hb stability or function is abnormal.

Hb defects can result from replacement of just a single amino acid (resulting from one DNA base substitution in the codon). Depending on the type and the position of the amino acid replacement, the effect on RBC survival may be different. Other Hb defects may be caused by amino acid deletion or nonhomologous crossover, resulting in a fusion Hb, such as Hb Lepore. In this hemoglobinopathy, the Hb synthesis, if impaired, can lead to a β-thalassemia-like syndrome. A different type of abnormality may result from an error in the termination codon. A classic example is Hb Constant Spring, frequent in Southeast Asia; it also leads to an α-thalassemia-like syndrome.

The most classic example of abnormal Hb resulting from a single base substitution is the replacement of glutamic acid with glycine in the sixth amino-acid position resulting in HbS (sickle). This single change results in a tendency of the HbS globin to polymerize into filamentous structure, especially with reduced oxygen or pH, leading to intracellular sickling. Heterozygous HbS, sickle trait, is asymptomatic under most physiologic conditions and does not cause anemia, hemolysis, or microcytosis. Where microcytosis is seen with sickle trait, most commonly there is concurrent α-thalassemia trait. When HbS is inherited in the homozygous state, this leads to a severe syndrome: HbSS, or sickle cell anemia. The effects of sickle cell anemia are profound on all body systems affected by the intravascular sickling and hemolysis and consequent tissue damage from hypoxia and inflammation. This condition is discussed in full in a separate chapter.

The replacement of glutamic acid with lysine in the same sixth amino acid position instead results in HbC, by itself a rather inoffensive alteration. In heterozygous individuals, HbC is only manifested by microcytosis and the diffuse presence of target RBCs (by microscopic evaluation) without anemia. The homozygous state, HbCC, or the compound heterozygote state of HbC and Hb β thalassemia (HbC-β thalassemia) can result in a modest asymptomatic anemia with mild hemolysis and diffuse target cells. When an individual is a compound heterozygote with both HbS and HbC, however, the resulting clinical manifestation is a form of sickle cell disease, HbSC.

Individuals who inherit the HbS gene and the gene for β thalassemia are also affected by a clinical syndrome (HbSβ-thalassemia zero, or HbSβ-thalassemia^0) of a severity comparable to homozygous sickle cell disease because no HbA is produced. The clinical severity of HbSβ-thalassemia correlates with the amount of normal β globin produced. HbSβ-thalassemia plus (HbSβ-thalassemia$^+$), where some HbA is produced, usually is a milder form of sickle cell disease.

6. Discuss hemoglobin variants with abnormal function.
Amino acid substitutions in unstable Hbs occur within the heme cavity of the α- or β-polypeptide chain. Unstable Hbs precipitate inside the red cells leading to intravascular hemolysis. Heinz bodies are often identified. Individuals with these defects are usually heterozygous because the homozygous state (extremely rare) would be incompatible with life.

Changes in the oxygen affinity have been found in some of the unstable Hbs and in the methemoglobinopathies (HbM) and can occur in variants of the α, β, or γ globins. An increased Hb oxygen affinity results in tissue hypoxia and an increased erythropoietic drive for a given level of anemia. In at least one hemoglobinopathy, Hb Chesapeake, the sole clinical manifestation is mild polycythemia.

The effects of hereditary HbM are similar to those unstable Hbs where the amino acid substitution is in the region of heme attachment. HbM results in increased susceptibility to oxidation of ferrous heme (Fe^{2+}) to ferric heme (Fe^{3+}) with consequent methemoglobin accumulation and cyanosis rather than hemolysis. Fresh blood can appear dark red or dark brown. Individuals with heterozygous HbM abnormalities have a high concentration of HbA and, apart from the cyanosis, are asymptomatic. The more common cause of congenital methemoglobinemia, however, reflects a defect in the enzyme methemoglobin reductase, not an Hb defect.

BIBLIOGRAPHY

1. Aher S, Kedar M, Kadam S. Neonatal anemia. *Semin Fetal Neonatal Med.* 2008;13(4):239–247.
2. Dame C, Juul SE. The switch from fetal to adult erythropoiesis. *Clin Perinatol.* 2000;27(3):507–526.

CHAPTER 3

SICKLE CELL SYNDROMES

Shipra Kaicker, MD and Margaret T. Lee, MD, MS

1. **What is sickle cell disease?**
   Sickle cell disease is an autosomal recessive inherited blood disorder caused by mutation in the ß-globin gene resulting in production of an abnormal hemoglobin (Hb), hemoglobin S (HbS), which polymerizes under deoxygenated conditions leading to formation of distorted "sickle-shaped" erythrocytes from which the disease derived its name. It is prevalent in individuals of African, Middle Eastern, Southern European, and Indian ethnicity. Globally, an estimated 300,000 babies are born with the disease annually, with 80% in Africa. In the United States, about 100,000 people are affected, primarily in the African American population and to a lesser degree in the Hispanic population of immigrants from the Caribbean.

2. **What are the different disorders covered by the term sickle cell disease?**
   The term *sickle cell disease* includes homozygous HbS (HbSS) and the compound heterozygous combination of HbS with another structural variant of ß globin, such as Hb C, D, E, O (HbSC, HbSD, HbSE, HbSO), or reduced production of ß globin as in β^0 and β^+ thalassemia (HbSß⁰thalassemia and HbSß⁺thalassemia). Although the clinical manifestations of these sickling syndromes are similar, there is wide heterogeneity and severity is variable. Typical findings in the common variants of sickle cell disease are shown in the following table.

| Disease | Clinical severity | Hematologic values | | | Hemoglobin electrophoresis (%) | | | | |
		Hb (g/dL)	MCV (fl)	Retic (%)	A	A2	F	S	C
HbSS	Usually severe	6–10	>80	5–20	0	<3.5	<10	>90	-
HbSC	Mild to moderate	10–15	75–95	5–10	0	-	<5	50	50
HbSß⁰thal	Moderate to severe	6–10	<80	5–20	0	>3.5	<20	>80	-
HbSß⁺thal	Usually mild	9–12	<75	5–10	20	>3.5	<20	>60	-

Hb, Hemoglobin; *HbSc*, HbS + HbC; *HbSS*, homozygous HbS; *HbSß⁰thal*, β^0 thalassemia; *HbSß⁺ thal*, β^+ thalassemia; *MCV*, mean corpuscular volume.
(Adapted from National Institutes of Health – National Heart, Lung and Blood Institute – NIH Publication No 96-2117. *The Management and Therapy of Sickle Cell Disease*. 3rd ed. 1995.)

3. **What is the underlying pathophysiology of sickle cell disease?**
   The pathophysiology of vaso-occlusion and sickle cell-related injury is complex and not simply obstruction by poorly deformable sickle erythrocytes within blood vessels under hypoxic conditions. Damaged sickle erythrocytes interact with the vascular endothelium causing upregulation of adhesion molecules such as E- and P-selectins, intercellular adhesion molecule 1 (ICAM-1), and vascular cell adhesion molecule 1 (VCAM-1). This leads to recruitment of neutrophils, platelets, and coagulation proteins contributing to worsening vascular stasis and vaso-occlusion. Chronic red cell hemolysis leads to release of free Hb and free heme into the circulation contributing further to endothelial dysfunction by creating reactive oxygen species and by depleting nitric oxide, an effective natural vasodilator. Ischemia-reperfusion injury and the presence of circulating free heme leads to a state of chronic "sterile inflammation."

4. **List some of the clinical manifestations of the disease.**
   Sickle cell disease can affect every organ of the body and presents with acute and chronic clinical manifestations:
   Acute:
   - Acute vaso-occlusive pain
   - Acute chest syndrome
   - Acute splenic sequestration
   - Aplastic crisis
   - Stroke
   - Priapism

   Chronic:
   - Chronic anemia and resultant complications (cardiomegaly, hypoxemia, stunted growth, and delayed sexual maturation)
   - Chronic hemolysis and consequent complications (gallstone formation, pulmonary hypertension)

- Functional asplenia and increased risk for bacterial infections (sepsis, osteomyelitis)
- Avascular necrosis (femoral and humeral heads)
- Nephropathy (glomerular hyperfiltration, microalbuminuria)
- Retinopathy
- Leg ulcers

5. What is acute chest syndrome?

Acute chest syndrome is a term used for the vaso-occlusive pulmonary complication of sickle cell disease. It is defined as an acute illness characterized by fever and/or respiratory symptoms, accompanied by a new pulmonary infiltrate on chest x-ray. Its causes are multifactorial, including hypoventilation, infection, asthma exacerbation, fat emboli from bone marrow necrosis, and pulmonary vascular microthrombi. Pathophysiology consists of massive inflammatory response leading to lung infarcts, hypoxia, and respiratory failure. Management includes monitoring for progression (because patients can demonstrate rapid clinical decompensation), respiratory support, broad-spectrum antibiotics including macrolides for atypical microorganisms, and red blood cell (RBC) transfusion. Transfusion can be either simple or exchange transfusion depending on Hb level and severity.

6. Define acute splenic sequestration.

Acute splenic sequestration is characterized by acute enlargement of the spleen, drop in Hb by at least 2 g/dL below baseline steady-state level, substantial reticulocytosis, and mild to moderate thrombocytopenia. It is commonly seen in young infants with HbSS or HbSβ⁰thalassemia and at times in older children and adolescents with HbSC or HbSβ⁺thalassemia, often associated with an infection. Patients should be closely monitored for severe anemia and hypovolemia. RBC transfusion, when indicated for severe anemia, is given in small aliquots of 5 mL/kg with the goal of partially correcting anemia while avoiding overtransfusion because erythrocytes sequestered in the spleen often re-enter the circulation and could lead to hyperviscosity. There is a high rate of recurrence after an initial episode. Splenectomy after age 2 years is recommended after two episodes of acute splenic sequestrations. Chronic RBC transfusions maintaining HbS less than 30% is often employed to prevent recurrent splenic sequestrations until splenectomy can be performed after age 2 years.

7. What is aplastic crisis?

Aplastic crisis is a transient abrupt cessation of erythropoiesis resulting in anemia with marked reticulocytopenia (<1%). Patients can present with fever, pallor, fatigue, lethargy, headache, and shortness of breath. It is almost exclusively caused by parvovirus B19. It is self-limited with resolution expected in 1 to 2 weeks. Recovery is heralded by an increase in circulating nucleated red blood cells (RBCs) and reticulocytes. Management is RBC transfusion for severe symptomatic anemia.

8. What are the strategies employed for infection prophylaxis in children with sickle cell disease?

Functional asplenia develops in almost all individuals with HbSS or HbSβ⁰thalassemia by age 3 to 5 years, making them susceptible to infections caused by *Streptococcus pneumoniae, Haemophilus influenzae,* and other encapsulated organisms. To decrease risk of sepsis, penicillin prophylaxis is started at 1 to 2 months of age or as soon as diagnosis is made for patients with HbSS and HbSβ⁰thalassemia. Penicillin prophylaxis can be discontinued at age 5 years unless the patient has a history of splenectomy or previous invasive pneumococcal infection. Although sometimes prescribed, the benefit of penicillin prophylaxis in less severe forms, such as HbSC and HbSβ⁺thalassemia, is less clear. Pneumococcal vaccines, including PCV-13 conjugate vaccine series in infancy and 23-valent polysaccharide vaccine at age 2 years, are administered to children with sickle cell disease to decrease the risk of pneumococcal bacteremia. Meningitis A, C, W, Y vaccines are recommended for children with functional asplenia by the Centers for Disease Control and Prevention (CDC) as early as 2 months of age, and meningitis B vaccine should be given after age 10 years.

9. List the indications for RBC transfusions in sickle cell disease.

Red blood cell transfusions are an important therapeutic intervention for sickle cell disease and should be used judiciously. Indications for RBC transfusion include:

For treatment:
- Acute stroke
- Acute chest syndrome with respiratory compromise
- Life-threatening anemia with reticulocytopenia (aplastic crisis)
- Splenic or hepatic sequestration and hypovolemic shock
- Multiorgan failure/hemodynamic compromise

For prophylaxis:
- Stroke prevention
- Preoperative preparation
- Recurrent severe acute chest syndrome despite hydroxyurea
- Severe recurrent vaso-occlusive pain despite hydroxyurea
- Recurrent priapism
- Progressive pulmonary hypertension
- Considered for silent cerebral infarcts
- Considered for recurrent splenic sequestration while waiting for splenectomy

10. **What are the different types of transfusions for patients with sickle cell disease?**
RBC transfusions can be provided by either simple red blood cell transfusion or exchange transfusion. In a simple red blood cell transfusion, the patient receives a prespecified volume of blood calculated to not exceed post-transfusion Hb/hematocrit (Hct) associated with hyperviscosity (e.g., Hb 10 g/dL [Hct 30%]). Exchange transfusion involves slowly removing the patient's blood and replacing it with donor blood. The decision between a simple or exchange transfusion depends on the Hb level, the percentage of HbS, and the clinical urgency to reduce the HbS percentage. Exchange transfusions are indicated when the baseline HbS percentage and Hb are too high to safely provide a simple RBC transfusion. In this setting, increasing the Hb too high confers a risk of hyperviscosity and potential risk of stroke and therefore sometimes an exchange is needed. For patients on chronic RBC transfusions, exchange transfusion offers the advantage of minimizing iron overload.

11. **What are the possible complications of red cell transfusions in sickle cell disease?**
RBC transfusions can be complicated by nonhemolytic febrile, allergic (urticarial or rarely anaphylactic), or hemolytic transfusion reactions. RBC transfusion in sickle cell disease is associated with a high incidence of allo-antibody formation arising from minor red cell antigen mismatch between donors and patients. Other complications include sepsis, transfusion-associated lung injury, transfusion-associated circulatory overload, and iron overload for those on chronic transfusion therapy. An acute transfusion reaction will present with fever, chills, flank pain, and oozing from intravenous (IV) sites. Transfusion should be stopped immediately, and the unit should be sent back to the blood bank along with samples of blood and urine from the patient for work up. Aggressive hydration and diuresis should be started. A delayed hemolytic transfusion reaction (DHTR) should be suspected in patients with sickle cell disease who develop worsening anemia within 1 to 4 weeks after a RBC transfusion. DHTR occurs because of development of red cell allo-antibodies in the patient against minor red cell antigens on the donor RBCs. Patients can present with new vaso-occlusive symptoms or acute chest syndrome and signs and symptoms of hemolysis such as icteric sclerae, jaundice, and dark urine because of hemoglobinuria from intravascular complement-mediated hemolysis. The initial Coombs test may be negative but subsequently become positive. Additional RBC transfusions can worsen ongoing hemolysis and need to be avoided unless there is life-threatening anemia (Hb <3g/dL). Management includes supportive care for potential renal and multiorgan failure, use of steroids, and early complement inhibition with eculizumab with or without rituximab.

12. **What are the central nervous system complications of the disease?**
Common cerebrovascular complications in sickle cell disease include acute stroke (ischemic and hemorrhagic), transient ischemic attack, silent cerebral infarct (small infarcts seen on magnetic resonance imaging [MRI] but without associated abnormal neurological findings), and neurocognitive impairment. Before preventive strategies, acute stroke occur in 11% of patients with HbSS by age 20 years, with peak incidence in children 2 to 9 years old. Patients with silent infarcts are at increased risk for progressive infarcts, acute stroke, and neurocognitive deficits. Neurocognitive impairments are seen in children and adults and include lower intelligence, visuo-motor impairments, and executive dysfunction.

13. **Are there strategies to predict and prevent stroke in sickle cell disease?**
Stroke risk can be predicted by transcranial Doppler (TCD), a noninvasive tool that measures blood flow velocities in the main cerebral arteries. A high-flow velocity indicates vascular stenosis and signifies high risk of stroke. Time-averaged mean maximum velocity (TAMMV) of at least 200 cm/sec is considered abnormal (i.e., high stroke risk), less than 170 cm/sec is normal, and 170 to 199 cm/sec is conditional. Annual screening is recommended for children 2 to 16 years old with HbSS and HbSβ^0-thalassemia; no standard recommendation exists for other genotypes (HbSC or HbSβ$^+$-thalassemia). Those with abnormal TCD velocities are placed on chronic monthly RBC transfusion, maintaining HbS of less than 30%, for primary stroke prevention. RBC transfusions are required indefinitely, but switching from RBC transfusions to hydroxyurea can be considered for some with milder cerebrovascular disease. After an acute stroke, the risk of stroke recurrence is high and chronic RBC transfusion therapy is needed to prevent secondary stroke.

14. **Are there pharmacological agents that can modify the clinical course of sickle cell disease?**
Hydroxyurea is the most widely used medication for sickle cell disease. It acts in a variety of ways, with fetal hemoglobin (HbF) induction as its main mechanism. High HbF percentage retards erythrocyte sickling. Regular hydroxyurea use is shown to reduce vaso-occlusive events, hospitalizations, acute chest syndrome, and the need for RBC transfusions. Its use has also been shown to have protective effects against silent organ damage in, for example, the kidneys, spleens, lungs, and brains of children with sickle cell disease and has demonstrated safety in infants as young as 6 to 9 months of age. Hydroxyurea use can cause myelosuppression and requires monitoring of blood counts at a minimum every 3 months while the patient is on a stable dose and more frequently during dose adjustments. Other Food and Drug Administration (FDA)–approved drugs include L-glutamine, crizanlizumab, and voxelotor. L-glutamine is an essential amino acid that decreases oxidative stress in sickle RBCs. Crizanlizumab is a P-selectin inhibitor that decrease adherence of sickle erythrocytes to the vascular endothelium and can reduce painful vaso-occlusive events. Voxelotor binds to sickle Hb and increases its oxygen affinity, keeping HbS in an oxygenated state, thus decreasing polymerization. It increases Hb and decreases markers of hemolysis.

15. What are some curative therapies for sickle cell disease?

Allogeneic hematopoietic stem cell transplant (HSCT) and gene therapy are the curative therapies for severe forms of sickle cell disease. HSCT from a matched sibling donor if done at a younger age ($<$13 years) and before the development of disease-associated comorbidities has the highest rate of success. HSCT using haploidentical and fully human leukocyte antigen (HLA)—matched unrelated donors should be done in the context of a clinical trial and with careful patient and donor selection given the higher rates of complications. Gene therapy is an emerging modality for cure. Mobilized hematopoietic stem cells from the patient are collected and ex vivo modified by either gene addition or gene editing and then infused back to the patient after a conditioning regimen. Gene addition introduces a nonsickling hemoglobin gene (e.g., β^{A-T87Q}) using a viral vector. Gene editing either repairs the defective gene or silences an active gene (e.g., *BCL 11a*, a normal repressor of HbF). Both approaches have been shown to effectively ameliorate the sickling phenotype.

BIBLIOGRAPHY

1. Linder GE, Chou ST. Red cell transfusion and alloimmunization in sickle cell disease. *Haematologica.* 2021;106(7).1805–1815.
2. Salinas Cisneros G, Thein SL. Recent advances in the treatment of sickle cell disease. *Front Physiol.* 2020;11:435.
3. Ware RE, de Montalembert M, Tshilolo L, Abboud MR. Sickle cell disease. *Lancet.* 2017;390(10091):311–323.

INTRINSIC AND EXTRINSIC RED BLOOD CELL DEFECTS

Angela Ricci, MD and Cindy Neunert, MD

CHAPTER 4

1. **What is hemolytic anemia?**
   Hemolytic anemia involves disorders originating from either inside the red blood cell (RBC; intrinsic) or outside of the RBC (extrinsic) that cause fragility and premature breakage and clearance of RBC.

2. **What is the typical presentation for hemolytic anemia?**
   - History and examination findings
     - Fatigue, pallor
     - Splenomegaly
     - Dark (tea/cola) urine
   - Laboratory findings
     - Low hemoglobin (Hb)
     - Elevated reticulocyte count
     - Elevated (indirect) bilirubin
     - Elevated lactate dehydrogenase (LDH)
     - Decreased haptoglobin
     - Hemoglobinuria
       Hemolysis can be classified as either intravascular or extravascular. Although clinical presentation and laboratory findings overlap, there are some key differences that can help in the diagnostic workup of hemolytic anemia. Intravascular hemolysis occurs, as its name suggests, within the blood vessels and is complement or shear mediated. Extravascular hemolysis occurs in the reticuloendothelial system (spleen or liver) as a result of macrophage digestion of RBC.
       Intravascular hemolysis typically causes more profound elevation of LDH and reduction of haptoglobin, as well as hemoglobinemia and hemoglobinuria. Conditions causing intravascular hemolysis include paroxysmal cold hemoglobinuria, cold autoimmune hemolytic anemia, paroxysmal nocturnal hemoglobinuria, and mechanical heart valves. Extravascular hemolysis typically leads to more modest changes in LDH and haptoglobin. Conditions causing extravascular hemolysis include hereditary spherocytosis (and other RBC membrane disorders), hemolytic disease of the newborn, and warm autoimmune hemolytic anemia. Overall, extravascular hemolysis is more common in pediatrics.

3. **What are the different intrinsic RBC disorders?**
   The intrinsic RBC disorders involve defects in normal RBC structure and function that lead to decreased RBC survival and hemolysis. They can be broadly categorized as they relate to major components of RBC:
   - Membrane disorder
   - Enzyme disorder
   - Hemoglobinopathies

4. **What is the normal structure of the RBC membrane?**
   The RBC membrane is made up of a lipid bilayer overlying a protein cytoskeleton. Channels function to maintain appropriate intracellular fluid content. Defects in any of these components can lead to altered RBC shape and anemia because of shortened RBC life span, increased cellular fragility, and removal in the reticuloendothelial system. Common RBC membrane defects include hereditary spherocytosis, hereditary elliptocytosis, and hereditary pyropoikilocytosis.

5. **What is the pathogenesis of hereditary spherocytosis (HS)?**
   Deficiency of RBC membrane proteins of spectrin, ankyrin, and band 3 lead to an abnormal vertical interaction of the membrane lipid bilayer to the underlying skeleton. This causes RBC to have a spherical shape rather than the normal biconcave disc. These cells have shortened life spans because of increased osmotic fragility and because they are trapped and selectively removed in the spleen. HS is the most common RBC membrane disorder. Although it is most commonly inherited in autosomal dominant fashion, HS can also be the result of autosomal recessive inheritance, which is the most common RBC membrane disorder.

6. **What is the typical presentation and diagnostic workup of a patient with HS?**

Typically children will present in the neonatal period with jaundice or in early childhood with hemolytic anemia with extravascular hemolysis. Because HS is most commonly autosomal dominant, there is often a positive family history of HS. Other suggestive family history could include splenectomy or early cholecystectomy.

Diagnostic workup would first identify features of hemolytic anemia. On the complete blood count (CBC), the mean corpuscular volume (MCV) is typically normal and there is a high mean corpuscular Hb concentration (MCHC). Peripheral smear will show abundant spherocytes. A typical clinical presentation, with spherocytes on smear in the setting of strong positive family history, may be adequate to confirm diagnosis. Confirmatory testing could include osmotic fragility and eosin-5'-maleimide (EMA) flow cytometric binding test. Diagnosis can also be confirmed with genetic testing for the most common genes involved: *ANK1*, *EPB42*, *SLC4A1*, *SPTA1*, and *SPTB*.

7. **What are common complications of HS?**
   - **Chronic hemolysis:** This is present for all patients, but there is significant variability from mild to severe chronic anemia.
   - **Aplastic crisis:** Given chronic hemolysis, patients are dependent on ongoing reticulocytosis to maintain their RBCs. Suppression of bone marrow production of reticulocytes, most commonly because of viral infection (often with parvovirus), can lead to a sudden drop in Hb and symptomatic anemia. Typical laboratory findings will be a decline in Hb compared with baseline in the setting of low or absent reticulocyte count. Patients may require supportive RBC transfusion for symptomatic anemia. Patients with HS should be counseled to obtain CBC if they develop fever or other signs of viral illness.
   - **Hemolytic crisis:** Similar to aplastic crisis, viral illness can lead to accelerated hemolysis. The bone marrow's normal reticulocyte production may not be able to keep up with increased hemolysis. Laboratory findings in this case would also include anemia with elevated reticulocyte count compared with baseline. This can also be managed with supportive RBC transfusion for symptomatic anemia.
   - **Splenomegaly:** This is related to chronic hemolysis. Patients with significant splenomegaly should be cautioned about high-risk contact activities.
   - **Cholelithiasis:** Chronic hemolysis can lead to development of gallstones, obstructive jaundice, and cholecystitis requiring cholecystectomy.

8. **What are the treatment options for HS?**

Typically patients are treated with supportive interventions for complications. Patients should also take folic acid supplementation. For patients with frequent complications or moderate to severe anemia, splenectomy can be considered. Although patients will have continued spherocytosis, splenectomy improves RBC survival to nearly normal, thereby decreasing RBC transfusion needs. The primary risk of splenectomy is lifelong increased risk for severe infection because of encapsulated bacteria. Before splenectomy, patients should receive full immunization series for pneumococcus and meningococcus, including B serotype. Typically lifelong penicillin prophylaxis is recommended, and patients should be promptly evaluated for fever. Partial splenectomy is more controversial but has the potential for some preservation of splenic function with regards to infections.

9. **What are other disorders associated with RBC structural membrane proteins?**
   - **Hereditary elliptocytosis (HE):** HE is caused by an abnormal RBC membrane cytoskeleton with impaired horizontal interaction. It is primarily because of autosomal dominant mutation in spectrin. This causes RBC to have an elliptical shape. Most patients are actually asymptomatic and have normal spleen size and Hb levels, although they may have a mild reticulocytosis consistent with small amount of compensated hemolysis. A small proportion of patients may experience symptoms similar to those seen in patients with HS. Infants may present with jaundice and hyperbilirubinemia. Osmotic fragility testing may be normal or abnormal. Peripheral smear will show characteristic elliptocytes. Genetic testing is now available to detect mutations in most commonly associated genes: *EPB41*, *GYPC*, *SPTA1*, and *SPTB*. Treatment is often not required for asymptomatic individuals. For symptomatic individuals, however, the same treatments paradigms used in HS could be applied.
   - **Hereditary pyropoikilocytosis (HPP):** HPP is a rare variant of HE associated with homozygous or compound heterozygous spectrin mutations. RBCs demonstrate a variety of morphologies (peripheral smear resembles that of a patient with severe thermal burn, hence the name). Osmotic fragility testing is markedly abnormal. Infants have evidence of significant jaundice and hemolytic anemia. In childhood, severe anemia can be associated with impaired growth and frontal bossing. Splenectomy can significantly improve anemia and hemolysis, although not as completely as it does for HS.

10. **What are disorders associated with red cell hydration defects?**

These are rare disorders. Hereditary stomatocytosis is characterized by abnormal cellular ion channel causing cellular swelling and rigidity. It is most commonly caused by a mutation in the gene *PIEZO1*. Peripheral smear is characterized by RBCs with "mouth-shaped" linear central clearing. It is most commonly autosomal dominant. Some patients are completely asymptomatic, whereas others may have the typical constellation of symptoms seen in other RBC membrane disorders including neonatal jaundice, anemia, and splenomegaly. Although splenectomy can reduce hemolysis, it is relatively contraindicated in hereditary stomatocytosis because of the high risk of thromboembolic events after splenectomy in these patients. Other disorders in this category include cryohydrocytosis and xerocytosis.

11. **Define RBC enzyme disorders**
    This group of disorders is characterized by hemolytic anemia in the setting of normal RBC morphology. They are caused by defects in enzymes that perform functions essential for RBC survival. The most common disorders in this category are gluose-6 phosphate dehydrogenase (G6PD) deficiency and pyruvate kinase deficiency.

12. **What is G6PD deficiency?**
    G6PD deficiency is the most common enzymopathy. Normal G6PD functions to protect RBCs from oxidative damage. With G6PD deficiency, RBCs are susceptible to damage from oxidative insults, leading to RBC destruction, intravascular hemolysis, and anemia. It is inherited as an X-linked disorder. It does confer some protection against malaria and thus more common in malaria-endemic regions. Clinical symptoms are related to the degree of enzyme deficiency. Thus males have a complete deficiency and therefore more severe disease. Females with heterozygous inheritance, because of X inactivation of one chromosome, have only a partial deficiency and therefore typically have no symptoms or only minor symptoms.

13. **What are the clinical manifestations of G6PD deficiency?**
    Most patients have no symptoms related to G6PD unless they are exposed to certain triggers. Important clinical considerations are described as follows:
    - **Neonatal jaundice:** G6PD deficiency is associated with increased incidence of neonatal jaundice, although it does not occur in all infants with G6PD deficiency. It is often not associated with evidence of significant hemolysis. Peak bilirubin typically occurs on day 2 to 3. Hyperbilirubinemia can be severe and lead to kernicterus, so it is crucial to have prompt evaluation and management with phototherapy and sometimes exchange RBC transfusion.
    - **Acute hemolytic anemia:** After exposure to a trigger, patients can develop moderate to severe hemolytic anemia. The most common triggers include fava beans, drugs, and certain infections. Of note, there are many drugs that have been described as triggers, including dapsone, rasburicase, and trimethoprim-sulfamethoxazole. After exposure, patients will develop symptoms of intravascular hemolysis, including dark urine and jaundice. The degree of symptoms and hemolysis is likely related to underlying patient characteristics and dose of exposure. Symptoms can range from mild compensated hemolysis that may not even present to care to life-threatening anemia. Rapid recovery occurs after removal of the exposure, and thus patients may only require supportive care. RBC transfusion can be given if hemolysis is severe.
    - **Chronic nonspherocytic hemolytic anemia (CNSHA):** This is a rare variant of G6PD deficiency where patients experience chronic hemolysis with symptoms similar to HS. These patients are also at risk for acute hemolytic crises after exposure. Like HS, splenectomy can improve symptoms.

14. **How is G6PD deficiency diagnosed?**
    Quantitative deficiency of G6PD is diagnostic. G6PD is normally present at higher levels in younger RBCs. In the setting of acute hemolysis, older RBCs with lower levels of G6PD will be most prone to lysis. Quantitative testing in this setting can be falsely normal because surviving RBCs and reticulocytes may have higher levels of G6PD. Thus testing in the setting of acute hemolysis is not recommended. During an acute hemolytic crisis, review of the peripheral blood smear will show characteristic bite cells. Genetic testing can also be done.

15. **What is pyruvate kinase deficiency (PKD)?**
    Pyruvate kinase is an enzyme in the glucolysis pathway, which is essential for generation of adenosine triphosphate (ATP) in RBCs. In PKD, individuals have decreased pyruvate kinase (PK) enzyme activity, which results in inadequate cellular energy production, leading to membrane defects, cellular dehydration, and shortened life span with destruction in the reticuloendothelial system. PKD is associated with severe hemolysis and reticulocytosis. It is a rare disorder and has autosomal recessive inheritance because of mutations in the *PKLR* gene.

16. **How is PKD diagnosed?**
    Generally patients present with typical symptoms of chronic hemolysis. PKD is usually considered once more common hemolytic anemias have been excluded. Diagnosis is confirmed with PK enzymatic assay and genetic testing.

17. **How is PKD treated?**
    Management depends on the severity of anemia and frequency of RBC transfusions. RBC transfusions may be used episodically for acute anemia or chronically, particularly if patients have chronic symptoms or impaired growth. Splenectomy generally reduces the severity of anemia and frequency of RBC transfusions. Reticulocyte count will increase after splenectomy, sometimes to much higher levels than baseline. Children must be carefully monitored for iron overload, which can develop even in the absence of significant RBC transfusion history. PK activators are a disease-modifying treatment that is currently in clinical development.

18. **What are the different causes of extrinsic RBC disorders?**
    - Immune-mediated hemolysis
      - Autoimmune hemolytic anemia
      - Paroxysmal cold hemoglobinuria (PCH)
      - Cold agglutinin disease
      - Neonatal alloimmune hemolytic anemia

- Mechanical hemolysis
  - Micro- or macroangiopathic hemolytic anemia
  - Thrombotic thrombocytopenia purpura (TTP)
  - Hemolytic uremic syndrome (HUS)
- Paroxysmal nocturnal hemoglobinuria
- Drug-induced hemolytic anemia
- Toxin-mediated hemolysis

19. **Define autoimmune hemolytic anemia (AIHA).**
AIHA is hemolysis that occurs as a result of premature destruction of RBCs by autoantibodies that bind antigens on the erythrocyte membrane. They can be classified as primary or secondary. Primary AIHA can be further classified based on type of autoantibodies as warm, cold, and PCH.

20. **Describe the difference between warm and cold AIHA.**
- Warm AIHA is the most common form of AIHA in children. It is caused by immunoglobulin G (IgG) antibodies that bind at warm temperatures (37°C). It results in extravascular hemolysis as RBCs are coated in IgG and removed in the reticuloendothelial system. It can cause brisk hemolysis leading to severe anemia. The typical course can be chronic, and medical therapies are indicated.
- Cold AIHA (also called cold agglutinin disease) is much less common in children and is mediated by antibodies that bind better at a cold temperature (~4°C). They are typically immunoglobulin M (IgM) and can fix complement, which results in intravascular hemolysis. The cause can be primary or secondary. Primary cold agglutinin disease is mainly seen in adults, whereas the secondary cause usually follows an infection, often mycoplasma pneumonia. Hemolysis and anemia are generally milder, and children can frequently be observed.

21. **What is the typical clinical presentation for AIHA?**
Patients will typically present with symptoms of acute anemia and hemolysis, including fatigue, pallor, and jaundice. Patients may also have tachycardia and flow murmur. Hepatosplenomegaly may also be present.

22. **What is the diagnostic workup for AIHA?**
Patients will have laboratory evidence of hemolysis including anemia, reticulocytosis, and elevated bilirubin and LDH. Thus the presence of hemoglobinuria consistent with intravascular hemolysis can be a helpful clue in suggesting underlying antibody type. Review of the peripheral blood smear may show spherocytes or, in the setting of cold agglutinin disease, the presence of agglutination can be appreciated.
Autoantibody identification using direct antiglobulin test (DAT; direct Coombs) is essential in the evaluation of AIHA. This tests for antibody and/or complement present on the surface of the patient's RBCs. The test is typically done at room temperature. Of note, a finding of complement alone suggests an IgM antibody that fixes complement at low temperature but binds poorly in warm temperature.

23. **What is a Donath-Landsteiner antibody?**
This is the antibody that causes PCH. It is an IgG antibody that binds at cold temperatures and, unlike other IgG, can fix complement. DAT may be negative or positive only for complement. Specific testing incubates the patient's serum with normal RBCs in the cold for 30 minutes and then warms the mixture to body temperature. Hemolysis in this "biphasic" test is considered diagnostic for PCH. Typically, hemolysis in PCH is mild.

24. **What is the treatment for AIHA?**
- **Observation:** Not all children with AIHA will require treatment. Patients with mild anemia and who are asymptomatic may be closely observed. Particularly cold AIHA is generally self-limited, although patients should be kept warm.
- **RBC transfusion:** For children with moderate to severe anemia or who are symptomatic, urgent RBC transfusion may be required. Particularly in warm AIHA, IgG may be panreactive, and thus a completely matched unit may not be possible. Nevertheless, excluding alloantibodies and giving the best matched unit should be done to prevent cardiovascular compromise. For patients with cold AIHA, a blood warmer can be used for RBC transfusions.
- **Corticosteroids:** Corticosteroids are important for the treatment of warm AIHA (and rarely for PCH). Generally children are started on methylprednisolone 1 to 2 mg/kg every 6 hours and then transitioned to oral prednisone 2 mg/kg/day. In adolescents, a lower dose of 1 mg/kg/day could be considered. Corticosteroids are continued for 2 to 4 weeks and then gradually weaned with close monitoring of Hb, LDH, and reticulocyte count. Stopping corticosteroids too abruptly can result in relapse.
- Therapies for patients who are refractory to corticosteroids or unable to wean off of corticosteroids include:
  - Rituximab
  - Intravenous immunoglobulin (IVIG; likely more effective for IgM-mediated AIHA)
  - Exchange RBC transfusion or plasmapheresis
  - Splenectomy (would be reserved for chronic, refractory AIHA)

25. **What are the causes of secondary AIHA?**
    - Autoimmune disease
    - Immunodeficiency
    - Lymphoproliferative disorder
    - Infections, including Epstein-Barr virus (EBV), mycoplasma, parvovirus, and cytomegalovirus (CMV)
    - Drugs, including piperacillin, cefotetan, and ceftriaxone; this should be suspected with recent drug exposure and requires communication with the blood bank to provide testing in the presence of the suspected drug if initial DAT is negative.

    All children with AIHA should be evaluated for systemic disease because AIHA may be a presenting phenomenon associated with another underlying disorder. Based on age, additional history or physical examination findings and family history additional screening testing can be undertaken.

26. **Describe thrombotic microangiopathic hemolytic anemias (TMAs)?**
    The TMAs represent a group of anemias that occur because of red cell shearing because of the formation of microthrombi. These include disseminated intravascular hemolysis (DIC), TTP, and HUS. Patients will present with a low platelet count because of microthrombi formation and hemolytic anemia. The peripheral smear will show schistocytes.
    - DIC is most commonly seen in individuals who are critically ill, and unlike TTP and HUS, patients will have additional coagulation defects, such as a prolonged prothrombin time and partial prothrombin time. Treatment is aimed at supportive care and treatment of the underlying condition.
    - Patients with TTP can present with the classical pentad of hemolytic anemia, thrombocytopenia, fever, acute kidney injury, and severe neurologic findings. It is because of a deficiency of the ADAMTS-13 metalloprotease either because of congenital absence or an acquired antibody. It is a medical emergency, and treatment is with rapid initiation of plasma exchange and corticosteroids. Rituximab and caplacizumab are additional treatments that can be added to plasma exchange and corticosteroids.
    - HUS is similar in presentation to TTP; however, the renal disease is the predominant feature and neurologic symptoms are uncommon. HUS can be classified as typical, after infection (most commonly with *Escherichia coli* or *Streptococcus pneumoniae*), or atypical because of complement overactivation. A mutation in complement factors can be found in about half of patients with atypical HUS, most commonly in complement factor H. Patients with typical HUS are managed with renal supportive care, and those with atypical HUS can receive treatment with eculizumab, a monoclonal inhibitor of complement activity.

BIBLIOGRAPHY

1. Chou ST, Schreiber AD. Autoimmune hemolytic anemia. In: Orkin SH, Nathan DG, Ginsburg D, et al. (eds). *Nathan and Oski's Hematology and Oncology of Infancy and Childhood.* 8th ed. Saunders, 2014:411–430.e6.
2. Grace RF, Barcellini M. Management of pyruvate kinase deficiency in children and adults. *Blood.* 2020;136(11):1241–1249.
3. Luzzatto L, Ally M, Notaro R. Glucose-6-phosphate dehydrogenase deficiency. *Blood.* 2020;136(11):1225–1240.
4. Lux SE. Disorders of the red cell membrane. In: Orkin SH, Nathan DG, Ginsburg D, et al. (eds). *Nathan and Oski's Hematology and Oncology of Infancy and Childhood.* 8th ed. Saunders, 2014:515–579.e21.
5. Mentzer WC. Pyruvate kinase deficiency and disorders of glycolysis. In: Orkin SH, Nathan DG, Ginsburg D, et al. (eds). *Nathan and Oski's Hematology and Oncology of Infancy and Childhood.* 8th ed. Saunders, 2014:580–608.e12.
6. Risinger M, Kalfa TA. Red cell membrane disorders: Structure meets function. *Blood.* 2020;136(11):1250–1261.

CHAPTER 5

THALASSEMIAS

Amy Tang, MD and Sujit Sheth, MD

1. **What is thalassemia?**

   Normal hemoglobin (Hb) is a heterodimer of two globins produced as a result of expression of genes from the alpha (α)-globin gene cluster on chromosome 16 and two globins produced as a result of expression of genes from the beta (β)-globin gene cluster on chromosome 11. Thalassemia refers to a group of congenital disorders of globin synthesis in which there is decreased or absent production of one of the two subunits of Hb. Thus it is a quantitative hemoglobinopathy. The most common thalassemias are α and β, with a reduction or absence of production of the respective globins. Other forms of thalassemia include gamma (γ)-β and delta (δ)-γ-β thalassemia, which are less common. The severity of thalassemia depends in large part on the degree of imbalance between α- and β-globin chains.

2. **Where are the thalassemia syndromes more commonly found?**

   The term thalassemia comes from the Greek words thalassa ("sea") and haema ("blood"), referencing the fact that these syndromes were first described in individuals living around the Mediterranean Sea. The β thalassemias are more common around the Mediterranean, including Europe and North Africa, and the Middle East, the Indian Subcontinent, and Southeast Asia, whereas α thalassemia occurs in high frequencies in the Far East and China.

3. **How are α thalassemia and β thalassemia different?**

   α thalassemia refers to decreased or absent α-globin synthesis, caused by deletions or mutations of one, two, three, or all four α-globin genes (two on each chromosome).

   β thalassemia refers to decreased or absent β-chain synthesis, resulting from any of over almost 300 gene defects, including point mutations and deletions in one or both of the β-globin genes. Point mutations have variable effects on gene regulation and expression. Completely absent expression of the β-globin gene is referred to as a β-zero (β^0) allele, whereas reduced or partial expression is classified as a β-plus (β^+) allele.

4. **What is thalassemia trait?**

   Thalassemia trait results from decreased, but not absent, production of either the α- or β-globin chain. In α-thalassemia trait, there is usually deletion of two of the four α-globin genes. In β-thalassemia trait, one of the two β-globin genes is abnormal. In either case, the decrease in globin production results in mild anemia, and affected individuals are generally asymptomatic without other complications of thalassemia.

5. **What are the characteristic complete blood cell (CBC) findings in thalassemia trait?**

   With both α- and β-thalassemia trait, there is usually a mild microcytic anemia with an increased red blood cell (RBC) count. Microcytic anemia is most commonly seen with iron deficiency. Thalassemia trait may be distinguished from iron deficiency by the increased RBC count, normal red cell distribution width values (RDW), and the Mentzer index. The Mentzer index is the mean corpuscular volume (MCV) divided by the RBC count (in millions). A Mentzer index of less than 12 suggests thalassemia trait, whereas an index of greater than 13 suggests iron deficiency, with an index between 12 and 13 requiring some additional testing.

6. **What is Hb Barts?**

   Fetal Hb is composed of two α-globin chains and two γ-globin chains. In α thalassemia, there is decreased α-globin chain production, and the excess γ chains in the developing fetus and newborn may form tetramers, resulting in **Hb Barts**. Fetal blood testing and newborn screening in offspring with α thalassemia may show the presence of this Hb, which is present in varying amounts correlating with the number of abnormal genes, being present in higher amounts in those with three or four deleted α-globin genes. Hb Barts will no longer be detected once Hb switching has occurred and γ-chain production declines.

7. **What are the different forms of α thalassemia?**

   The clinical severity of α thalassemia depends on the number of genes affected. When a single α-globin gene is abnormal, this results in the α-**thalassemia silent carrier state** (α-/$\alpha\alpha$), which is asymptomatic and is typically associated with normal CBC findings or mild microcytosis without anemia. When two genes are abnormal, the phenotype is α-**thalassemia trait**, which is also asymptomatic and associated with mild microcytic anemia. The two deleted genes can be inherited in a *cis* formation with both deletions on the same gene (-/$\alpha\alpha$), more common in Southeast Asia, or a *trans* formation with one deletion on each gene (α-/α-), more common in Africa. When three genes are abnormal (α -/-), the result is **HbH disease,** which is associated with a moderate microcytic anemia. Finally, when all four genes are nonfunctional (-/-), no α globin is produced, resulting in the absence of fetal Hb (HbF) in the second trimester of pregnancy, with resulting severe anemia and **hydrops fetalis**, termed α thalassemia major.

α-Thalassemia-Hemoglobin Patterns

Deletion	Genotype	Disease	Clinical	MCV	Electro.	% Bart's
0	αα/αα	None	Normal	Normal	Normal	0%–2%
1	-α/αα	Silent Carrier	Normal	Normal	Normal	1%–2%
2	-α/-α	α$^+$ Thal Trait	Mild Anemia	Low	Normal	5%–10%
	- -/αα	α° Thal Trait	Mild Anemia	Low	Normal	5%–10%
3	- -/- α	HbH	Mod Anemia	Low	Bart's Hb H	20%–40%
4	- -/ - -		Death in utero	Low	Bart's	>80%

Hb Barts normally disappears postnatally but is replaced by HbH in HbH Disease.
-α/-α: more common in African descent; - -/αα: more common in Asian descent
Hb, Hemoglobin; MCV, mean corpuscular volume; Thal, thalassemia.

8. Describe HbH disease.
   HbH disease is caused by three dysfunctional α-globin genes and produces a moderate hemolytic anemia. The clinical phenotype is variable, but most individuals are moderately anemic, with some evidence of chronic hemolysis, and develop some degree of splenomegaly. HbH is a tetramer of β-globin chains that forms in the setting of excess β chains relative to α chains; this is an unstable Hb and a poor oxygen transporter. Although very small amounts may form in individuals with α thalassemia trait, this usually precipitates in precursors and is not detected on electrophoresis. When three α-globin genes are deleted (α-/- -), this is termed deletional HbH disease. Such individuals are also susceptible to increased hemolysis with exposure to oxidant stress, similar to what is seen in glucose-6-phosphate dehydrogenase (G6PD) deficiency. They are generally transfusion-independent but may need episodic RBC transfusions during periods of increased hemolysis. If two α-globin genes are deleted and another is mutated, the result is nondeletional HbH disease, which may have a more severe phenotype.

9. What is HbH-Constant Spring?
   HbH-Constant Spring (HbH-CS) is a form of nondeletional HbH disease in which a two-gene deletion α thalassemia is coinherited with a nondeletional α-globin gene mutation (in this instance, the CS variant). This combination (α α^{CS} /-) results in less α-globin production by the remaining functional α-globin gene. Patients with HbH-CS have more severe anemia, more inefficient erythropoiesis, and are more likely to require regular RBC transfusions and/or splenectomy compared with those with deletional HbH disease.

10. What is hydrops fetalis?
   Hydrops fetalis is a condition of extreme fluid buildup and edema in fetal tissues and organs associated with congestive heart failure; α thalassemia major, where all four α-globin genes are nonfunctional, results in severe anemia and heart failure in the second trimester of pregnancy and a hydrops fetalis phenotype. Most of these pregnancies will result in intrauterine fetal demise. If this condition is recognized sufficiently early, however, intrauterine RBC transfusions can be initiated, which may be able to allow the fetus to reach viability. Postnatally, these infants will require lifelong regular RBC transfusions.

11. What are the different forms of β thalassemia?
   In β thalassemia, the clinical severity depends on the number and type (β° or β $^+$) of gene defects, the coinheritance of other abnormal β-globin genes such as β^E, and the presence or absence of concomitant α-globin gene mutations. Decreased β-globin synthesis results in excess α-globin chains, which precipitate within erythroid precursors and maturing RBCs, leading to intramedullary apoptosis, causing ineffective erythropoiesis and hemolysis.
   At one end of the spectrum of severity is (β°/β°) thalassemia or β thalassemia major. With the inability to make any normal HbA, these individuals are transfusion dependent from early infancy. Individuals with less severe genotypes (β$^+$/β$^+$, β°/β$^+$), in which some functional β globin is produced, have an intermediate phenotype (β thalassemia intermedia) with variable severity of anemia and transfusion requirements, depending on the particular combination of mutations and the presence of coinherited α-globin mutations, among other factors. These individuals may not be transfusion dependent early in life but may become transfusion dependent over time as their Hb drops or they develop complications related to the rampant ineffective erythropoiesis. In HbE/β thalassemia (β^E/β$^+$, β^E/β°), a β-thalassemia mutation is coinherited with the structural variant HbE, producing a variable degree of decreased β-globin synthesis. The phenotype can range from mild or moderate to severe, with the severe form being transfusion dependent. At the other end of the spectrum is β-thalassemia trait (β/β° or β/β $^+$), or minor, where individuals have an asymptomatic mild microcytic anemia and no other complications.
   When a β-thalassemia mutation is coinherited with a sickle mutation (HbS), this produces a form of sickle cell disease (HbS/β° or HbS/β$^+$). Sickle cell disease is discussed in a separate chapter.

12. What is the role of regular RBC transfusion therapy in the management of thalassemia?
   Aside from thalassemia silent carrier or trait, the thalassemias are broadly classified into transfusion-dependent thalassemias (TDTs) and nontransfusion-dependent thalassemias (NTDTs). The role of RBC transfusions is twofold: to supply normal erythrocytes needed for tissue oxygenation and to suppress ineffective erythropoiesis, which

would otherwise lead to bone marrow expansion with bone deformities and reduced bone mass, extramedullary hematopoiesis leading to hepatosplenomegaly, vascular disease caused by the abnormal red cells that are released from erythropoiesis, and increased enteric iron absorption.

Patients who have TDT, including β thalassemia major, severe forms of HbE/β thalassemia, severe HbH-CS, and α thalassemia major surviving beyond the neonatal period, require RBC transfusions to sustain tissue oxygen delivery. These individuals are generally transfused every 2 to 4 weeks, with a pretransfusion Hb goal of 9.5 to 10.5 g/dL to improve activity levels and quality of life, maintain normal growth and development (children), and suppress ineffective erythropoiesis. Certain complications such as heart failure, continued evidence of extramedullary hematopoiesis, fatigue, or bone pain may warrant a higher pretransfusion Hb target.

Patients with NTDT, although not requiring lifelong RBC transfusion therapy, may still require sporadic or regular RBC transfusions for certain periods of time to prevent or manage certain disease complications, such as leg ulcers, splenomegaly, and extramedullary hematopoiesis in the spine, around infections or surgery, or during pregnancy. NTDT includes β thalassemia intermedia, mild to moderate forms of HbE/β thalassemia, mild to moderate HbH-CS, and HbH disease.

The decision of when to initiate regular RBC transfusion therapy should take into account the patient's age, growth velocity, achievement of puberty, presence of hepatosplenomegaly and other extramedullary hematopoiesis, degree of anemia, and clinical symptomatology resulting in impaired quality of life.

13. **How does iron overload occur in β thalassemia?**
Iron overload and its complications in β thalassemia occur both through iron loading from repeated RBC transfusions and from abnormal iron metabolism caused by **ineffective erythropoiesis,** which downregulates **hepcidin** through increased **erythroferrone**. Inappropriately low hepcidin levels lead to increased intestinal iron absorption, increased release of iron from the reticuloendothelial system, and uptake of this iron into the tissues. Therefore iron overload can be a significant problem in NTDT even in the absence of regular RBC transfusions.

With TDT, iron loading occurs more rapidly with the addition of transfusional iron. Each packed RBC (PRBC) unit contains approximately 200 mg of iron, compared with the approximately 1 to 2 mg of iron that the body loses daily. There is no physiologic mechanism to excrete this excess iron, and the progressive accumulation of iron, especially into the heart and endocrine organs, leads to heart disease and a variety of endocrinopathies including insulin-dependent diabetes, hypothyroidism, and hypogonadism. In the absence of measures to remove excess iron, heart failure leading to death occurs in the second decade of life.

14. **How are patients with β thalassemia screened for the development of iron overload?**
Iron accumulation in both TDT and NTDT leads to iron deposition in the liver, heart, and endocrine organs, leading to complications such as hepatic fibrosis and cirrhosis, heart failure and arrhythmias, and endocrinopathies. Routine monitoring of iron status is a key component of disease management. The most reliable means of assessing the body iron burden is to measure tissue iron levels. **Magnetic resonance imaging (MRI) assessment** of hepatic iron after individuals have received 12 to 15 RBC transfusions generally detects iron levels indicating the need for chelation therapy.

Liver iron concentration (LIC) measurements were previously obtained by liver biopsy but are now usually measured by an MRI-based techniques using **R2 or R2*** sequences. The LIC should be obtained on initiation of chelation and annually to monitor iron overload and compliance with chelation. In thalassemia, ideally the LIC should be maintained in the 2 to 5 mg/g dry weight (dw) range. An LIC of 5 to 10 mg/g dw indicates moderate iron overload, and an LIC greater than 10 mg/g dw indicates severe iron overload, which would require intensification of chelation.

Cardiac iron is measured by **cardiac T2* MRI**, with values in milliseconds (ms) correlating inversely to the severity of cardiac iron overload. Normal cardiac T2* is over 20 milliseconds (ms). Cardiac T2* values between 10 and 20 ms (mild cardiac iron overload) are associated with declining left ventricular ejection fraction and associated with arrhythmias, whereas cardiac T2* values less than 10 ms (severe cardiac iron overload) are associated with clinical symptoms of heart failure and increased mortality. Cardiac MRI is recommended annually after age 10 years to assess cardiac function and iron deposition.

Serum ferritin is easy to measure but is not a reliable indicator of body iron burden and may underestimate the severity of iron overload, especially in NTDT. Ferritin is also prone to fluctuations with inflammation, illness, or other factors, so ferritin trends over time are more useful than single measurements. Ideally, the serum ferritin should be periodically correlated with the liver iron concentration by MRI measurement.

15. **What are the different types of iron chelation therapy used in TDT?**
There are three iron chelators that are currently available for treatment of iron overload in thalassemia: deferasirox (Exjade, Jadenu), deferoxamine (Desferal), and deferiprone (Ferriprox).

Deferasirox is an oral chelator that is available as a dispersible tablet, a film-coated tablet, or sprinkles administered once daily. This is currently the most commonly used chelator because of ease of administration and wide therapeutic index. Side effects can include gastrointestinal (GI) upset, transaminitis, and renal toxicity in the form of Fanconi syndrome. Monthly monitoring of a complete metabolic profile and urinary protein excretion is recommended.

Deferoxamine is administered as subcutaneous (SQ) or intravenous injection and was the first available chelator, approved in 1968. It has a very short half-life, requiring administration by SQ infusion for 8 to 10 hours, 5 to 7 nights a week. There is a high degree of noncompliance because of the difficulty of this regimen. Side effects can include infusion-site reactions, high-frequency hearing loss, vision changes, and growth plate issues in young children 2 to 3 years of age. This agent is now used mostly in combination with an oral chelator either when there is a need for intensification or when there is a dose-limiting toxicity.

Deferiprone is available in tablet or solution and is the most effective chelator at removing cardiac iron. Nevertheless, it requires two- or three-times-a-day dosing and is associated with neutropenia and even rare agranulocytosis, so a CBC with differential is recommended every 7 to 10 days for monitoring. Other side effects include GI upset, liver toxicity, and arthralgia.

Combinations of the aforementioned chelators can be used depending on the severity and pattern of iron overload and side effect profile in the individual patient.

16. **What is the role of hematopoietic stem cell transplant and gene therapy in thalassemia?**
Allogeneic hematopoietic stem cell transplant (HSCT) remains the only curative therapy for thalassemia. HSCT after myeloablative conditioning corrects defective erythropoiesis and has high rates of disease-free survival, particularly when using human leukocyte antigen (HLA)–matched sibling donors. In the absence of an HLA-matched sibling donor, alternative donor transplants (matched unrelated donor, haploidentical donor, or cord blood transplants) are an option but carry a much higher risk of adverse outcomes. Consideration must be given to the risk to fertility, particularly in prepubertal children where fertility preservation is still uncertain, and to the risk for development of clonal disease or a secondary malignancy related to the myeloablative conditioning regimen.

17. **What are some of the novel approaches to the management of thalassemia?**
    1. Several potential targets have been used to advance noncurative intent therapy for thalassemia. The goal of these is improvement of ineffective erythropoiesis primarily, leading to reduced RBC transfusion requirement in TDT and higher hemoglobin levels in NTDT. These are in clinical trials for β thalassemia, except as noted, and broadly categorized as:
        a. **Erythroid maturation agent:** Luspatercept has been approved for adults with transfusion-dependent (TD) β thalassemia.
        b. Pyruvate kinase activators (mitapivat- also for α thalassemia, and etavopivat)
        c. Fetal hemoglobin inducers (benserazide, IMR-687, thalidomide)
        d. Hepcidin mimetics and stimulators
    2. Curative intent therapies (all in clinical trials) leading to transfusion independence in TDT include:
        a. Gene addition (*BB305* and Globe vectors) seeking to introduce a copies of the normal β globin into autologous CD34$^+$ cells, which are introduced after myeloablative conditioning
        b. Gene editing (*CTX001*, and others), which turn off *BCL11A* suppression of γ-globin synthesis and increase HbF production

BIBLIOGRAPHY

1. Chonat S, Quinn C. Current standards of care and long term outcomes for thalassemia and sickle cell disease. *Adv Exp Med Biol.* 2017;1013:59–87.
2. Khandros E, Kwiatkowski J. Beta thalassemia: monitoring and new treatment approaches. *Hematol Oncol Clin North Am.* 2019;33:339–353.
3. Sheth S, Thein SL. Thalassemia: A disorder of globin synthesis. *Williams Hematology.* 10th ed. McGraw Hill, 2021.
4. Singer S, Kim HY, Olivieri N, et al. Hemoglobin H-constant spring in North America: An alpha thalassemia with frequent complications. *Am J Hematol.* 2009;84(11):759–761.
5. Taher A, Weatherall D, Cappellini M. Thalassaemia. *Lancet.* 2018;391:155–167.
6. Vichinsky E. Non-transfusion-dependent thalassemia and thalassemia intermedia: Epidemiology, complications, and management. *Curr Med Res Opin.* 2016;32(1):191–204.

CHAPTER 6

NUTRITIONAL ANEMIA

Lia N. Phillips, MD, MPH and Gary M. Brittenham, MD

1. **What is nutritional anemia?**
Anemia develops when a pathological decrease in the circulating red blood cell (RBC) mass reduces the oxygen-carrying capacity of blood below the physiologic requirements of the body. Anemia is clinically assessed by measuring the hemoglobin (Hb) concentration, hematocrit (packed cell volume), or RBC count in the peripheral blood. Nutritional anemia develops as a result of a deficiency of one or more essential nutrients, regardless of the underlying cause of such deficiency.

2. **Worldwide, what are the predominant causes of pediatric nutritional anemia?**
Globally, iron deficiency is by far the most common cause of nutritional anemia in infants, children, and adolescents. Deficiencies of vitamin B_{12} (cobalamin) and folate are much less common but account for most other nutritional anemia. In low- and middle-income countries, vitamin A deficiency, the leading cause of pediatric blindness and a major nutritional risk factor for severe infection and death, is a cause of anemia that interferes with iron utilization and immune responsiveness. Deficiencies of thiamine (vitamin B_1), riboflavin (vitamin B_2), niacin (vitamin B_3), pantothenic acid (vitamin B_5), pyridoxine (vitamin B_6), vitamin C, vitamin E, copper, and selenium are recognized but uncommon or rare causes of nutritional anemia.

IRON DEFICIENCY: MICROCYTIC ANEMIA

3. **Describe the pathways of body iron absorption, utilization, and storage, in the absence of inflammation and infection.**
The amount of body iron is determined by careful control of gastrointestinal (GI) absorption. Humans have no way to regulate iron excretion to avoid iron excess, and the minimal mandatory daily losses, less than 0.05% of the total body iron, are matched by daily absorption. Iron is efficiently recycled with approximately 80% of the flux carried by transferrin in plasma to the erythroid marrow for incorporation into Hb. Senescent RBCs, at the end of their life span of about 120 days, are phagocytized by specialized macrophages within the spleen, bone marrow, and liver (Kupffer cells), which rapidly recycle most of the iron back to plasma transferrin for return to the erythroid marrow. Any excess iron is stored within ferritin and hemosiderin in macrophages and hepatocytes. Transferrin-bound iron delivery to nonerythroid tissues in the body is balanced by the return from cellular turnover.

4. **How does the body regulate the amount, absorption, utilization, and storage of iron?**
The hepatic iron regulatory hormone hepcidin governs the amount and distribution of body iron by controlling the entry of iron into plasma for transport by transferrin (Figure 6.1). Hepcidin binds to the sole known cellular iron exporter, ferroportin, and induces its occlusion or internalization, ubiquitination, and degradation, resulting in sequestration of iron within iron-exporting cells (enterocytes, macrophages, hepatocytes).
   - Hepcidin increases with inflammation and iron loading, thereby inhibiting iron absorption by GI enterocytes, iron recycling by macrophages, and iron release from hepatocyte stores. Inflammation can increase circulating hepcidin to concentrations that critically restrict iron recycling and absorption and can cause severe anemia.
   - Hepcidin decreases with reduced or absent body iron stores, increased erythropoietic demand, and hypoxemia. When inflammation and iron deficiency coexist, the increase from sufficiently severe inflammation can overwhelm the effect of absent body iron stores.

5. **Describe the epidemiology of iron-deficiency anemia worldwide.**
It is estimated that 25% of the global population is anemic, with more than 60% of the anemia caused by iron deficiency, which affects almost 2 billion people. Worldwide, the highest rates of iron deficiency are found among infants, preschool-aged children, and females of reproductive age.

6. **Distinguish absolute from functional iron deficiency.**
Absolute iron deficiency is a deficit in total body iron with absent or reduced iron stores that cannot meet iron requirements (Figure 6.2). Functional iron deficiency develops with sufficient or increased body iron stores that are unable to meet iron requirements because of (1) iron sequestration produced by increased hepcidin or (2) increased erythropoietic demand resulting from endogenous (hemolysis) or exogenous (erythropoiesis-stimulating agents) causes. Absolute and functional iron deficiency may coexist.

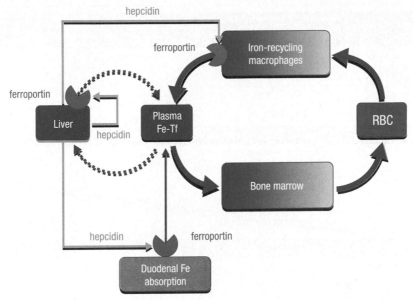

Figure 6.1 The movement of iron into plasma is regulated by the interaction of hepcidin with ferroportin, the iron export protein, on iron-recycling macrophages, duodenal enterocytes, and hepatocytes. *Fe,* Ferroportin; *RBC,* red blood cell. (Figure reproduced from Nemeth E, Ganz T. Hepcidin-ferroportin interaction controls systemic iron homeostasis. *Mol Sci.* 2021;22:6493.)

7. **Describe the successive stages of absolute iron deficiency.**
   The successive stages of absolute iron deficiency traditionally have been defined by the effects on the Hb concentration:
   1. *Storage iron depletion:* Body iron stores are exhausted, but the iron supply for erythropoiesis is maintained and the Hb concentration is not decreased.
   2. *Iron-deficient erythropoiesis:* Body iron stores are exhausted and limit the iron supply for erythropoiesis, but the resulting decrease in Hb concentration is insufficient to be detected by the standard used to diagnose anemia.
   3. *Iron-deficiency anemia:* Body iron stores are exhausted and limit the iron supply for erythropoiesis sufficiently to decrease the Hb concentration below the standard used to diagnose anemia.

      In addition to the effects on erythropoiesis, iron deficiency is a multisystem disorder with a variety of clinical manifestations, including signs and symptoms of adverse effects on developmental, neurological, cardiac, GI, and immunological functions (Box 6.1).

8. **How should iron deficiency and iron-deficiency anemia be prevented in infants, toddlers, school-age children, and adolescents?**
   - **Neonates:** Delayed cord clamping may help prevent iron deficiency.
   - **Preterm infants** (<37 weeks gestational age): If receiving full enteral feeds, premature infants should have an iron intake of at least 2 mg/kg/day, beginning by 2 weeks of life.
   - **Term infants:**
     - If exclusively breastfed, supplement 1 mg/kg/day beginning by 4 months of age and continuing until iron-containing complementary foods are introduced.
     - If formula-fed, supplemental iron is generally not needed because standard formulas are iron-fortified.
     - Cow's milk, as a substitute for breast milk or formula, should not be given to any infant before 1 year of age.
   - **Toddlers (1–4 years of age):** Iron supplementation should be considered if the diet does not contain iron-rich foods, which may include sources of heme iron.
   - School-age children and adolescents should have diets that contain a diversity of iron-rich foods.

9. **Compare breast milk and cow's milk with respect to iron content, absorption, and effects on GI mucosa.**
   - Both breast milk and cow's milk contain low amounts of iron (0.5–1.5 mg/L), but GI absorption of iron from breast milk (~50%) far exceeds the absorption of cow's milk (~5% to 10%).
   - Cow's milk contains proteins that can damage the intestinal mucosa and cause iron loss through microvascular bleeding. Breast milk contains proteins, lipids, oligosaccharides, and a variety of other bioactive components that help protect the mucosa against infection and inflammation.

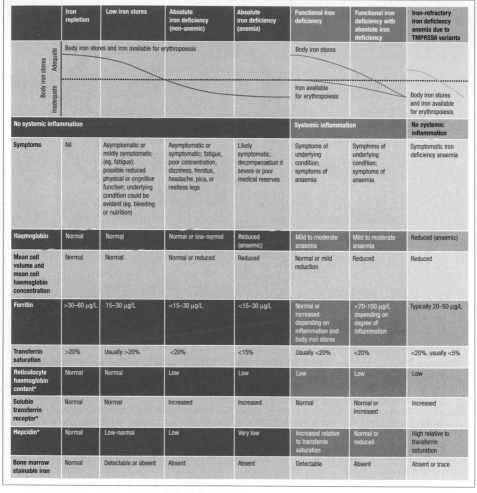

	Iron repletion	Low iron stores	Absolute iron deficiency (non-anemic)	Absolute iron deficiency (anemia)	Functional iron deficiency	Functional iron deficiency with absolute iron deficiency	Iron-refractory iron deficiency anaemia due to TMPRSS6 variants
Symptoms	Nil	Asymptomatic or mildly symptomatic (eg, fatigue); possible reduced physical or cognitive function; underlying condition could be evident (eg. bleeding or nutrition)	Asymptomatic or symptomatic; fatigue, poor concentration, dizziness, tinnitus, headache, pica, or restless legs	Likely symptomatic, decompensation if severe or poor medical reserves	Symptoms of underlying condition; symptoms of anaemia	Symptoms of underlying condition; symptoms of anaemia	Symptomatic iron deficiency anaemia
Haemoglobin	Normal	Normal	Normal or low-normal	Reduced (anaemic)	Mild to moderate anaemia	Mild to moderate anaemia	Reduced (anaemic)
Mean cell volume and mean cell haemoglobin concentration	Normal	Normal	Normal or reduced	Reduced	Normal or mild reduction	Reduced	Reduced
Ferritin	>30–60 μg/L	15–30 μg/L	<15–30 μg/L	<15–30 μg/L	Normal or increased depending on inflammation and body iron stores	<70-100 μg/L depending on degree of inflammation	Typically 20–50 μg/L
Transferrin saturation	>20%	Usually >20%	<20%	<15%	Usually <20%	<20%	<20%, usually <5%
Reticulocyte haemoglobin content*	Normal	Normal	Low	Low	Low	Low	Low
Soluble transferrin receptor*	Normal	Normal	Increased	Increased	Normal	Normal or increased	Increased
Hepcidin*	Normal	Low-normal	Low	Very low	Increased relative to transferrin saturation	Normal or reduced	High relative to transferrin saturation
Bone marrow stainable iron	Normal	Detectable or absent	Absent	Absent	Detectable	Absent	Absent or trace

Figure 6.2 Laboratory evaluation of absolute and functional iron deficiency. Characteristic changes in indicators of absolute and functional iron deficiency are shown, both for established measures and for some tests in development. (Reprinted with permission from Elsevier, Pasricha SR, Tye-Din J, Muckenthaler MU, Swinkels DW. Iron deficiency. *Lancet.* 2021;397:233–248.)

10. How and when should the pediatrician screen for iron deficiency?

At all ages, clinical evaluation should include screening for the symptoms and signs of the causes of absolute iron deficiency (Table 6.1).

- A full CBC and serum ferritin are optimal for screening for iron deficiency, with or without anemia.
- **Infants:** Universal screening for iron deficiency, with or without anemia, is suggested at 9 to 12 months of age, especially for all premature infants and for term infants for whom breast milk is the primary source of nutrition.
- **Toddlers:** Rescreening for iron deficiency, with or without anemia, is suggested at 15 to 18 months of age, especially for those at heightened risk for iron deficiency.
- **School-aged children:** Screening should be considered if risk factors, such as poor dietary intake, low socioeconomic status, or special healthcare needs, are present.
- **Adolescents:** Universal screening for iron deficiency, with or without anemia, is suggested (1) for females at about age 14 for those who are at least 1 year postmenarche and (2) for males during their peak growth period. Additional screening should be considered for those with heightened risk of iron deficiency, such as low iron diets, blood donation, and females with increased menstrual losses

Box 6.1 Manifestations and Multisystem Sequelae of Iron Deficiency

Nutritional
Pica, pagophagia

Neurocognitive
Reduced mental and motor function
Poorer outcomes in executive function and recognition memory
Visual and auditory systems' functioning

Neurologic
Restless leg syndrome
Neuronal hypomyelination
Decreased neurotransmitter production

Cardiac
Impaired myocyte function

Immunologic
Impaired resistance to bacterial, viral and parasitic infections

Gastrointestinal
Epithelial tissue injury (glossitis; angular stomatitis)
Esophageal web or stricture, gastric atrophy
Microvillus damage; protein-losing enteropathy

Hematologic
Anemia (fatigue; diminished exercise tolerance and productivity)

Hb, Hemoglobulin.
(Box adapted from Powers JM, Buchanan GR. Diagnosis and management of iron deficiency anemia. *Hematol Oncol Clin North Am.* 2014;28:729-45.)

Table 6.1 Pediatric Causes of Absolute Iron Deficiency Anemia

INADEQUATE INTAKE OR ABSORPTION (TOO LITTLE IN)	LOSS OF BODY IRON STORES (TOO MUCH OUT)	INCREASED REQUIREMENTS (MORE NEEDED)
Inadequate dietary intake • For premature infants, lack of supplemental iron • Low iron formula • Overconsumption of cow's milk • Insufficient bioavailable iron in diet Poor absorption • Obesity • Chronic inflammation • Malabsorption syndromes • Celiac disease • Inflammatory bowel disease • *Helicobacter pylori* infection • Antacids, proton-pump inhibitors, and H2 blockers • Bariatric and other gastric surgery • Genetic (iron-refractory iron-deficiency anemia [IRIDA]).	Chronic blood loss • Gastrointestinal • Gynecological • Urinary • Respiratory • Blood donation	High growth velocity • Premature infants • First year of life • Adolescent growth spurt • Pregnancy & lactation

11. Which laboratory studies are used in the diagnosis of absolute and functional iron deficiency?
   - **Bone marrow examination:** Bone marrow examination with staining for iron is considered the reference method for the diagnosis of absolute iron deficiency, with or without functional iron deficiency, but is rarely needed clinically.
   - **Serum ferritin concentration:** World Health Organization (WHO) guidelines recommend thresholds of less than 12 μg/L in children under 5 years of age and less than 15 μg/L in older children and adolescents who are apparently healthy, and in the presence of inflammation, less than 30 μg/L and less than 70 μg/L, respectively. Higher thresholds, with and without inflammation, are suggested in some clinical laboratories and by some other authorities. Ferritin is an acute phase reactant that may be elevated in the setting of inflammation. If ongoing inflammation is suspected, ferritin is best interpreted in conjunction with inflammatory indicators and other iron studies.
   - **Other iron studies:** Figure 6.2 summarizes the patterns of change in other iron studies in the various stages of absolute iron deficiency, functional iron deficiency, and coexisting absolute and functional iron deficiency.

12. How should iron deficiency be treated?
   Before treatment of iron deficiency, the most important task is to identify and, if possible, remedy the underlying cause.
   Oral iron therapy: The goal of oral iron therapy is to supply sufficient iron to correct anemia, if present, and to replenish iron stores. For most pediatric patients, oral iron is the treatment of choice for iron deficiency and is indicated with or without anemia. Oral iron is better absorbed when given on an empty stomach or with water or fruit juice. Iron absorption will be diminished with milk and other dairy products, tea, coffee, and solid foods. Generally, the effectiveness of iron therapy should be assessed with a CBC and serum ferritin at 1 month and 3 months; treatment should continue until the serum ferritin is within the normal range.
   - **Infants and young children:** In infants and young children with nutritional iron deficiency, limiting cow milk intake to less than 24 ounces per day and increasing iron-rich foods in the diet should be recommended. Although definitive clinical trials in children are lacking, limited pediatric data and extrapolation from adult studies suggest that for infants and young children, elemental iron, 3 mg/kg, as ferrous sulfate, administered once daily may be used as initial therapy. Conventionally, higher doses of elemental iron (3–6 mg/kg) given in divided doses two or three times daily as an iron salt (ferrous sulfate, ferrous fumarate, ferrous gluconate) or iron polysaccharide preparation have been recommended but may be no more effective and less acceptable to patients.
   - **Adolescents:** As for children, definitive clinical trials are lacking but limited data and extrapolation from adult studies suggest that elemental iron, 65 mg, as ferrous sulfate, given once daily, may be used as initial therapy. Conventional adult therapy has been a ferrous iron salt taken separately from meals in three divided doses that supply a daily total of 200 mg or more of elemental iron, but single daily dosing may be equally as effective.
   Intravenous (IV) iron therapy: Although data for the use of IV iron in pediatric populations is limited, current IV iron products seem much safer than those originally available. Nonetheless, patients requiring IV iron are best treated in pediatric centers experienced in IV iron therapy. Patients to be considered for IV iron administration include those in whom oral iron therapy has been unsuccessful or cannot be tolerated, those with continuing blood losses that cannot be controlled, those unable to absorb sufficient amounts of iron from the diet because of malabsorption disorders or surgery, and those with the rare genetic disorder iron-refractory iron-deficiency anemia (IRIDA).

FOLATE AND VITAMIN B$_{12}$ (COBALAMIN) AND DEFICIENCY: MEGALOBLASTIC ANEMIA

13. Describe the pathways of folate and vitamin B$_{12}$ absorption.
   - **Folate:** Tetrahydrofolate (THF) polyglutamates, the form of folate in dietary sources, are hydrolyzed to THF monoglutamates and then absorbed in the upper small intestine by the proton-coupled folate transporter. The THF monoglutamates enter and circulate in plasma to be taken up by cellular folate receptors.
   - **Vitamin B$_{12}$:** Most B$_{12}$ is absorbed through an active receptor-mediated pathway; less than 2% passively is absorbed. After release in the low pH of the stomach, dietary B$_{12}$ binds to salivary R-binder (haptocorrin). The R-binder-B$_{12}$ complex and intrinsic factor (IF; produced by parietal cells) are transported to the upper small intestine, where the higher pH results in the release of B$_{12}$ from the R-binder. The B$_{12}$ then binds to IF. In the terminal ileum, the IF- B$_{12}$ complex enters the ileal enterocyte via receptor-mediated endocytosis. followed by the release of B$_{12}$ into plasma, where the B$_{12}$ binds to transcobalamin for transport.

14. How do deficiencies of either folate or vitamin B$_{12}$ interfere with hematopoiesis?
   Vitamin B$_{12}$ is required for the methionine synthesis reaction that regenerates folate, present as 5-methyltetrahydrofolate (5-methylene-THF), to THF, which is then metabolized to 5,10-methylene-THF. In turn, 5,10-methylene-THF is required for the methylation of deoxyuridylate (dUMP) to form thymidylate (dTMP), which is then metabolized to thymidine triphosphate (dTTP) for incorporation into DNA (Figure 6.3). Folate is also needed for de novo synthesis of purines and for the methylation of cytosines in DNA. Without sufficient B$_{12}$ or folate, these reactions cannot proceed, interfering with the production and metabolism of the DNA needed for hematopoiesis. Peripheral macrocytosis may be masked by iron deficiency or other causes of microcytic anemia.

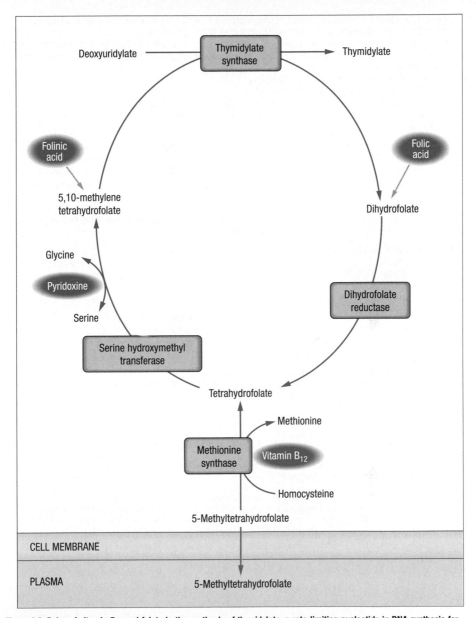

Figure 6.3 Roles of vitamin B$_{12}$ and folate in the synthesis of thymidylate, a rate-limiting nucleotide in DNA synthesis for hematopoiesis. Folate enters the cell from plasma as 5-methyltetrahydrofolate (5-methyl-THF) and is demethylated to tetrahydrofolate (THF) by methionine synthase, a vitamin B$_{12}$-dependent enzyme. THF is then methylated to 5,10-methylene tetrahydrofolate (5,10-methylene-THF). The methyl group is subsequently added to the 5-carbon of uridylate to form thymidylate (thymidine monophosphate), resulting in the formation of dihydrofolate. Dihydrofolate can then be reduced by dihydrofolate reductase to regenerate THF. If vitamin B$_{12}$ is deficient, the conversion of methyl-THF to THF is inhibited (the so-called "folate trap") and the methyl-THF accumulates and cannot serve as a substrate for thymidylate synthesis. (Figure reproduced from Hesdorffer CS, Longo DL. Drug-induced megaloblastic anemia. *N Engl J Med.* 2015;373:1649–1658.)

15. Which laboratory studies are used in the diagnosis of nutritional megaloblastic anemia?

Both serum folate and vitamin B_{12} concentrations should be measured before therapy of megaloblastic anemia because hematological abnormalities caused by B_{12} deficiency may be partially corrected by therapy with folate alone and result in irreversible neurologic damage. Laboratory reference ranges should be used for diagnosis; typical concentrations are shown as follows:

- Initial screening: serum B_{12} less than 200 pg/mL
- Initial screening: serum folate less than 3 ng/mL
- Further evaluation: Methylmalonic acid: increased in B_{12} deficiency but not in folate deficiency.
- Further evaluation: Homocysteine: Invariably increased in folate deficiency; may also be increased with B_{12} deficiency

16. What are the clinical signs and symptoms of vitamin B_{12} deficiency?

Mild deficiency is characterized by megaloblastic anemia and fatigue without neurologic findings. *Moderate* deficiency is characterized by macrocytic anemia with mild neurologic impairment. *Severe* deficiency is characterized by obvious neurologic impairment and risk for cardiomyopathy. In addition to anemia, thrombocytopenia or neutropenia may be present.

Neurologic symptoms can occur in the absence of anemia and include motor and sensory disturbances, cognitive impairment, abnormal coordination, and memory loss. Subacute combined degeneration of the spinal cord may be present and is irreversible even with treatment of B_{12} deficiency.

17. How do you treat vitamin B_{12} deficiency?

Correction of B_{12} deficiency may be given with daily high-dose oral replacement or with less frequent intramuscular injection (monthly). Depending on the mechanism of deficiency, some patients may require supplementation for life. If both B_{12} and folic acid deficiencies are identified together, B_{12} must be corrected first to avoid precipitating catastrophic neurologic injury.

18. What are the clinical signs and symptoms of folate deficiency?

Folate deficiency causes megaloblastic anemia. Signs and symptoms include fatigue, glossitis, mouth sores, and GI manifestations (nausea, vomiting, diarrhea, abdominal pain), but neurological abnormalities are absent. Pregnant females with folate deficiency have an increased risk of fetal neural tube defects.

19. How do you treat folate deficiency?

Correction of deficits in the diet should be recommended, and oral folate supplementation can be given to correct deficiency. If combined B_{12} deficiency and folate deficiency are present, B_{12} deficiency must be corrected before treatment of folate deficiency to avoid neurological harm.

BIBLIOGRAPHY

1. Allen LH, Miller JW, de Groot L, et al. Biomarkers of Nutrition for Development (BOND): Vitamin B-12 review. *J Nutr.* 2018;148(suppl allen4):1995s–2027s.
2. Bailey LB, Stover PJ, McNulty H, et al. Biomarkers of Nutrition for Development-folate review. *J Nutr.* 2015;145:1636s–1680s.
3. Lynch S, Pfeiffer CM, Georgieff MK, et al. Biomarkers of Nutrition for Development (BOND)-iron review. *J Nutr.* 2018;148 (suppl_1):1001s–1067s.
4. Pasricha SR, Tye-Din J, Muckenthaler MU, Swinkels DW. Iron deficiency. *Lancet.* 2021;397:233–248.
5. Powers JM, Buchanan GR. Disorders of iron metabolism: new diagnostic and treatment approaches to iron deficiency. *Hematol Oncol Clin North Am.* 2019;33:393–408.

CHAPTER 7

GRANULOCYTES

Jill S. Menell, MD and Mary Ann Bonilla, MD

1. **What are the signs and symptoms suggestive of a defect in neutrophil number or function?**
   The skin and mucous membranes are the first line of defense against infection. Once these barriers are broken, the white blood cells (WBCs), specifically neutrophils, come into play. When neutrophil counts are low or defective, the most common sites of infection are the skin and mucous membranes. Common presentations include cellulitis, superficial or deep abscesses, furunculosis, pneumonia, and septicemia. Also common are gingivitis, aphthous ulcers, perirectal inflammation, and otitis media. Recurrent respiratory infections, such as pneumonia or sinusitis, also raise suspicion of a WBC disorder. With profound neutropenia (<200 cells/μL), patients may present with high fevers and no obvious focus of infection. The usual inflammatory signs may be absent because the neutrophils normally release cytokines to mediate an inflammatory response. Infants with frequent infections should be evaluated for an underlying problem in the neutrophils or other branches of the immune system.

2. **What are the common pathogens noted in patients with neutrophil disorders?**
   Common infections arise from skin and gut flora. Patients with additional underlying immune defects (such as lymphocytes) or those who are neutropenic secondary to chemotherapy are also at risk for viral, fungal, and parasitic pathogens because of a more global immunodeficiency. Individuals with chronic granulomatous disease (CGD) are unable to mount a respiratory burst to destroy organisms. Common infections include *Staphylococcus aureus,* but there are also unusual pathogens, such as *Burkholderia cepacia, Serratia marcescens, Candida species,* and *Aspergillus fumigatus.*

3. **What are normal values for white blood cells and neutrophil counts?**
   WBC and neutrophil counts vary with age and race. Newborns have high WBC counts of 10,000 to 30,000 cells/μL with predominantly neutrophils. These numbers drop sharply after the first few days of life. An infant's WBC count after the first month is slightly higher than older children and adults (6,000–17,000 cells/μL), and the differential is predominantly lymphocytes, 60% to 70%, with 20% to 30% neutrophils. The toddler and preschool-aged child have approximately equal numbers of lymphocytes and neutrophils. The older child and adolescent have predominantly neutrophils with WBC counts similar to adults (5,000–11,000 cells/μL).

   Neutropenia is defined as an absolute neutrophil count (ANC) less than 1,000 cells/μL for infants less than 1 year of age and 1,500 cells/μL for individuals greater than 1 year of age. The ANC is calculated by multiplying the total WBC count by the percentage of neutrophils plus bands. People of African or Caribbean ancestry have 200 to 600 neutrophils/μL fewer compared with Caucasians.

   The severity and duration of neutropenia correlate with risk of infections. Neutropenia is graded according to ANC as follows:
   - Mild neutropenia: ANC 1,000 to 1,500 cells/μL
   - Moderate neutropenia: ANC 500 to 1,000 cells/μL
   - Severe neutropenia: ANC less than 500 cells/μL

4. **What are the clinical features of alloimmune and autoimmune neutropenia?**
   Neonatal alloimmune neutropenia is analogous to Rh hemolytic disease in that maternal antibodies directed against paternal antigens expressed on the surface of the neonate's neutrophils cross the placenta and mediate immune destruction. The mother lacks the fetal WBC antigens that are inherited from the father. The most common antigens are NA1 and NA2, which are isotypes of the Fcγ receptor IIIB (FcγRIIIB). The infants may be quite ill with infections secondary to profound neutropenia, or they may be asymptomatic. Omphalitis, skin infections, pneumonia, sepsis, and meningitis are the most common infections. The diagnosis of alloimmune neutropenia is established by detecting antineutrophil antibodies in the mother that react with paternal cells.

   Autoimmune neutropenia of childhood is generally a benign disorder. Affected individuals are often found incidentally with a routine blood count or when diagnosed with a minor infection. Despite ANCs of less than 500 cells/μL, 80% to 90% of patients do not have severe infectious complications. The total WBC count is normal. Some patients exhibit increased numbers of monocytes and eosinophils. The median age at diagnosis is 8 months with a range of 3 to 30 months. Other signs of autoimmune disease are absent. The disease is self-limited, often resolving by 4 years of age. Granulocyte colony-stimulating factor (G-CSF) can be used for those patients with severe infections.

   Autoimmune neutropenia in adolescents and adults may be associated with systemic disease, such as systemic lupus erythematosus (SLE), rheumatoid arthritis, common variable immunodeficiency, hyper immunoglobulin M (IgM) syndrome, and immunoglobulin A (IgA) deficiency.

5. **What would be the approach to evaluating a patient with neutropenia?**

The history should focus on the duration of neutropenia, recent viral infections, past bacterial infections, growth and development, congenital anomalies, medication history or toxic exposures, ethnicity, and a family history of neutropenia or unexplained infant deaths.

The physical examination should focus on signs of underlying disease (i.e., growth and development, phenotypic abnormalities, lymphadenopathy, organomegaly, pallor, bruising, petechiae). Sites of infection should be evaluated carefully, including mucous membranes, gingiva, skin, ears, lungs, and perianal area.

Laboratory testing should be based on the history and physical examination. If the child is well and the past medical history unremarkable, then the likely diagnosis is an intercurrent viral illness. In this case, a complete blood count (CBC) with peripheral smear may be the only test indicated. If there are no abnormal cells on review and the other cell lines are normal, then it is reasonable to repeat the count in 3 to 4 weeks to document recovery of normal counts. Serum B_{12} and red blood cell (RBC) folate levels may be indicated based on dietary history and high mean corpuscular volume (MCV) or other changes in the CBC. A bone marrow aspirate is not indicated in the child who is not having frequent infections. Antineutrophil antibodies are not always detected or may be falsely positive and are not currently recommended for a work up of neutropenia.

After assessing the severity and duration of neutropenia, causes of acquired neutropenia should be excluded. Genetic testing should be considered for suspected congenital neutropenia (CN) patients. Currently, next-generation sequencing panels are commercially available that include genes for known CN, such as *ELANE*, *HAX1*, *CXCR4*, *TAZ*, *WAS*, *JAGN1*, and others that are added continuously. Genetic testing is vital for diagnosis, treatment, and determining the risk of myelodysplastic syndrome (MDS)/acute myeloblastic leukemia (AML). This will guide decisions regarding hematopoietic stem cell transplantation (HSCT).

Children with a significant infectious history associated with chronic neutropenia (>3 months) require more extensive evaluation. CBCs should be obtained three times per week for 4 to 6 weeks to document whether or not there is cycling of the blood cells. Children with malabsorption/diarrhea should be assessed for pancreatic exocrine function and skeletal survey to evaluate for metaphyseal chondrodysplasia.

Bone marrow aspirate and biopsy are indicated for any child with more than isolated neutropenia (i.e., anemia, high MCV with normal B_{12}/ folate levels, or thrombocytopenia). The bone marrow should be sent for cytogenetics, fluorescent in situ hybridization (FISH), and flow cytometry studies as indicated. Bone marrow should be performed before use of G-CSF.

6. **What are the different forms of congenital neutropenia?**

CNs are very rare. They should be considered in children presenting during the first year of life with recurrent fevers or severe infections. Findings on physical examination may include cardiac, urogenital, skeletal, or skin abnormalities leading to the diagnosis. Family history may be helpful but will be negative in de novo mutations. The *ELANE* gene mutation was the first described and is the most common cause of severe CN and cyclic neutropenia. Now, however, there are many other genes that have been detected with various CN syndromes. See Table 7.1.

Severe CN or Kostmann syndrome is characterized by a maturational arrest of bone marrow at the promyelocyte stage. Patients have profound neutropenia (less than 200 cells/μL) and develop fever, skin infections (omphalitis), stomatitis, and perirectal abscesses. There is high incidence of evolution to AML (30% over 10 years).

Cyclic neutropenia is a disorder of neutrophil production where the neutrophils and other cells oscillate in number every 21 days (give or take 3 days). The ANC nadir is usually less than 200 cells/μL and generally persists for 3 to 5 days. At nadir, oral symptoms including aphthous ulcers and gingivitis/periodontitis can occur. Patients have increased risk of peritonitis, vaginal or rectal ulcerations, and pneumonia. Treatment with G-CSF does not eliminate cycling but decreases the length from 21 to 14 days and decreases serious infections.

Table 7.1 Congenital Neutropenia

DISEASE	INHERITANCE	GENE	OTHER FEATURES
Ethnic neutropenia	?	*DARC*	
Severe congenital neutropenia	AD	*ELANE* *HAX1* and *G6PC3*	Secondary AML or MDS
Cyclic neutropenia	AD	*ELANE*	Cyclic hematopoiesis
Barth syndrome	X-linked	*TAZ*	Cardiomyopathy, proximal skeletal myopathy, growth retardation
Glycogen Storage disease 1b	AR	*SLC37A4*	Hypoglycemia, hepatosplenomegaly, seizures and failure to thrive in infants
WHIM/ Myelokathexis	AD	*CXCR4*	Warts, Hypo-immunoglobulin (Ig), leukopenia, infections, myelokathexis

AD, Autosomal dominant; *AML*, acute myeloblastic leukemia; *AR*, autosomal recessive; *MDS*, myelodysplastic syndrome; *WHIM*, warts, hypogammaglobulinemia, infections, and myelokathexis.

Glycogen storage disease 1b is characterized by severe hypoglycemia, hepatomegaly, enterocolitis, and neutropenia. There is both neutrophil and monocyte dysfunction increasing the risk of infections. Inflammatory bowel disease is also a common feature.

Barth syndrome is caused by a phospholipid mitochondrial membrane defect. Clinical features include cardiomyopathy, proximal myopathy, delayed motor development, growth delay, and stable or oscillating neutropenia. Because of the cardiomyopathy, patients are less able to tolerate the stress of sepsis.

WHIM syndrome is a congenital immunodeficiency associated with severe neutropenia. "WHIM" is short for warts, hypogammaglobulinemia, infections, and myelokathexis. Myelokathexis (sequestration of mature neutrophils in the bone marrow) is due to mutations in the *CXCR4* chemokine receptor gene. Severe lymphopenia is also noted. *CXCR4* controls the trafficking of neutrophils. A novel *CXCR4* agonist is presently in clinical trials.

Bone marrow failure syndromes may present as isolated neutropenia and include reticular dysgenesis, Shwachman-Diamond syndrome, cartilage-hair hypoplasia, dyskeratosis congenita, and Fanconi anemia. Some of these are discussed in the bone marrow failure chapter.

7. **What is the most common congenital neutropenia?**
Benign ethnic neutropenia can occur commonly in individuals of African, Caribbean, Middle Eastern, and West Indian descent. Most patients have an ANC between 1000 to 1500 cells/μL. There is an association with the *DARC* gene polymorphism on chromosome 1. The mechanism of neutropenia is unclear, but most suggest that it results from a defect in the release of mature granulocytes from the bone marrow. This will also result in patients being negative for the Duffy antigen on their red cells. Work-up can be based on at least 3 blood counts at more than 2-week intervals showing stable counts with no additional changes to the CBC. No further investigations are indicated, and these patients are not at higher risk of infection.

8. **What are acquired causes of neutropenia?**
Infection is the most common cause of acquired neutropenia, with viruses being most frequent. There may be a history of a nonspecific viral illness in the preceding days to weeks before presentation. Viral causes of neutropenia include cytomegalovirus, Epstein-Barr virus, hepatitis, herpes simplex, human immunodeficiency virus (HIV), influenza A and B, measles, mumps, parvovirus, respiratory syncytial virus (RSV), roseola, and varicella, SARS-CoV-2, and others. Bacterial causes of neutropenia include gram-negative sepsis, para-typhoid and typhoid fever, brucellosis, tuberculosis, and tularemia. Other rare infectious causes of neutropenia include histoplasmosis, which is fungal; leishmaniasis and malaria, which are protozoan; and rickettsialpox, Rocky Mountain spotted fever, and typhus fever, which are rickettsial diseases.

Many medications can either affect bone marrow production or cause an immune-mediated destruction of the neutrophil. The broad categories of medications that may cause neutropenia include chemotherapy, heavy metals, analgesics/anti-inflammatories, antipsychotics/antidepressants, anticonvulsants, antithyroids, cardiovascular medications, antihistamines, antimicrobials, antiretrovirals, and other miscellaneous medications. It is important to review a medication history before doing an extensive work-up.

Immune mechanisms, either alloimmune or autoimmune, may be a cause of an acquired neutropenia as previously discussed. Nutritional causes of neutropenia include severe generalized deficiencies (such as starvation, anorexia nervosa, or marasmus), megaloblastic (vitamin B_{12} or folic acid), or copper deficiency. Splenomegaly may cause neutropenia because of sequestration. Infiltration of the bone marrow by leukemia or extrinsic tumor cells (e.g., neuroblastoma) may be associated with neutropenia. Nutritional deficiencies, splenomegaly, and bone marrow infiltration are often associated with involvement of more than one cell line (i.e., thrombocytopenia, anemia).

9. **What are the clinical features of leukocyte adhesion disorder?**
Leukocyte adhesion disorder presents in infancy with recurrent bacterial pulmonary and skin infections. Classic features include omphalitis, delayed umbilical cord separation, and poor wound healing. Despite marked leukocytosis (50,000–100,000 cells/μL), there is an absence of pus formation. Neutrophils have a complete or partial deficiency in the CD11/CD18 family of integrins responsible for adhesion of the neutrophils to vasculature. Neutrophils are unable to exit from the circulation to sites of inflammation. Individuals die in early childhood without HSCT.

10. **Describe the clinical features, diagnosis, and management of a patient with chronic granulomatous disease (CGD)?**
CGD is a qualitative disorder of the neutrophil. The neutrophils have normal chemotactic and phagocytic function but are unable to kill catalase positive organisms because of an inability to generate reactive oxygen species. Defects in cellular oxidative burst are caused by mutations in the genes involved in the NADPH oxidase system. Approximately two-thirds of cases are inherited in a X-linked recessive fashion involving the membrane protein, cytochrome oxidase b_{558} (91 kDa protein). The others are inherited in an autosomal recessive pattern with involvement of cytosolic proteins 22, 47, or 67 kDa.

Patients present with severe recurrent bacterial or fungal purulent disease. The common sites of infection are lungs, skin, gastrointestinal (GI) tract, liver, and lymph nodes. Generalized lymphadenopathy and hepatosplenomegaly are common. The infections often involve bacteria and fungi not ordinarily considered pathogens. The common offending organisms are catalase positive and include *Staphylococcus aureus, Burkholderia cepacia, Serratia marcescens, Nocardia, Candida species,* and *Aspergillus fumigatus.* Dysregulated inflammation seen in CGD can result in inflammatory bowel disease, granulomas in lungs, bowel and bladder, and macrophage activation syndrome.

The diagnosis is established with flow cytometry with dihydrorhodamine[123] or the nitroblue tetrazolium test (NBT). Patients with abnormal screening for CGD should undergo genetic testing for confirmation.

Management includes antibiotic and antifungal prophylaxis with trimethoprim-sulfamethoxazole and itraconazole. Interferon (IFN)-γ can result in decreased infections. HSCT remains the only curative modality with new trials of gene therapy underway.

11. **What are the general guidelines for the treatment of patients with disorders of neutrophil number and function?**

Individuals with neutropenia without recurrent infections should be monitored periodically, but no specific therapy is indicated. General precautions include a heightened awareness of the danger of fevers with prompt evaluation by a physician. Good oral hygiene and avoidance of rectal temperatures should be reviewed with the family. Patients with fever and severe neutropenia (ANC less than 500 cells/μL) should be treated as bacterial sepsis until proven otherwise. Bacterial sepsis occurs in approximately 20% of patients with severe neutropenia. Broad-spectrum antibiotics to cover skin and GI flora are indicated until bacterial cultures are negative. Patients in septic shock should receive a beta-lactamase resistant antibiotic and an aminoglycoside for gram-negative organisms. A rapid response time is imperative.

G-CSF has been proven to reduce the rate of infections in a number of inherited and acquired disorders of neutropenia. These include severe congenital neutropenia (Kostmann syndrome), cyclic neutropenia, Shwachman-Diamond syndrome, and dyskeratosis congenita. G-CSF is useful with severe infections associated with immune neutropenia as well.

HSCT is the only cure for the severe congenital neutropenias and bone marrow failure states.

12. **What are causes of eosinophilia?**

Degrees of eosinophilia are defined as mild (500–1,500 cells/μL), moderate (1,500–5,000 cells/μL), and severe (>5,000 cells/μL). An underlying allergy is the most common cause of eosinophilia in children from the United States. Acute allergic reactions can be associated with counts exceeding 20,000 cells/μL. Chronic allergies are associated with more modest increases in eosinophils to approximately 2,000 cells/μL. Outside of the United States, the most common cause of eosinophilia is parasitic infestation. See Table 7.2 for a list of causes of eosinophilia.

Table 7.2 Causes of Eosinophilia

Allergic conditions	Parasitic infections	Immune dysregulation
Asthma	Amebiasis	Autoimmune lymphoproliferative disorder
Allergic bronchopulmonary aspergillosis	*Ascaris lumbricoides*	Collagen vascular disease (e.g., systemic lupus erythematosus [SLE])
Drug reaction	Echinococcus	Hyper immunoglobulin E (IgE) syndrome
Episodic angioedema	Filariasis	IPEX
Hay fever	Flukes	Omenn syndrome
Dermatologic conditions	Hookworm	Wiskott-Aldrich syndrome
Acute urticaria	Malaria	ZAP-70 deficiency
Atopic dermatitis	Pneumocystis	
Eczema	Schistosomiasis	**Other**
Pemphigus	Strongyloides	Abdominal radiation
Scabies	*Toxocara canis/Toxocara cati*	Chronic peritoneal or hemodialysis
Toxic epidermal necrolysis	Toxoplasmosis	Congenital heart disease
Gastrointestinal disorders	Trichinosis	Sarcoidosis
Chronic hepatitis	Visceral larval migrans	Thrombocytopenia with absent radii (TAR) syndrome
Crohn disease	**Other infections**	
Food allergy	Cat scratch fever	
Eosinophilic gastritis	Coccidiomycosis	
Ulcerative colitis	Fungal rhinosinusitis	
	Infectious mononucleosis	
	Scarlet fever	
	Tuberculosis	
	Malignancy	
	Brain tumors	
	Hodgkin and Non-Hodgkin lymphoma	
	Leukemia	
	Myeloproliferative disorders	

13. **What is hypereosinophilic syndrome (HES)?**

HES is rare in children. It is defined as persistent eosinophilia of greater than 1,500 cells/μL for longer than 6 months, no evidence of malignancy, or other cause of the increased count with signs and symptoms of organ involvement with infiltration of eosinophils. The bone marrow shows increased numbers of eosinophils but no immature forms to suggest leukemia. Nonspecific symptoms include fever, weight loss, and fatigue. Cardiac damage by the eosinophils and their byproducts may be fatal. Chronic hypereosinophilia without organ involvement is called idiopathic hypereosinophilia. Patients with chronic severe eosinophilia should be monitored with periodic physical examinations and echocardiograms to monitor for organ toxicity.

BIBLIOGRAPHY

1. Arnold DE, Heimall JR. A review of chronic granulomatous disease. *Adv Ther.* 2017;34:2543–2557.
2. Atallah-Yunes SA, Ready A, Newburger PE. Benign ethnic neutropenia. *Blood Reviews.* 2019;37, 100586.
3. Dinauer MC. The phagocyte system and disorders of granulopoiesis and granulocyte function. In: Orkin SH, Fisher DE, Ginsburg D, Look AT, Lux SE, Nathan DG (eds). *Nathan and Oski's Hematology and Oncology of Infancy and Childhood.* 8th ed. Elsevier/Saunders, 2015:773–847.
4. Furutani E, Newburger PE, Shimamura A. Neutropenia in the age of genetic testing: advances and challenges. *Am J Hematol.* 2019;94 (3):384–393.
5. Gotlib J. World Health Organization-defined eosinophilic disorders: 2017 update on diagnosis, risk stratification and management. *Am J Hematol.* 2017;92:1243–1259.
6. Skokowa J, Dale DC, Touw IP, et al. Severe congenital neutropenias. *Nat Rev Dis Primers.* 2017;3:10732.
7. Liapis K. Approach to eosinophilia. *HAEMA.* 2019;10(2):116–127.

CHAPTER 8

DISORDERS OF PLATELETS

Manpreet Kochhar, MD and Cindy Neunert, MD, MSCS

1. **What is pseudothrombocytopenia?**
   Pseudothrombocytopenia, or spurious thrombocytopenia, is a falsely low automated platelet count that occurs secondary to in vitro platelet clumping. This is generally an incidental finding in an otherwise asymptomatic patient and can be confirmed by observation of platelet clumping on the peripheral smear. Pseudothrombocytopenia can be caused by a poorly collected specimen that has clotted, the presence of ethylenediaminetetra-acetic acid (EDTA)–dependent antibodies against platelets, or platelet satellitism (platelets around neutrophils or monocytes). An accurate platelet count can be obtained by doing a manual count on a freshly collected sample or by collecting the sample in a tube with a different anticoagulant, such as citrate.

2. **Differentiate the signs and symptoms of bleeding secondary to a platelet disorder from that of a coagulation disorder.**
   Bleeding because of a platelet disorder typically consists of skin and mucous membrane bleeds, such as petechiae, small ecchymoses, gum bleeding, epistaxis, gastrointestinal (GI) bleeding, and menorrhagia. Petechiae is a rather specific finding for thrombocytopenia and should prompt checking a platelet count. Deep subcutaneous muscle and joint bleeds are more characteristic of coagulation disorders, although they can also occur in rare disorders of platelet dysfunction.

3. **Discuss the mechanisms and causes of thrombocytopenia in the newborn.**
   Mechanisms of thrombocytopenia in the newborn can be broadly categorized as those with decreased bone marrow production, increased peripheral destruction, or consumption. In many conditions, it is not easy to delineate the exact mechanism, and a combination of mechanisms occurs. The best approach to identify the etiology is to look for the most common causes in the particular setting, whether the infant is well or sick, and search for any relevant maternal factors and significant family history. Box 8.1 enumerates the many possible causes of neonatal thrombocytopenia.

4. **What is the treatment for neonatal thrombocytopenia?**
   Except in cases of maternal autoimmune thrombocytopenia, platelet transfusion with cytomegalovirus-negative, white blood cell (WBC)–depleted platelet concentrate remains the treatment of choice for severe thrombocytopenia in the neonate. The primary aim for platelet transfusion is to maintain a platelet count that will prevent the risk of significant hemorrhage, particularly intracranial bleeding.
   There is no general consensus as to a "safe" platelet count in the neonate and no true "threshold" that should be maintained because lower platelet count is not a strong predictor of increased bleeding. Gestational age less than 34 weeks, early-onset severe thrombocytopenia (in 10 days from birth), sepsis, and illnesses like necrotizing enterocolitis are factors for increased risk of bleeding events and may be conditions where vigilance for increased bleeding risk should be maintained and platelets transfused based on clinical concern. A randomized controlled trial that compared platelet transfusion thresholds in preterm infants with severe thrombocytopenia noted that a higher rate of death or major bleeding was seen within 28 days after randomization in patients assigned to receive platelet transfusions at a platelet-count threshold of 50×10^9/L, as opposed to those at 25×10^9/L. A dose of 10 mL/kg of platelet concentrate should raise the platelet count to 75×10^9/L to 100×10^9/L.

5. **Define neonatal alloimmune thrombocytopenia (NAIT).**
   NAIT is thrombocytopenia in the neonate resulting from immune-mediated platelet destruction caused by alloantibodies produced and transferred by the mother against a specific fetal platelet antigen that the baby inherited from the father and that is absent in the mother.
   This is the platelet equivalent of Rh hemolytic disease of the newborn, although it can occur during the first pregnancy. This should be suspected in an otherwise healthy full-term newborn with no other obvious causes for thrombocytopenia who presents with petechiae, GI bleeding, or, in as many as 20% of cases, intracranial hemorrhage. The diagnosis is confirmed by determination of platelet alloantigen phenotype of the parents and detection of maternal antibody with specificity for paternal or fetal platelet antigen. The most common platelet antigen involved is the human platelet antigen (HPA)-1a, or HPA-4 in those of Asian background.

6. **Discuss the management of NAIT.**
   NAIT is a self-limiting condition with eventual recovery of the platelet count in 2 to 4 weeks. Until the platelet count recovers, however, the neonate is at an increased risk for life-threatening hemorrhage because of severe thrombocytopenia in the immediate newborn period. It is recommended that infants with NAIT be transfused to maintain a platelet count greater than 30×10^9/L in the absence of bleeding, and higher based on clinical bleeding

Box 8.1 Causes of Neonatal Thrombocytopenia

- Increased platelet destruction
  a. Immune-mediated
     Neonatal alloimmune thrombocytopenia
     Maternal immune thrombocytopenic purpura
     Maternal autoimmune diseases
     Maternal drug ingestion
  b. Nonimmune mediated
     Birth asphyxia
     Disseminated intravascular coagulation
     Necrotizing enterocolitis
     Giant hemangiomas (Kasabach-Merritt syndrome)
     Thrombosis
     Cardiac anomalies
     Hypersplenism
- Decreased platelet production
  a. Bone marrow aplasia
     Thrombocytopenia with absent radii
     Amegakaryocytic thrombocytopenia
     Fanconi anemia
     Trisomy syndromes and other chromosomal abnormalities
  b. Bone marrow replacement
     Congenital leukemia
     Neuroblastoma
     Osteopetrosis
     Histiocytosis
- Mixed or uncertain etiology
  a. Congenital intrauterine infections
  b. Maternal preeclampsia
  c. Phototherapy
  d. Rh hemolytic disease
  e. Polycythemia
  f. Genetic disorders (Alport's, metabolic disorders)
  g. Other hereditary thrombocytopenias

symptoms. The gold standard of treatment is transfusion with maternal platelets; however, this is often not a practical option. If transfusions are needed, then random donor platelets can be given and HPA-1a can be requested. Additionally, intravenous immunoglobulin (IVIG) 1 gram/kg for 1 to 2 days can be given along with random donor platelets. Antenatal management should be considered for subsequent at-risk pregnancies in conjunction with high-risk obstetric care.

7. Differentiate neonatal autoimmune thrombocytopenia (NITP) from NAIT.
   In NITP, immunoglobulin G (IgG) autoantibodies from the mother who has an underlying immune thrombocytopenia or other autoimmune diseases, such as systemic lupus erythematosus, are passively transferred to the baby who may subsequently develop thrombocytopenia secondary to immune destruction of platelets. The antibodies are directed against antigens common to both mother and baby, unlike in NAIT, in which the antibodies are only directed against the baby's platelets. Therefore in NITP, the mother has a low platelet count, whereas in NAIT, maternal platelet count is normal. The platelet count in NITP can be normal at birth, with nadir at 2 to 5 days after delivery. Bleeding problems in utero or during delivery are rare. This is also a self-limiting condition, with platelet recovery in 2 to 3 months. Treatment options in cases of severe thrombocytopenia ($<50 \times 10^9$/L) include IVIG and corticosteroids.

8. What is the differential diagnosis of acquired thrombocytopenia in children?
   a. Destruction (i.e., immune- or nonimmune-mediated)
   b. Sequestration (i.e., hypersplenism)
   c. Dilution (i.e., massive transfusion)
   d. Decreased production (i.e., bone marrow infiltration, injury, or failure)

9. Describe the pathophysiology of immune thrombocytopenia (ITP) and how to make the diagnosis.
   ITP is defined as isolated low platelet count (<100 x10^9/L) in the absence of other etiologies for thrombocytopenia. Thrombocytopenia results from both increased platelet destruction and decreased platelet production. Platelet destruction is because of IgG antibodies against platelet receptors, which come from autoreactive B cells

and are aided by cytotoxic T cells that have escaped negative selection. Further evidence has accumulated to suggest that the autoreactive B cells also produce antibodies against megakaryocytes in the bone marrow, leading to impaired platelet production.

The diagnosis of ITP is highly clinical and is also one of exclusion. A good and thorough history and physical examination, along with a complete blood count (CBC) and review of the peripheral smear, can confirm the diagnosis. In newly diagnosed ITP, the presenting history is typically brief and the physical examination only significant for the bleeding signs and symptoms that are related to the degree of thrombocytopenia. The CBC shows a low platelet count and normal WBC count, important for distinguishing this from an acute leukemia. The hemoglobin/hematocrit is generally normal but may be low in the case of severe bleeding from thrombocytopenia. On the peripheral smear the platelets are reduced, and many appear large, indicating an active bone marrow that is trying to compensate for the increased peripheral destruction. Additionally, the WBC and red blood cell (RBC) morphologies will be normal. A bone marrow examination is not necessary unless the patient has other atypical findings on presentation or laboratory evaluation. Antiplatelet antibody testing is not crucial in making the diagnosis, and these tests are not commonly done because of their lack of sufficient sensitivity and specificity.

10. **Define the different stages of ITP.**
ITP can be thought of as newly diagnosed, persistent, or chronic. Each diagnosis consists of having a platelet count of less than 100 x10^9/L, for varying durations of time.

ITP	*Platelet count <100 x10^9/L for:*
Newly diagnosed	<3 months
Persistent	3–12 months
Chronic	>12 months

"Nonresponsive" or "refractory" ITP includes acute ITP that does not respond to initial treatment (either ongoing thrombocytopenia or bleeding symptoms) and all persistent and chronic ITP diagnoses.

11. **Discuss the treatment of ITP in children.**
ITP in children is most often acute and self-limited. The goal of treatment is to cease active bleeding, minimize side effects from medication, and allow the child to live comfortably with maximal quality of life. In children with a history of bleeding, avoidance of future episodes may also influence the need for treatment. The decision to treat is based on severity of bleeding symptoms, lifestyle and activity of the patient, and other comorbidities that may increase the risk of bleeding. The platelet count alone should not be used as a reason to treat in a child with no or mild bleeding because this value does not actually correlate with the degree of bleeding. The currently available treatment options for upfront management of acute ITP include observation, corticosteroids, IVIG, and anti-Rh(D) antibody. For the majority of children with no or mild bleeding, treatment with observation alone may be sufficient given that there are no concerns for lack of follow-up, distance to the hospital, parental anxiety, upcoming procedures, or other factors that increase the child's risk for bleeding. If treatment is needed, corticosteroids are the preferred first-line treatment with IVIG and anti-D being reserved for children with more significant bleeding that requires a more rapid increase in the platelet count.

12. **Describe the mechanism of action and side effects of IVIG in the treatment of ITP.**
IVIG works by blocking the Fc receptors on macrophages, thereby sparing destruction of the IgG-coated platelets and allowing them to remain in the circulation. It also contains anti-idiotypic antibodies that can bind to circulating antibodies, thereby rendering them ineffective in binding to platelets. The major side effect of IVIG is headache, which can be severe and usually occurs 24 hours after the infusion. Additional side effects include infusion reactions, aseptic meningitis, thrombosis, and renal failure.

13. **How does anti-D immunoglobulin work in the treatment of ITP? What are the potential side effects?**
Intravenous anti-D immunoglobulin can be used to treat ITP in patients who are Rh(D)-positive. The patient's Rh (D)-positive RBCs are coated by the anti-Rh(D) antibodies. These antibody-coated RBCs are then destroyed by the reticuloendothelial system, occupying the Fc receptor on these macrophages and thereby sparing the destruction of the antibody-coated platelets. Of note, this treatment can only be used in patients who are Rh(D)-positive and have an intact spleen. Additionally, it can lead to a decrease in hemoglobin concentration of up to 2 gm/dL. Other side effects include infusion reactions and, rarely, life-threatening disseminated intravascular coagulopathy (DIC).

14. **What options are there for failed first-line therapy in (acute) ITP, and what are their mechanisms?**
Second-line treatment options for ITP include immunosuppressive agents (i.e., rituximab, mycophenolate mofetil, 6-mercaptopurine), surgical splenectomy, and thrombopoietin receptor agonists (TPO-RAs; i.e., eltrombopag, romiplostim).

Immunosuppressive therapy aims to inhibit different functions of the immune system so that it can no longer produce antibodies against platelets or megakaryocytes. Surgical splenectomy is used to prevent destruction of antibody-coated platelets by splenic macrophages, although this practice is usually reserved for highly refractory patients because it confers a lifelong risk of sepsis. TPO-RAs work to stimulate the thrombopoietin receptor, leading to increased platelet production in the bone marrow.

15. **What are some drugs that can cause immune-mediated thrombocytopenia?**
    - Heparin
    - Valproic acid
    - Digoxin
    - Penicillin
    - Cimetidine
    - Quinine
    - Quinidine

16. **What are some causes of nonimmune platelet destruction?**
    - DIC
    - Infection
    - Thrombotic thrombocytopenic purpura (TTP)/hemolytic uremic syndrome (HUS)
    - Mechanical destruction
    - HELLP (hemolysis, elevated liver enzymes, and low platelets)
    - Kasabach-Merritt syndrome

17. **What is thrombotic thrombocytopenic purpura, and how is it managed?**
    TTP is a condition caused by a deficiency of ADAMTS13, a metalloprotease that cleaves von Willebrand factor (VWF) into smaller multimers. The uncleaved factor forms multimers that attract platelet aggregation in the endothelium and can lead to microthrombotic disease. This generally presents with the classic pentad of microangiopathic hemolytic anemia, thrombocytopenia, neurologic findings, renal complications, and fever. Peripheral smear demonstrates schistocytes and thrombocytopenia. Other laboratory markers of hemolysis are also elevated, such as lactate dehydrogenase, reticulocyte count, and bilirubin. Although patients may be critically ill, this condition can be distinguished from DIC because prothrombin time (PT)/partial thromboplastin time (PTT) are normal in TTP.

    Treatment of TTP is immediate plasmapheresis, even while confirmatory testing is pending, because untreated disease is often fatal. The goal of plasmapheresis is to remove the circulating anti-ADAMTS13 antibody from circulation. In addition, patients are started on corticosteroids, and it is suggested that they also receive rituximab (a B cell-depleting therapy). An anti-VWF agent that blocks the aggregation of platelets (caplacizumab) is now available, although it is not clear if this should be used upfront or reserved for patients with relapsing disease. Of note, there is also a congenital form of TTP in which there is a deficiency of ADAMTS13 without the presence of antibodies. The treatment for congenital TTP is regularly scheduled fresh frozen plasma (FFP) transfusions because this product contains ADAMTS13 and can replace the deficiency.

18. **Name some of the hereditary disorders of platelet number, their mode of inheritance, and clinical features.**

Disorder	Inheritance	Platelets	Clinical features
Wiskott Aldrich syndrome/X-linked thrombocytopenia	XLR	Small size, low count	Associated with B- and T-cell defects (immunodeficiency), eczema, and recurrent infections. Confirmatory testing looks for *WASP* gene.
MYH9-RD	AD	Large size, low count	Associated with renal failure, sensorineural hearing loss, cataracts; leukocyte inclusions on peripheral smear (Dohle bodies).
TAR (thrombocytopenia absent radii)	AR	Normal size, low count	Absent radii but with present thumbs (differentiates from Fanconi anemia); elevated thrombopoietin levels; often have cow milk intolerance.
CAMT (congenital amegakaryocytic thrombocytopenia)	AR	Normal size, low count	Because of mutation in the C-MPL receptor; often progresses to aplastic anemia.

AD, Autosomal dominant; *AR*, autosomal recessive; *XLR*, X-linked recessive.

19. Name some of the hereditary disorders of platelet function, their mode of inheritance, platelet aggregation defects, and pertinent clinical features.

Disorder	Inheritance	Platelets	Platelet defect and aggregation studies	Bleeding symptoms	Associated clinical features
Glanzmann's thrombasthenia	AR	Normal size and count	• Deficiency in GPIIb-IIIa platelet receptor • ↓ to all agonists except ristocetin (normal)	Moderate to severe	None
Bernard-Soulier syndrome	AR	Large size, low count	• Absent GP1b platelet receptor • ↓ to ristocetin secondary to reduced membrane GP1b-V-IX complex	Moderate to severe	DiGeorge/Velocardial facial syndrome
Gray platelet syndrome	AR	Large size, normal count, pale-staining	• Mild defects with ADP and epinephrine	Mild to moderate	Myelofibrosis, splenomegaly
Hermansky Pudlak / Chediak-Higashi (CH)	AR	Normal size and count, giant granules in CH	• Absent dense granules on EM • Absent second wave with all agonists	Mild to moderate	Oculocutaneous albinism and strabismus, neutropenia, risk of pulmonary fibrosis
Platelet-type von Willebrand disease	AD	Variable size and platelet count	• Defect of GP1b, increased binding of VWF • ↑ to ristocetin	Moderate	Absence of high molecular weight VWF multimers

AD, Autosomal dominant; *ADP*, adenosine diphosphate; *AR*, autosomal recessive; *EM*, electron microscopy; *VWF*, von Willebrand factor.

20. What are the options for treatment of platelet function disorders?
Bleeding episodes in patients with known hereditary platelet function disorders can be managed with local measures and platelet transfusions. Platelet transfusions should be given with caution in patients with receptor defects because antibodies can develop that render the patient platelet transfusion refractory. Recombinant factor VIIa can be used in patients who are refractory to platelet transfusions with severe bleeding. Desmopressin (DDAVP) infusions may also be used. The potential role of DDAVP is to stimulate the release of VWF, enhancing platelet adhesion and aggregation. Adjunctive treatment with an antifibrinolytic agent, such as epsilon-amino-caproic acid or tranexamic acid, is also helpful. The treatment for the acquired platelet function disorders is generally management of the primary disease or etiology. For patients with uremia-induced platelet dysfunction, estrogens have shown to be useful, although the mechanism of action is unclear. RBC transfusions can correct anemia and increase viscosity, which may also lead to decreased bleeding.

21. List some other diseases or conditions that are associated with platelet function defects.
   • Uremia
   • Liver disease
   • Leukemia
   • Glycogen storage diseases
   • Valvular heart defects
   • Cardiopulmonary bypass
   • Nephrotic syndrome
   • Infections: human immunodeficiency virus (HIV), infectious mononucleosis
   • Medication-induced platelet disorders.

22. **Name some drugs that are known to cause platelet dysfunction.**
    - Dextran
    - Antihistamines
    - Phenothiazines
    - Tricyclic antidepressants
    - Propranolol
    - Targeted antiplatelet therapies (i.e., aspirin, ibuprofen)

23. **Describe the differences between antiplatelet effects of different anti-inflammatory agents.**
    - Reversible effects: Indomethacin, ibuprofen, phenylbutazone, sulfinpyrazone
    - Irreversible effect: Aspirin

24. **Describe the different oral antiplatelet therapies and their mechanisms of action.**
    - Aspirin: Irreversibly inhibits prostaglandin synthase in platelets and megakaryocytes
    - Thienopyridines (Clopidogrel, Prasugrel): Reversibly inhibits P2Y12 at a site other than the adenosine diphosphate (ADP) binding site
    - Ticagrelor: Reversibly inhibits P2Y12 at a site other than the ADP binding site
    - Dipyridamole: Reversibly causes inhibition of platelet cyclic adenosine monophosphate (cAMP) and potentiation of adenosine inhibition of platelet function

25. **Discuss the difference between primary and secondary thrombocytosis.**
    Thrombocytosis is defined as a platelet count above the upper limit of normal value ($>450 \times 10^9$/L). This can be further classified as either essential (primary) or reactive (secondary) thrombocytosis. Reactive thrombocytosis is the most common cause of an elevated platelet count in children. Platelets are an acute phase reactant and therefore reactive thrombocytosis arises as a "reaction" to a predisposing condition, such as hypoxia, inflammation, autoimmune disorders, or platelet loss. This is fairly common in children, particularly in young infants. Marked thrombocytosis can also be seen in patients who have had splenectomy, regardless of the reason for removal. Thrombocytosis can also be seen in patients with hepatoblastoma.

    Essential thrombocytosis results from a stem cell defect and is very rare in children. This is generally seen with myeloproliferative disorders such as polycythemia vera, chronic myelogenous leukemia, and idiopathic myelofibrosis. An underlying mutation in JAK2, CALR, or MPL can be seen in patients with essential thrombocytosis.

26. **What are the indications for treatment of thrombocytosis?**
    Complications from secondary thrombocytosis are extremely rare, and the increased platelet count is generally transient. Except in Kawasaki disease, in which there is a known risk for thrombotic complications, reactive thrombocytosis generally does not require treatment. Antiplatelet prophylaxis with aspirin can be considered when there are other existing risk factors for thrombosis, such as immobilization, vessel damage, or hyperviscosity.

    Essential thrombocytosis is associated with elevated platelet count and bleeding complications from disturbed platelet function. Treatment options include myelosuppressive agents (i.e., hydroxyurea, busulfan, interferon), platelet pheresis, and platelet aggregation inhibitors (i.e., aspirin, dipyridamole). For high-risk disease, cytoreductive treatment with hydroxyurea is recommended for patients of any age, particularly with a prior history of thrombosis. Lower risk disease can be managed with aspirin alone or even just observation. It is important to note that patients with essential thrombocytosis can developed an acquired von Willebrand disease that places them at risk for bleeding; therefore VWF levels should be checked in all patients at diagnosis or any time they have bleeding symptoms, and the use of antiplatelet therapy must be balanced against the risk of bleeding.

BIBLIOGRAPHY

1. Blanchette V, Carcao M. Approach to the investigation and management of immune thrombocytopenic purpura in children. *Semin Hematol.* 2000;37:299–314.
2. Hathaway WE, Goodnight SH. Hereditary function defects. In *Disorders of Hemostasis and Thrombosis: A Clinical Guide.* McGraw-Hill, Inc., 1993:94–102.
3. Hathaway WE, Goodnight SH. Acquired platelet function disorders. In *Disorders of Hemostasis and Thrombosis: A Clinical Guide.* McGraw-Hill, Inc.; 1993:94–102.
4. Neunert C, Noroozi N, Norman G, et al. Severe bleeding events in adults and children with primary immune thrombocytopenia: a systematic review. *J Thromb Haemost.* 2015;13(3):457–464.
5. Neunert C, Terrell DR, Arnold DM, et al. American Society of Hematology 2019 guidelines for immune thrombocytopenia. *Blood Adv.* 2019;3(23):3829–3866.
6. Saes JL, Schols EM, Van Heerde WL, Nijziel MR. Hemorrhagic disorders of fibrinolysis: a clinical review. *J Thrombosis and Hemostasis.* 2018;16:1498–1509.
7. Smith OP. Inherited and congenital thrombocytopenia. In: Lilleyman J, Hamn I, Blanchette V (eds). *Pediatric Hematology.* Churchill Livingstone; 1999:419–435.
8. Sutor AH. Thrombocytosis in childhood. Semin Thrombosis Hemostasis. 1995;21:330–339.

CHAPTER 9

BONE MARROW FAILURE SYNDROMES

Megan Askew, MD and Staci D. Arnold, MD, MBA, MPH

1. **Describe the three main pathophysiological mechanisms of aplastic anemia.**
   a. Direct damage to bone marrow
      i. Typically iatrogenic because of cytotoxic drugs/chemotherapy, radiation therapy, and other myelosuppressive medications. Has also been seen with environmental toxins, including benzene (workplace toxin), now more common in low-income countries.
      ii. Effects are dose-dependent and often associated with spontaneous recovery.
   b. Immune-mediated
      i. Acquired aplastic anemia, when severe and acute, is most often associated with immune-mediated process as evidenced by response of blood counts to immunosuppressive therapies and dependence of counts after recovery on maintenance immunosuppression.
      ii. This immune-mediated process is believed to be because of an aberrant T-cell immune response; as such, treatment designed to suppress T-cell response has been shown to be effective. This may have an identifiable viral trigger or can be associated with typable and nontypable hepatitis; however, in most cases, no trigger can be identified.
   c. Constitutional genetic defects
      i. Less often, bone marrow failure is associated with genetic defects. Factors that suggest an inherited bone marrow failure syndrome include macrocytosis; physical anomalies; failed response to immunosuppressive therapy; past history of moderate, chronic pancytopenia; significant infectious history or family history of cytopenias; early death; myelodysplastic syndrome (MDS)/acute myelogenous leukemia (AML), or early cancer.
      ii. Screening for causes of constitutional marrow failure is indicated for patients with aplastic anemia. If pancytopenia is severe and acute with no family history or clinical features on examination, screening is less likely to be positive.

2. **What are the treatment options for idiopathic severe aplastic anemia?**
   In children, if a human leukocyte antigen (HLA)–matched, related donor is available, the treatment of choice is hematopoietic stem cell transplant (HSCT). If no such donor is available, patients can be treated with immunosuppressive therapy.
   Immunosuppressive therapy has typically included horse antithymocyte globulin (ATG) and cyclosporine. In a randomized study, horse ATG was found to be superior to rabbit ATG in treatment of severe aplastic anemia based on improved hematological response and survival. Additionally, new trials have shown improved response in approximately 60% of patients with the addition of eltrombopag to an upfront immunosuppressive regimen.
   If immunotherapy fails, matched unrelated donor transplant is a suitable option. Alternatively, haploidentical transplant or second-line immunosuppressive therapy can be used if an unrelated transplant donor is unavailable.

3. **What is the underlying defect of paroxysmal nocturnal hemoglobinuria?**
   Paroxysmal nocturnal hemoglobinuria (PNH) is a clonal hematopoietic stem cell disease that is the result of an acquired defect in the *PIG-A* gene necessary for the synthesis of glycosylphosphatidylinositol, which anchors proteins to the surface of cells. The mutation leads to the loss of CD55 and CD59, inhibitors of the complement system, thereby leading to uncontrolled complement activation and both intravascular and extravascular hemolysis.
   Patients with classic PNH present with symptoms of intravascular hemolysis, including elevated reticulocyte count, large population of PNH cells, elevated lactate dehydrogenase (LDH), hemoglobinuria, fatigue, smooth muscle dystonias, and thrombosis. More common to pediatric patients, an expanded PNH clone may be found in patients with acquired aplastic anemia. These patients may present with aplastic anemia and often a smaller number of PNH clones. Nevertheless, some will experience expansion of *PIG-A* mutation mutant clone and progress to classical PNH.

4. **What is the therapy of choice for classical PNH and/or PNH complications?**
   In patients with classical PNH, HSCT and complement inhibition therapy are the only proven effective therapies. Complement inhibition therapy is the current first-line treatment of choice for severe classical PNH in children. It is highly effective in reducing intravascular hemolysis and reducing risk of thrombosis; however, it does not treat bone marrow failure. Patients with severe aplastic anemia should be considered for allogeneic transplant or immunosuppressive therapy if no HLA-matched sibling donor is available. Additionally, HSCT may be considered in patients with severe classical PNH with suboptimal response to complement inhibition therapy.

5. Describe the inheritance patterns, common genetic mutations, and treatment options associated with inherited bone marrow failure syndromes.

Syndrome	Genetics	Common Gene Mutations	Clinical Features	Treatment
Fanconi anemia	AR X-LR AD	BRCA1, FANC genes except FANCB RAD51	Short stature, café-au-lait spots, skeletal and urogenital anomalies	Oxymetholone HSCT
Dyskeratosis congenita	X-LR AD AD/AR	DKC1 TINF2 TERC, TERT	Lacy reticular skin, nail dystrophy, oral leukoplakia, hepatic and pulmonary fibrosis	Danazol HSCT
Diamond-Blackfan anemia	AD	RPS19, RPL5, RPL11	Short stature, thumb anomalies (triphalangeal), cleft palate/lip	Supportive care[a] Corticosteroids HSCT
Schwachman-Diamond syndrome	AR	SBDS	Malabsorption, short stature, metaphyseal dysostosis, thoracic abnormalities, developmental delay	G-CSF Supportive care HSCT
Thrombocytopenia absent radii syndrome	AR	RBM8A	Bilateral absent radii with presence of thumbs, other skeletal anomalies, cow's milk intolerance	Supportive care
Congenital amegakaryocytic thrombocytopenia	AR	MPL	Petechiae or more serious hemorrhages in infancy	Supportive care HSCT
Severe congenital neutropenia	AD AR	ELA-2 HAX1, G6PC3, JAGN1	Severe infections (abscesses, pneumonia) often during infancy	G-CSF HSCT

[a]Supportive care may include transfusion and antibiotic treatment or prophylaxis.

AD, Autosomal dominant; *AR*, autosomal recessive; *GCSF*, granulocyte colony-stimulating factor; *HSCT*, hematopoietic stem cell transplant; *X-LR*, X-linked recessive.

6. What test is necessary to make the diagnosis of Fanconi anemia?

Fanconi anemia (FA) is characterized by abnormal chromosomal breakage because of a defective DNA repair pathway. Clastogenic studies, in which agents such as diepoxybutane (DEB) and mitomycin-C are used to induce chromosomal breaks, are reliable in assessing whether breakage is increased and are diagnostic of FA. Chromosomal breakage testing is recommended for all patients with congenital malformations known to be associated with FA, aplastic anemia at any age, or with MDS with complex cytogenetic abnormalities. If chromosomal breakage studies are inconclusive, but there is high suspicion for FA, testing should be performed on skin fibroblasts. Although genetic testing exists for known FA mutations, not all mutations resulting in FA have been identified, and thus genetic testing is not required for diagnosis in the presence of abnormal chromosomal breakage studies and other clinical criteria.

7. What are the most common physical anomalies in Fanconi anemia?

Approximately 60% of patients with FA are reported to have at least one physical abnormality.

System	Anomaly
Skin	Café-au-lait spots, hyper/hypopigmented lesions
Skeletal	• Head: Microcephaly, hydrocephaly • Upper limbs: Absent/hypoplastic radii and/or thumbs[a] • Axial: Vertebral anomalies, spina bifida, Klippel-Feil, Sprengel deformity • Lower limbs: Congenital hip dislocation, abnormal toes
Eyes	Microphthalmia, epicanthal folds, hyper/hypotelorism, strabismus, cataracts
Ears	Deafness (usually conductive), abnormally shaped/positioned ears, microtia, abnormal middle ear
Cardiopulmonary	Congenital heart disease, patent ductus arteriosus, ventricular septal defect
Renal	Ectopic, horseshoe, hypoplastic, or absent kidney, hydronephrosis, hydroureter
Genital	• Males: Micropenis, undescended or absent testes • Females: Hypogenitalia, bicornate uterus, small ovaries

Endocrine	Short stature, growth hormone (GH) deficiency, hypothyroidism, abnormal glucose/insulin metabolism, dyslipidemia
Gastrointestinal	Atresia (esophagus, duodenum, jejunum, anal), tracheoesophageal fistula, annular pancreas, malrotation
Central nervous system	Small pituitary, absent corpus callosum, neural tube defects, cerebellar hypoplasia

[a]Absence of thumb associated with abnormal or absent radius in Fanconi anemia is different than triphalangeal thumb with normal radius, as seen in Diamond-Blackfan anemia (DBA).

8. **Describe treatment options and their associated risks in Fanconi anemia.**
   The only curative option for hematological complications of FA is HSCT. FA patients have historically had poorer outcomes compared with other aplastic anemia patients because of hypersensitivity to cytotoxic agents used in conditioning regimens (i.e., cyclophosphamide, irradiation). Significantly improved outcomes, however, have been seen with the advent of reduced intensity conditioning regimens, the use of fludarabine, and T-cell depletion of donor grafts. Although best outcomes are still seen in patients transplanted early with HLA-matched sibling donors, patients with HLA-matched unrelated donors can also have excellent outcomes.
   Alternatively, patients have historically been treated with androgen therapy (i.e., oxymetholone) to promote hematopoiesis with response rates over 50%. Unfortunately, patients often become refractory, and androgen use can be complicated by virilization, premature fusion of growth plates, hepatic adenomas, and/or hypertension.

9. **What is the risk of malignancy in Fanconi anemia? How is malignancy risk related to treatment options?**
   Patients with FA are at increased risk for MDS, AML, squamous cell carcinoma (SCC), liver tumors, and brain tumors. The development of MDS or AML is an indication for HSCT; however, these patients have worse outcomes than if undergoing HSCT without preexisting diagnosis of MDS or AML. Unfortunately, HSCT does not decrease the risk of solid tumors in patients with FA, and therefore patients require ongoing surveillance. In addition, the development of post-transplant graft versus host disease (GVHD) further increases the risk of solid tumors and secondary malignancy among FA patients.

10. **What is the diagnostic triad of dyskeratosis congenita? What are other associated clinical features?**
    Dyskeratosis congenita (DKC) has historically been characterized by the mucocutaneous triad of lacy reticular skin pigmentation, nail dystrophy, and oral leukoplakia. Although it is now known that disease manifestations are variable, this triad is reported in approximately 50% of patients and, when present, is highly suggestive of DKC. Other associated clinical features include epiphora (excessive lacrimation), developmental delay, pulmonary disease, periodontal disease, esophageal stricture, premature hair graying or loss, hyperhidrosis, osteoporosis, liver disease, and bone marrow failure.

11. **What is the underlying defect in DKC, and how does it aid in diagnosis?**
    DKC is a disease of defective telomere maintenance resulting in premature telomere shortening, replicative senescence, and premature stem cell exhaustion and tissue failure. Telomere length less than first percentile for age in the majority of lymphocyte subsets as measured by flow cytometry and fluorescence in situ hybridization (FISH) has been found to be both sensitive and specific for diagnosis of DKC in conjunction with clinical sequelae of the disease.

12. **How do complications of DKC affect treatment options?**
    In childhood, the most frequent complication of DKC is bone marrow failure. Later complications include pulmonary and hepatic fibrosis, including cirrhosis. The only curative option for hematologic complications of DKC is HSCT; however, patients are at increased risk of transplant complications because of existing or treatment-related hepatic and pulmonary fibrosis as well as late-onset sinusoidal obstruction syndrome. Reduced intensity preparation regimens have been used with improved survival. Similar to FA, development of graft-versus-host disease (GVHD) also increases malignancy and end-organ complications. Additionally, patients with DKC have been reported to have good response to androgen therapy (i.e., danazol); however, they need close monitoring of liver function because of the risk of hepatotoxicity.

13. **What are the clinical and lab features characteristic of Diamond-Blackfan anemia?**
    DBA is a pure red cell aplasia that commonly presents before 12 months of age with severe macrocytic anemia with reticulocytopenia, normal platelet and leukocyte counts, and congenital anomalies (~50% of patients). The characteristic feature of DBA is erythroid hypoplasia in the bone marrow. In addition, patients may present with elevated fetal hemoglobin, erythropoietin, and erythrocyte adenosine deaminase activity (eADA). Absence of these lab findings does not preclude a DBA diagnosis because recent red blood cell transfusions may alter results.

14. **What inherited bone marrow failure syndromes are associated with exocrine pancreatic insufficiency?**
    Schwachman-Diamond syndrome (SDS) and Pearson syndrome are two inherited bone marrow failure syndromes associated with exocrine pancreatic insufficiency. SDS typically presents in early infancy with

malabsorption because of exocrine pancreatic dysfunction with neutropenia noted later. It may progress to aplastic anemia in approximately 20% of patients. Unlike SDS, Pearson syndrome is associated with mitochondrial DNA abnormalities and sideroblastic anemia as well as exocrine pancreatic dysfunction.

15. **What are the long-term malignancy risks associated with inherited bone marrow failure syndromes?**
Inherited bone marrow failure syndromes (IBMFS) are often linked to increased risk of MDS and AML. In particular, patients with FA, SDS, and DKC have significantly higher risk of MDS and/or AML transformation by 30 years of age. Patients with DBA are also at increased risk compared with the general population; however, there is less pediatric risk relative to other IBMFS, with many patients surviving to over 40 years of age without developing MDS and/or AML. Rather, DBA has been associated with a higher risk of early-onset gastrointestinal cancers, primarily of the colon. Also previously noted, patients with both DKC and FA are at increased risk of solid tumors, particularly SCCs.

BIBLIOGRAPHY

1. Auerbach AD. Fanconi anemia and its diagnosis. *Mutat Res.* 2009;668(1-2):4–10.
2. Brodsky RA. Paroxysmal nocturnal hemoglobinuria. *Blood.* 2014;124(18):2804–2811.
3. Brodsky RA. Eculizumab: another breakthrough. *Blood.* 2017;129(8):922–923.
4. Da Costa L, et al. Diamond-Blackfan anemia, ribosome and erythropoiesis. *Transfus Clin Biol.* 2010;17(3):112–119.
5. Ebens CL, MacMillan ML, Wagner JE. Hematopoietic cell transplantation in Fanconi anemia: current evidence, challenges and recommendations. *Expert Rev Hematol.* 2017;10(1):81–97.
6. Farruggia P, Di Marco F, Dufour C. Pearson syndrome. *Expert Rev Hematol.* 2018;11(3):239–246.
7. Fernandez Garcia MS, Teruya-Feldstein J. The diagnosis and treatment of dyskeratosis congenita: a review. *J Blood Med.* 2014;5:157–167.
8. Gadhiya K, Budh DP. Diamond Blackfan anemia. In *StatPearls.* Treasure Island (FL), 2020.
9. Khincha PP, Savage SA. Neonatal manifestations of inherited bone marrow failure syndromes. *Semin Fetal Neonatal Med.* 2016;21(1):57–65.
10. Nelson AS, Myers KC. Diagnosis, Treatment, and molecular pathology of Shwachman-Diamond syndrome. *Hematol Oncol Clin North Am.* 2018;32(4):687–700.
11. Shimamura A, Alter BP. Pathophysiology and management of inherited bone marrow failure syndromes. *Blood Rev.* 2010;24(3):101–122.
12. Townsley DM, Scheinberg P, Winkler T, et al. Eltrombopag added to standard immunosuppression for aplastic anemia. *N Engl J Med.* 2017;376(16):1540–1550.
13. Young NS. Aplastic anemia. *N Engl J Med.* 2018;379:1643–1656.

CHAPTER 10

HEMATOLOGICAL MANIFESTATIONS OF SYSTEMIC DISEASE

Angela Ricci, MD and Cindy Neunert, MD

1. **Describe the systemic diseases that have hematological manifestations.**

   Almost all systemic conditions can result in some degree of derangement of the hematological system. Conditions associated with inflammation can cause increase in platelets, which are an acute phase reactant, as well as anemia, typically because of impaired iron metabolism. Other disruptions in nutrients critical to hematologic system can also cause derangements. In other cases, particular organ dysfunction, such as liver and kidney disease, can disrupt production and regulation of blood cells and factors. Lastly, some conditions can result in impairment of blood cell function. For these reasons, hematological manifestations of disease can be seen with cardiac, pulmonary endocrine, gastrointestinal, rheumatological, metabolic, nervous system, renal, and liver conditions.

2. **What hematological disorders are seen in cardiac disease?**
   - Polycythemia is a well-known consequence of cyanotic heart disease as a compensatory mechanism to increase oxygen-carrying capacity.
   - Coagulation abnormalities appear to be associated with the degree of polycythemia. The exact cause is not clear; however, it has been postulated that the tissue hypoxia that results from the hyperviscosity may cause a consumptive process.
   - Thrombocytopenia is also related to cyanotic heart disease. The degree of thrombocytopenia correlates with the severity of the polycythemia and with ongoing hypoxia. Platelet production in the bone marrow has been demonstrated to be normal; however, platelet survival is diminished. These patients may additionally have platelet aggregation defects.
   - Individuals who have prosthetic heart valves generally have some hemolysis of red blood cells (RBCs) because of direct mechanical injury. The degree of hemolysis may or may not be severe enough to cause anemia.

3. **Discuss the hematological disorders seen in renal disease.**
   - Renal disease is most commonly associated with anemia. This anemia is classified as normocytic, normochromic anemia. The anemia is caused by a deficiency of erythropoietin, which is primarily produced in the kidney. RBC survival also may be decreased because of uremia when renal disease is severe.
   - Uremia also has an effect on the clotting factor levels, specifically factors V, VII, IX, and X. In addition, patients with renal protein losses may be prothrombotic because of losses of protein C and S.
   - Platelet survival and platelet function also may be diminished in renal disease.
   - Patients on dialysis often become deficient in folic acid and can have transient sequestration of granulocytes, resulting in granulocytopenia.
   - In terms of management, patients demonstrating anemia should be on erythropoietin replacement, plus daily folate and iron supplementation.

4. **What hematological disorders are seen in liver disease?**
   - Liver disease has most commonly been associated with coagulation abnormalities. The liver is involved in the synthesis of many of the clotting factors; therefore when there is liver dysfunction, factor levels are diminished. The vitamin K–dependent factors are the factors that are most affected: factors II, VII, IX, and X. Factor VII is the most severely and acutely affected factor because its synthesis takes place almost entirely in the liver and it has a very short-half life. Factor VIII is generally unaffected in liver disease or is elevated because it is produced by the endothelium and is an acute phase reactant. For these reasons, the prothrombin time (PT) may be prolonged before the activated partial prothrombin time (PTT) in patients with early liver disease. When the liver damage is caused by obstruction, fibrinogen may be elevated, as may factors XI and XII and antithrombin III. Additionally, proteins C and S are also low in patients with liver disease. Therefore patients with liver disease have a "balanced" coagulopathy that is prone to both bleeding and clotting.
   - Anemia associated with liver disease is multifactorial. It is typically macrocytic, which is because of folate deficiency. There is also decreased RBC survival, which is probably because of dysfunction of the antioxidant system. Patients who develop portal hypertension may develop hypersplenism and subsequent splenic sequestration. Additionally, patients may have varices, which are prone to bleeding, leading to the development of iron-deficiency anemia.
   - If patients are folate deficient or iron deficient, they should be on daily supplementation. Vitamin K supplementation may help transiently correct the coagulation defects.

5. **What pulmonary diseases are associated with abnormal hematological findings?**
   - Hypoxia leads to polycythemia and, in severe instances, thrombocytopenia.
   - Pulmonary hemosiderosis is a condition that results in recurrent hemorrhage into the lungs and should be considered in any individual with iron-deficiency anemia of unclear etiology that has a history of pulmonary infections, which could be misdiagnosed hemorrhages. This condition may be secondary to collagen vascular disease, glomerulonephritis, or systemic lupus erythematosus (SLE), or it may be idiopathic.

6. **How are endocrine disorders associated with hematological abnormalities?**
   - Hyperthyroidism causes increased RBC mass and therefore a macrocytic anemia. Although it affects some of the metabolic functions of the RBC, this does not adversely affect the cell's life span. Occasionally associated neutropenia and thrombocytopenia are present.
   - Hypothyroidism, on the other hand, can cause a normocytic normochromic anemia. Some patients with hypothyroidism also have low levels of factors VIII, VII, IX, and XI and diminished platelet function.
   - Anemia is also associated with both hypopituitarism and adrenal insufficiency. The latter is probably because of an overall reduction in basal metabolism.

7. **What hematological abnormalities are associated with diabetes mellitus?**
   - The most common finding is the hemoglobin (Hb) A_{1c}, which is a glycohemoglobin (fusion between Hb and an aldehyde or a ketone). It is also present in the normal population but markedly increased in people with diabetes and is an important marker of diabetic control.
   - Diabetic control is also important for RBC survival. Acidosis also increases oxygen delivery and 2,3-diphos-phoglycerate levels. Frequently, anemia of chronic disease occurs.
   - The function of the neutrophils is usually impaired.
   - Patients with diabetes also have increased risk of thrombosis. This is multifactorial in origin. There is increased platelet aggregation, increased factor VIII, XI, XII and decreased angiotensin III and fibrinolysis. The increased risk of thrombosis is also well described in infants of diabetic mothers.

8. **What is anemia of chronic disease?**
   This form of anemia is common in any condition, acute or chronic, that results in inflammation and is also known as anemia of inflammation. The primary cause is disruption in iron metabolism caused by inflammation. With inflammation, there is an increase in a peptide called hepcidin. Hepcidin regulates iron metabolism controlling movement of iron from iron absorbing intestinal cells to the macrophages and hepatocytes by binding to and blocking the ferroportin receptor. Additionally, inflammation can lead to decrease RBC production and increased turnover depending on the underlying etiology.

9. **Describe the laboratory findings typical of the anemia of chronic disease.**
   The anemia is usually normochromic and normocytic; it is occasionally hypochromic and microcytic, in which case the differential diagnosis with iron-deficiency anemia can be difficult. Plasma iron, total iron binding capacity, and transferrin saturation are usually diminished, whereas the ferritin can be normal or increased. This is the main difference compared with iron deficiency, which will have low ferritin.

10. **What other hematological findings are seen in rheumatological conditions?**
    - Iron-deficiency anemia is frequently seen in rheumatological conditions because of decreased iron absorption and microscopic gastrointestinal bleeding secondary to nonsteroidal anti-inflammatory drug intake. In an uncontrolled disease state, patients may have anemia of chronic disease and elevated factor VIII levels as an acute-phase reactant.
    - Autoimmune hemolytic anemia can be seen in SLE.
    - Aplastic anemia has been associated with scleroderma.
    - Leukocytosis or leukopenia can be present as a result of inflammation, immune destruction, or bone marrow depression.
    - Thrombocytopenia is common, usually because of autoimmune destruction. Nevertheless, because platelets are an acute-phase reactant, there can also be thrombocytosis in the setting of inflammation.
    - Patients with SLE can present with prolonged PTT because of the presence of a lupus anticoagulant, which is discussed further in the thrombosis chapter.

11. **What are the hematological manifestations of common infections?**
    - Infections in children cause abnormalities in all of the three cell lines, sometimes as a complication of infectious process, other times as the necessary response of the immune system to infectious pathogen.
    - RBCs: There may be anemia of inflammation, as previously described. Hemolytic anemia may also be seen in the setting of certain infections. The degree of hemolysis is dependent on the pathogen and the severity of the infection. Severe hemolytic anemia is seen in bacterial sepsis (especially from *Clostridium, Pneumococcus, Meningococcus,* and *Hemophilus*). Mild anemia because of suppression is more commonly seen in viral infections. Parvovirus infection is a very well-known cause of anemia, mostly from bone marrow suppression. This is especially true in patients with congenital hemolytic anemia (including sickle cell, thalassemia, G6PD deficiency), in whom it can cause aplastic crises.

- White blood cells: Leukocytosis and neutrophilia is a "healthy" response to infections, particularly bacterial infections. Usually the degree of neutrophilia, as well as the degree of bandemia, correlates with the severity of the infections. Neutropenia in the setting of a bacterial infection is an ominous sign, often indicating overwhelming sepsis or inability to mount an adequate response, as in newborns or preemies. Lymphocytosis is common in viral infections, particularly infectious mononucleosis and pertussis. Eosinophilia is frequent in parasitic infections.
- Platelets: Both thrombocytopenia and thrombocytosis are common findings during infections because they are an acute-phase reactant. It usually resolves once the infection is under control, but it may take a few weeks. One should always check a coagulation profile in the setting of a severe infectious process, particularly when thrombocytopenia is present because of the possibility of associated disseminated intravascular coagulation (DIC).

12. **When is treatment indicated for patients with hematological manifestations of infection warranted?**

In general, the most effective treatment of the hematological abnormalities associated with any condition is the treatment of the condition itself. Transfusion of packed RBCs is indicated only when the child is symptomatic from the anemia. Iron may be provided orally if the patient has associated iron deficiency or parentally if the patient has an underlying condition that affects absorption. Platelet transfusion is indicated when the degree of thrombocytopenia represents a significant risk of hemorrhage based on additional comorbidities or if the patient has bleeding symptoms. Secondary thrombocytosis is not associated with increased thrombotic risk; therefore it does not require any intervention. The same is true for secondary elevation of factor VIII in the absence of a thrombosis. Treatment for DIC is indicated only in the presence of bleeding or when the laboratory parameters are significantly abnormal in coexistence of other risk factors for bleeding. The treatment is supportive and requires replacement of platelets, fresh frozen plasma, and cryoprecipitate.

BIBLIOGRAPHY

1. Abshire TC. The anemia of inflammation: a common cause of childhood anemia. *Pediatr Clin North Am.* 1996;43:623–637.
2. Lanzkowsky P. *Manual of Pediatric Hematology and Oncology.* 2nd ed. Churchill Livingstone, 1995:104–111.
3. Nathan DG, Orkin SH. *Nathan and Oski's Hematology of Infancy and Childhood.* Vol. 1. 5th ed. W. B. Saunders Company, 1998:544–664.

II

ONCOLOGY

CHAPTER 11

EPIDEMIOLOGY

Michael Weiner, MD

1. **Internationally there are approximately 300,000 cases of child and adolescent cancer diagnosed annually. What variables exist in childhood cancer incidence and outcome when comparing high-income countries with low-income countries?**

   The difference in high-income versus low-income countries resides in the inability of so-called "third-world countries" to make a proper, timely diagnosis; obstacles also exist in accessing care, abandonment of treatment, lack of supportive care, and death from toxicity. These factors contribute to higher rates of relapse and mortality. The overall cure rate of childhood cancer in high-income countries approaches 80%, but in low- and middle-income countries, only about 20% of children and adolescents are cured.

   Additionally, there are differences in risk among different ethnic or racial population subgroups. Burkitt lymphoma, a type of non-Hodgkin lymphoma, affects 6 to 7 children per 100,000 in parts of sub-Saharan Africa, where it is associated with a history of infection by both Epstein-Barr virus (EBV) and malaria, whereas in industrialized countries, Burkitt lymphoma is not associated with these infectious conditions.

2. **Describe the variables that distinguish cancer in children and adolescents from cancers recognized in adults.**

   Many studies have sought to identify the causes of childhood cancer, but unlike cancer in adults, the vast majority of childhood cancers do not have a known cause. In children, approximately 5% to 10% have an identified familial or genetic etiology and less than 5% to 10% have known environmental exposures or exogenous factors. Nevertheless, it has been established that lifestyle-related factors such as poor nutrition, alcoholism, high fat diets, tobacco use, lack of physical activity, and environmental exposure to radon, ultraviolet light, asbestos, benzene, and radioactive material predispose adults to cancer. In general, childhood cancers cannot be prevented or screened and are assumed to involve multiple risk factors and variables.

   Approximately 90% of adult cancers are carcinomas derived from ectodermal epithelial tissue of the prostate, breast, lung, colorectum, uterus, and ovaries. In contradistinction, childhood malignancies are of mesenchymal origin, bone marrow, lymph glands, bone, and muscle and are almost exclusively leukemias, lymphomas, sarcomas, and cancers of the central nervous system (CNS). National Cancer Institute (NCI) SEER (Surveillance, Epidemiology, and End Results) data indicate the incidence of cancer from birth through 14 years of age is 14 cases per 100,000 per year. For patients between 15 and 19 years, the incidence approaches 20 cases per 100,000 per year. Thus there are approximately 15,000 to 16,000 new cases of cancer per year diagnosed in children and teenagers. In the United States, there are between 1.7 to 1.8 million cases of adult cancer diagnosed each year; thus, for every case of childhood cancer, there are approximately 110 to 115 cases diagnosed in adults.

   Child and adolescent cancer remains the leading cause of disease-related mortality in the United States with between 2500 to 3000 deaths per year.

3. **What are the genetic and congenital disorders that predispose patients to developing pediatric malignancies?**

   Historically approximately 15% of the cases of childhood cancer have been associated with a genetic and/or congenital condition. Genetic disorders that have gene alterations that disrupt normal mechanisms of genomic repair, such as xeroderma pigmentosa, Bloom syndrome, and ataxia telangiectasia, are associated with skin cancer, leukemia, and lymphoma, respectively. Beckwith-Wiedemann syndrome, multiple endocrine neoplasia, and neurofibromatosis are congenital conditions with dysfunctional cellular growth and proliferation and are associated with Wilms tumor, hepatic tumors, adrenal cancers, and CNS tumors, respectively.

   Recently, the Precision in Pediatric Sequencing (PIPseq) program at Columbia University Irving Medical Center has found using whole-exome and RNA sequencing of malignant tissue that approximately 90% of more than 550 cases of pediatric cancer have evidence of sequence variants, mutations, fusion transcripts, and/or copy number variation. It is thought that there are sequencing identified genes of diagnostic or prognostic significance in 45% of cases and identified genes associated with drug resistance in 5% of patients. The determination of whether these genetic alterations represent driver mutations of malignancy remains to be determined.

4. **How is epidemiological data collected? What are the contemporary public health surveillance processes followed by population scientists and investigators?**

   Public health surveillance involves the collection, analysis, and interpretation of health data to prevent and treat disease. In the United States, cancer statistics are compiled by the NCI's Surveillance, Epidemiology and End Results (SEER) program (http://www.seer.cancer.gov); in addition, all states have cancer registries and report data to the North American Association for Central Cancer Registries that is supported by the Centers for Disease Control and Prevention. More recently, the Children's Oncology Group (COG) initiated a volunteer Childhood Cancer Research Network (CCRN) and Project Every Child, which not only collects data but also extends the efforts of CCRN to allow specimen collection. Collectively, because 90% of children in the United States are treated on COG protocols, the CCRN and Project Every Child make it feasible to perform population-based research on the etiology of cancer in children and adolescents.

5. **According to statistics from the SEER database, what is the age distribution by percentages for child and adolescent cancers?**

Percentage Distribution of Specific Cancer Diagnoses by Age

Diagnosis	Age 0–14 years	Age 15–19 years
Acute lymphoblastic leukemia	25	8
Acute myelogenous leukemia	5	4
Central nervous system	21	10
Neuroblastoma	7	1
Wilms tumor	5	1
Non-Hodgkin lymphoma	6	8
Hodgkin disease	4	16
Rhabdomyosarcoma	3	2
Soft tissue sarcoma	7	6
Osteosarcoma	3	4
Ewing sarcoma	2	2
Germ cell tumors	4	14
Retinoblastoma	3	
Hepatocellular	1	
Melanoma		7
Thyroid carcinoma		9

Incidence data from Surveillance, Epidemiology, and End Results (SEER) and percent distribution based on the International Classification of Childhood, which reflects the most prevalent tumor types.

6. **Delineate the incidence disparities of child and adolescent cancer by sex and race.**
For patients younger than 15 years of age, there exists a male predominance for acute lymphoblastic leukemia (ALL), Hodgkin disease, non-Hodgkin lymphoma (NHL), Ewing sarcoma, and rhabdomyosarcoma. In adolescents, osteosarcoma, Ewing sarcoma, and germ cell tumors are more prevalent in males, whereas Hodgkin disease and germ cell tumors were distributed equally. In the 15- to 19-year-old age group, the risk of thyroid cancer, melanoma, and Wilms tumor is greater.

Adult Black Americans have a higher risk of cancer than adult White Americans; however, White children have a 50% increased incidence compared with children of color. The higher rate in White children may be attributable to increased rates in ALL (34 per million White children versus 17 per million Black children). The rates for acute myelogenous leukemia (AML) are identical. The incidence of Ewing sarcoma, however, is six times greater and of melanoma is 22 times greater in White children than Black children. Interestingly, and worth noting, the incidence of ALL in Hispanic children is greater than White children (45 per million vs. 34 per million, respectively).

7. **Describe the historical origins of cancer.**
The earliest description of cancer, although the word was not used, is found in fossilized bones suggestive of osteosarcoma by the Egyptians in 3000 BC. Also, in a textbook on surgery referred to as the Edwin Smith Papyrus, several cases of breast tumors are described.

Hippocrates (460–370 BC), first used the words "cancinos" and "carcinoma" to designate ulcer-forming tumors. These words in Greeks refer to a crab secondary to finger-like projections from a cancer. Galen (130–200 AD) coined the term "oncos," which is Greek for swelling. This term is now used to define cancer specialists as oncologists.

Galileo and Newton, Renaissance scientists in the 15th century, developed the scientific method to study the human body. In 1628, autopsies performed by Harvey, although not focused on cancer, enhanced understanding of the heart and circulatory system.

The field of cancer epidemiology began during the 18th century when Bernardino Ramazzini in 1713 observed the high incidence of breast cancer and the virtual absence of cervical cancer in nuns secondary to sexual abstinence. In 1761, John Hill wrote a treatise that described the association of tobacco in snuff and cancer and Percival Pott in London described the association of scrotal cancer in chimney sweeps in 1775; these observations led to the observation of occupational carcinogenic exposures.

In 1761, Giovanni Morgagni of Padua laid the foundation for scientific oncology by performing autopsies to relate the patient's illness to pathologic findings after death. John Hunter, a Scottish surgeon in the mid 18th century, introduced surgical extirpation as treatment for cancerous tumors.

In the 19th century, Rudolf Virchow introduced the field of cellular pathology and correlated microscopic pathology to disease. These methods permitted an understanding of cancer and the ability to make accurate diagnoses.

8. **Briefly define survival rates for children and adolescents with cancer.**
Survival rates for children and adolescents have improved dramatically in the last half century. In the 1960s, the overall survival rate for all diagnoses was less than 30%; in the 21st century, 3- and 5-year survival outcome exceeds 80%. Survival data is comparable for children 0 to 14 years, as well as for teenagers (15 to 19 years of age). The best outcomes are realized for Hodgkin disease, thyroid cancer, germ cell tumors, and ALL, whereas for rhabdomyosarcoma, osteosarcoma, Ewing sarcoma, and brain tumors, the outcome appears to have plateaued and has not improved appreciatively.

With respect to cancer deaths, one-third are attributable to ALL, one-third to CNS tumors, and one-third is secondary to neuroblastoma and sarcomas of bone and soft tissues.

9. **Briefly describe the history of the child and adolescent cooperative groups.**
The history of the cooperative group dates back to 1948 with two seminal, historic findings; first, Dr. Sidney Farber at the Boston Children's Hospital reported temporary remissions in children with leukemia with folic acid antagonists. Second, Dr. Joseph Burchenal reported the effect of nitrogen mustard compounds on mouse leukemia. Subsequently, investigators identified beneficial effects of antipurine analogs and hormonal agents, including adrenocorticotropic hormone (ACTH; cortisone) to induce temporary remissions in children with acute lymphocytic leukemia. By the mid-1950s, the median survival improved from 8 moths to 22 months.

In 1955 the Cancer Chemotherapy National Service Center of the National Institute of Health sponsored programs to organize institutions to cooperate in evaluating new potential antileukemic agents for children. This initiative led to the founding of the Acute Leukemia Chemotherapy Cooperative Study Group A (ALCCSGA). The original members included Dr. Frank Bethell of the University of Michigan; Dr. Joseph H. Burchenal of Memorial Hospital Sloan Kettering and Cornell University Medical College; Dr. Byron Hall of Stanford University Medical School; Dr. Charles D. May of State University of Iowa; Dr. E. Clarence Rice of the Children's Hospital of the District of Columbia; Dr. Carl Smith of The New York Hospital; Dr. Phillip Sturgeon of the Children's Hospital Society of Los Angeles; and Dr. James Wolff of Babies Hospital in New York.

The ALCCSGA evolved to become the Children's Cancer Group (CCG) and in 1998 merged with the other legacy groups the Pediatric Oncology Group, National Wilm's Tumor Group, and the Intergroup Rhabdomyosarcoma to create a single cooperative group called the Children's Oncology Group (COG). The spirit of collaboration signified by this event remains visible through the continued involvement of clinical investigators, laboratory scientists, patients, parents, and other advocates. The COG has treated more children with cancer than any other organization in history and has been responsible for many advances during the past 50 years.

The COG has had numerous accomplishments. First, there is the prognostic significance of minimal residual disease (MRD) in ALL and its relationship to other prognostic variables such as cytogenetics and molecular diagnostics to more accurately define risk group assignment. Second, the COG established the use of computed tomography (CT) and positron emission tomography (PET) scan response to determine the duration and aggressiveness of subsequent therapy for patients with Hodgkin disease. Third, the COG has fostered enhanced collaboration with European cancer cooperative groups and the launch of an international protocol for the treatment of osteosarcoma.

10. **Briefly describe the future direction of the pediatric and adolescent oncology community of investigators and scientists.**
The last 50 years have witnessed scientific discoveries and accomplishments in the treatment of childhood cancer. The emphasis for the next half century will be on incorporating the many discoveries in translational research, developing a pediatric cancer registry and a long-term survivor registry, and improving the quality of life for survivors of childhood cancer.

The 21st century will usher in a new era, an era that will focus on reducing therapy to lessen long-term effects in diseases with high cure rates such as ALL, Hodgkin disease, Wilms tumor, and some types of non-Hodgkin lymphoma. Newly designed clinical trials will attempt to improve outcomes for patients with high-risk diseases such as neuroblastoma, CNS tumors, relapsed acute lymphocytic leukemia, infant leukemia, and AML in those lacking stem cell donors.

COG investigators are committed to looking at the biologic parameters of the cancers and evaluating gene expression signatures in leukemia and solid tumors. Recent evidence exists to demonstrate that gene expression patterns can refine diagnosis and predict outcome. Another area of interest is pharmacogenomic investigations to predict toxicities, which may lead to individualized therapy models. The COG participates in the NCI collaboration with the Cancer Genome Atlas and Cancer Genome Anatomy Project through the TARGET (Therapeutically Applicable Research to Generate Effective Treatments) initiative. Ultimately, this endeavor should identify sequenced genes that may direct potential novel therapeutic targets.

11. **Describe the meaning of the evolving field of molecular epidemiology.**
Molecular epidemiology refers to the interrelationship between epidemiology and molecular biology. The technology incorporates molecular and biologic markers into studies to identify, validate, and incorporate endogenous and

exogenous factors into a comprehensive approach to characterize cancer risk, etiology, and potential strategies for prevention.

12. **Describe the factors that contribute to risk of child and adolescent cancer.**
The carcinogenic processes that contribute to cancer in adults and children are different. In the former, environmental exposures have long latency periods. For example, cigarette smoking begins in the second or third decade of life, and the associated malignancy is not apparent for decades after the initiation of smoking. In childhood cancers, the relevant environmental exposure history of the mother of the patient and the maternal genotype are often of greater influence and importance. Data exist that maternal and paternal smoking increase the risk of cancer in their offspring. In addition, increasing maternal age has been associated with an increased risk of childhood leukemia, lymphoma, neuroblastoma, Wilms tumors, and bone cancers. Paternal occupational exposures to paint, solvents, and benzene increases risk in their children. Interestingly, the notion that exposure to magnetic fields and high power electrical lines can cause cancer has been debunked and not established.

In addition, the carcinogenic process in children is significantly shorter in time; embryonal neoplasms predominate in early childhood, and one may surmise that pediatric cancers result from abnormalities in early development.

State and national childhood cancer registries have identified birth defects and congenital malformations as a strong risk factor for malignancy. Reports in the literature indicate that the risk of developing cancer in the first years of life is sixfold greater in children with major and minor congenital malformations than in age-matched controlled contemporaries (Table 11.1).

Table 11.1 Known Risk Factors Associated With Childhood Cancer

DISEASE	RISK FACTOR
Acute lymphoblastic leukemia	Ionizing radiation White children: Twofold greater risk Down syndrome: 20-fold greater risk Neurofibromatosis type 1 Bloom syndrome Ataxia telangiectasia Langerhans cell histiocytosis
Acute myelogenous leukemia	Chemotherapy exposure: alkylating agents, epipodophyllotoxins Down syndrome Neurofibromatosis type 1 Familial monosomy 7
Brain tumors	Ionizing radiation Neurofibromatosis type 1: optic glioma Tuberous sclerosis
Hodgkin disease	Epstein-Barr virus exposure/infection Monozygotic twins
Non-Hodgkin lymphoma	Immunodeficiency: congenital and acquired Immunosuppressive therapy
Osteosarcoma	Ionizing radiation Chemotherapy exposure: alkylating agents Li-Fraumeni syndrome Hereditary retinoblastoma
Ewing sarcoma	White children: ninefold greater risk
Retinoblastoma	Hereditary: bilateral disease
Wilms tumor	Aniridia Beckwith-Wiedemann syndrome
Rhabdomyosarcoma	Congenital anomalies Li-Fraumeni syndrome Neurofibromatosis type 1
Hepatoblastoma	Beckwith-Wiedemann syndrome Hemihypertrophy Gardner syndrome Familial adenomatous polyposis
Germ cell tumor	Cryptorchidism

13. **How has study of the human genome contributed to our understanding of childhood cancer susceptibility?**

Genome-wide studies and the expanding field of molecular epidemiology are increasingly used to investigate rare and common childhood cancers, particularly in the setting of relapse or recurrence in the latter. A number of genes have been identified and have been found to be associated with an increased risk of childhood cancer. The potential use of genome-wide sequencing is being incorporated into population-based studies and is beginning to allow insights into tumor biology and the initiation of therapeutic and preventive measures.

In general, childhood cancers exhibit a lower overall mutational burden than adult cancers, and recent sequencing studies have revealed that the genomic events central to childhood oncogenesis include mutations resulting in broad epigenetic changes or translocations that result in fusion oncoproteins. Similarly, fusion genes are also more common than in adult cancers, and the specific mutations found in pediatric cancers are rare in adult malignancies. Rather than the numerous mutational "hits" frequently observed in adult cancers, the emerging theme is that epigenetic dysregulation is central to many forms of childhood cancer.

In a report by Grobner et al. in *Nature,* commonalities and differences in 961 childhood children, adolescents, and young adults, involving 24 distinct molecular types of cancer, were examined. They concluded that commonalities and differences among various cancer types have emerged as a powerful way to obtain novel insights into cancer biology. Genetic alterations in 149 putative cancer driver genes were of two classes: small mutation and structural/copy-number variant. The latter were strongly linked to *TP53* mutation. The authors conclude that 7% to 8% have an unambiguous predisposing germline variant and that nearly 50% of childhood neoplasms possess a potentially druggable event, which is highly relevant for the design of future clinical trials.

Studies of children with B-ALL have provided the first evidence that the initial genetic event is of fetal origin. At the time of the leukemia diagnosis, clonal fusion genes corresponded to gene sequence findings identified on archived newborn fetal blood spots collected on Guthrie cards used to screen for metabolic disease years before the malignancy occurred. Recently in a review of cord blood samples from healthy children, the incidence of the *ETV6-RUNX1* fusion was about 100-fold higher than the incidence of *ETV6-RUNX1* fusion-positive B-ALL in children, suggesting that additional genetic events or a specific microenvironmental context are necessary to turn preleukemic cells into overt leukemia. This phenomenon (the presence of gene fusions like *ETV6-RUNX1*) is consistent with the Knudson two-hit hypothesis on the origin of childhood ALL, indicating that a preleukemia pool is present in hematopoietic stem cells, but a second event is required for the development of overt leukemia.

14. **What are the challenges faced by childhood cooperative groups in the design of clinical trials?**

The major challenge is the number of cases diagnosed each year. Child and adolescent cancer is a relatively unusual disease, with approximately 15,000 patients annually. This necessitates cooperative group collaboration because single institutions infrequently have sufficient numbers of subjects to run independent trials. Small numbers also influence negatively the ability to conduct randomized trials to identify small but significant incremental improvement. The increasing use of molecular diagnostics has demonstrated the heterogeneity of childhood cancer that mitigates against precise classification and risk-group assignment. Another important issue is that pharmacokinetic tolerability, drug metabolism, immune system variability, and the microenvironment can differ dramatically from infants to children to adolescents to young adults.

Most clinical trials, new agents, and novel therapeutics are developed for adults and repurposed for children. Therapeutics developed for the often-unique pathophysiology of childhood cancers are needed.

Monitoring long-term sequelae of childhood cancer therapies such as development, cognitive issues, organ dysfunction, and second malignant neoplasms are extremely important and require ongoing and decades-long observation.

BIBLIOGRAPHY

1. Brookmeyer R, Stroup DF. *Monitoring the Health of Populations: Statistical Principles and Methods for Public Health Surveillance.* Oxford University Press, 2004.
2. Filbin M, Monje M. Developmental origins and emerging therapeutic opportunities for childhood cancer. *Nat Med.* 2019;25(3):367–376.
3. Grobner SN, Worst BC, Pfister SM. Landscape of genomic alterations across childhood cancers. *Nature.* 2018;555:321–327.
4. Hammond GD, Nixon DW, Nachman JB, et al. American Cancer Society Workshop on Adolescents and Young Adults with Cancer. Workgroup #4: clinical research implications. *Cancer.* 1993;71:2423.
5. Koepsell TD, Weiss NS. *Epidemiologic Methods: Studying the Occurrence of Illness.* Oxford University Press, 2003.
6. O'Leary Krallo, M, Anderson, JR, Reaman, GH. Progress in childhood cancer: 50 years of research collaboration, a report from the Children's Oncology Group. *Semin Oncol.* 2008;35:484–493.
7. Reaman GH, Haase GM. Quality of life research in childhood cancer. The time is now. *Cancer.* 1996;78:1330–1332.
8. Rothman K, Greenland S, Lash T, eds. *Modern epidemiology.* 3rd ed. Lippincott Williams & Wilkins, 2008.

CHAPTER 12

PRINCIPLES OF CHEMOTHERAPY

Julia Glade Bender, MD

1. **What is the single most important determinant when choosing a treatment using anticancer drugs (chemotherapy) and what is the concept of "risk stratification"?**
   Before embarking on a treatment plan that involves the use of anticancer drugs, every effort should be made to ascertain an accurate histologic and molecular diagnosis. This involves pathologic examination and molecular testing of tumor tissue after surgical excision or a well-planned biopsy. Empiric therapy, before pathologic diagnosis, is permissible only in the rare setting of a true oncologic emergency (see Chapter 17). Because chemotherapy is highly toxic, with both acute and long-term side effects, it is imperative that the choice of treatment be correct for the diagnosis and that the intensity and risk of the regimen be well-aligned with the prognosis of the disease. Most pediatric cancers can be divided into standard, intermediate, and high-risk categories, where the goals are to minimize risk and maintain excellent outcomes for lower risk patients and to augment therapy and improve survival for higher risk patients. Critical factors beyond pathologic diagnosis determining the appropriate risk stratification include:
   - Patient age
   - Disease stage: extent of disease
   - Histologic subtype (e.g., favorable or unfavorable in Wilms tumor, T or B cell leukemia/lymphoma)
   - Biological and molecular features (e.g., *MYC-N* amplification in neuroblastoma, *BCR-ABL1* fusion, *KMT2A* rearrangement or additional adverse cytogenetics in acute lymphocytic leukemia [ALL], and molecular subtype in medulloblastoma)

2. **What is meant by *adjuvant* and *neoadjuvant chemotherapy*, and what is the rationale behind them?**
   Adjuvant chemotherapy is given to patients without evidence of residual disease after local control of a malignant tumor has been achieved with surgery and/or radiation. Historically, patients treated with local measures alone had a high risk (60%–95%) for tumor recurrence with distant metastases. The goal of adjuvant chemotherapy is to eliminate microscopic spread of the tumor or micrometastasis, which is assumed to have already occurred by the time of diagnosis. This strategy has been successful in the treatment of most pediatric solid tumors including Wilms tumor, Ewing sarcoma, osteosarcoma, rhabdomyosarcoma, medulloblastoma, and anaplastic astrocytoma.

   Neoadjuvant chemotherapy, or primary chemotherapy, is given to patients before surgical resection or radiation to the primary site. Neoadjuvant chemotherapy has been used to decrease tumor bulk, thereby making the primary more amenable to surgery. Other rationales include the early eradication of micrometastasis, preempting costly delays in systemic therapy from surgical or radiation-related morbidity, and the ability to assess tumor responsiveness to initial therapy, both clinically and histologically. The neoadjuvant strategy has been particularly important in the treatment of bone tumors. Orthopedic surgeons can offer a larger number of limb-sparing procedures, in part because of tumor shrinkage and the extra time available to plan and obtain individualized prosthetic devices. Additionally, the histologic tumor response to initial therapy (extent of necrosis) has proven to be a potent prognostic factor of relapse-free survival in osteosarcoma and is being studied in other diseases.

3. **What does history tell us about the overall efficacy of single-drug regimens?**
   In the late 1940s and early 1950s, ALL was universally and rapidly fatal. The first single-agent trials were able to induce remarkable results with impressive complete remission rates of up to 60%. Nevertheless, remissions were short lived, lasting only 6 to 9 months, despite continued therapy with the agent. Today, outside of a few molecularly targeted agents like the ABL1 tyrosine kinase inhibitors (TKIs) in chronic myeloid leukemia (CML) or a TRK/ROS/ALK or RET inhibitor before surgery in a few low-grade malignancies like infantile fibrosarcoma, it is understood that curative therapy requires combination chemotherapy. In patients with refractory disease and no curative options, single agent trials are still used in early drug development to determine the safety profile, dose, and single agent anticancer activity across tumor types.

4. **What is the rationale behind the use of combination chemotherapy?**
   The rationale behind combination chemotherapy is twofold.

   First, combination chemotherapy may be used to overcome inherent tumor resistance to a particular single agent. Because it is neither feasible nor scientifically valid to test each individual tumor against a panel of cytotoxic agents, the concept is to treat with a combination of the most active agents for a given histologic diagnosis to increase the likelihood that any individual tumor will respond.

   Second, combination chemotherapy may be used to prevent acquired resistance in an initially sensitive tumor. The assumption is that large, heterogeneous tumors harbor small populations of cells that are either naturally resistant or have undergone de novo mutation to acquire resistance. Single-agent therapy places selective positive pressure on these populations, whereas concurrent administration of other active drugs with different mechanisms of action may allow for independent cell killing.

5. **What constitutes the ideal combination of agents for the treatment of a given neoplastic disease?**
The ideal combination of agents includes the following:
- Drugs that are the most active in the disease
- Drugs that have different, nonantagonistic, and preferably additive or synergistic mechanisms of action
- Drugs that are non–cross-resistant (i.e., are subject to different mechanisms of resistance)
- Drugs that have nonoverlapping toxicities so that each can be delivered at the dose and schedule that optimizes efficacy

6. **Define dose intensity.**
The concentration of a drug given over a specified time is dose intensity. Many chemotherapeutic agents have a very steep dose-response curve, and even small escalations in dose can have a profound effect on tumor cell kill. This is especially true of drugs that are not cell cycle dependent, particularly the alkylating agents, for which it has been shown that a twofold increase in the dose of cyclophosphamide can increase therapeutic efficacy up to 10-fold. Increased dose intensity can also be achieved by decreasing the time interval between cycles. Numerous clinical studies have demonstrated that patients who receive greater dose intensity have superior response rates and disease-free survival. Nevertheless, these gains must always be balanced against morbidity and mortality from drug toxicity.

7. **What is the fractional or log cell kill hypothesis?**
The fractional cell kill hypothesis states that a given drug or drug combination at a given dose intensity kills a constant fraction of the tumor cell population, regardless of overall tumor burden. Thus each cycle of chemotherapy will diminish the remaining tumor cell population by a fixed percent. The objective of curative therapy is complete eradication, which results in zero tumor cells. Thus if there are 10^{11} tumor cells, and each cycle has a 99% cell kill, it will theoretically take six cycles to diminish the tumor cell population to less than one cell, assuming no regrowth between cycles. Although this hypothesis was initially derived for treatment of leukemia and lymphoma and may not be directly applicable to slow-growing solid tumors or treatment with cell cycle–dependent agents, the general principle regarding the need for frequent, repetitive therapy is a well-established paradigm.

8. **What is the difference between traditional chemotherapy and targeted therapy?**
Traditional chemotherapy is most commonly "cytotoxic" (capable of killing cells) and cannot discriminate between cancer and normal dividing cells because they cause DNA damage or interfere with global mechanisms involved in cell replication, cell division, and protein synthesis. Targeted therapies are more able to differentiate cancer cells from normal cells either by recognizing a specific cell surface marker (monoclonal antibody or antibody drug conjugate) or by blocking a growth pathway upon which the cancer cell is uniquely dependent, often by virtue of a molecular change or mutation specific to the cancer cell. Growth pathway inhibitors are often "cytostatic" (prevent new growth), trigger apoptosis (programmed cell death), or induce terminal differentiation.

9. **List the most common classic cytotoxic chemotherapeutic agents used to treat pediatric cancers by class and describe their mechanisms of action.**

Table 12.1 Classes of Traditional Cytotoxic Chemotherapeutic Agents

DRUG CLASS	EXAMPLES	MECHANISM OF ACTION
Alkylating agents		Cross-link DNA thereby preventing replication of DNA and transcription of RNA
	Cyclophosphamide, ifosfamide, melphalan (nitrogen mustards)	DNA cross-linking via classic covalent bond of alkyl group to DNA template
	Carmustine (BCNU), lomustine (CCNU) (nitrosoureas)	DNA cross-linking and inhibition of DNA repair
	Cisplatin, carboplatin, oxaliplatin (platinum analogs)	DNA cross-linking by platination
	Busulfan, thiotepa, dacarbazine, procarbazine, temozolomide	DNA cross-linking
Antimetabolites		Structural analogs of key molecules involved in DNA/RNA synthesis

Table 12.1 Classes of Traditional Cytotoxic Chemotherapeutic Agents (*Continued*)

DRUG CLASS	EXAMPLES	MECHANISM OF ACTION
	Methotrexate	Structural analog of folic acid; inhibits dihydrofolate reductase (DHFR), depleting tetrahydrofolate and precursors for the synthesis of purines and thymidine
	6-Mercaptopurine (6MP), 6-thioguanine (6TG)	Purine analogs; compete with endogenous purine bases
	Cytarabine	Pyrimidine analog (deoxycytosine); incorporates into DNA and inhibits DNA polymerase leading to chain termination
Antitumor antibiotics		Naturally occurring products with various mechanisms
	Doxorubicin, daunomycin, idarubicin (anthracyclines)	DNA intercalation and inhibition of topoisomerases I and II, altering the three-dimensional shape of DNA/RNA during replication and transcription, leading to double- and single-strand breaks; free radical formation; interaction with cell membranes
	Dactinomycin	DNA intercalation and inhibition of topoisomerase II
	Bleomycin	Induction of DNA strand breaks by free radicals
Plant alkaloids		Derived from plant extracts
	Vincristine, vinblastine (vinca alkaloids)	Inhibitors of mitosis; bind to tubulin, interfering with microtubule assembly and formation of the mitotic spindle
	Paclitaxel, docetaxel (taxanes)	
	Etoposide (epipodophyllotoxins)	Topoisomerase II inhibitor
	Topotecan, irinotecan (camptothecin analogs)	Topoisomerase I inhibitors
Miscellaneous	Prednisone, dexamethasone (corticosteroids)	Lympholysis, probably via binding of steroid receptor complex; also used as anti-inflammatory, immunosuppressant, and antiemetic
	L-asparaginase	Enzyme that depletes asparagine in cells

10. Describe the cell cycle and its critical phases. Which chemotherapy agents are cell cycle dependent, and in which phase are they most active?

The growth and division of cells must proceed through an orderly series of events termed the cell cycle. Normally, cell proliferation is regulated by checkpoints that control entry into the following phase. At each checkpoint, the cell undergoes a genome survey to see whether the DNA is adequately intact to proceed to the next stage of cell division. Under normal circumstances, an altered genome will activate the DNA damage response if repair is possible or trigger apoptosis and undergo programmed cell death. One such checkpoint is the *P53* gene that controls progression from the G1 to S phase (Figure 12.1).

11. What are the implications for treatment with agents that are cell cycle dependent?

- Cell kill is limited with bolus dosing: Generally speaking, only those cells active in the specific phase of the cell cycle at the time of drug exposure will be killed.
- Prolonged continuous infusion or frequent intermittent dosing at a fixed, effective dose represents a more rational intensification strategy than dose escalation because cumulatively more cells will be exposed to the drug during the sensitive phase of the cell cycle.
- "Recruitment" may increase cell kill: If more cells can be recruited into or arrested at the phase in which an agent is active, a greater number of cells will be killed.

12. Why is drug toxicity such a major problem in traditional cancer chemotherapy? Describe the most common side effects of the major classes of chemotherapy agents.

Because the mechanisms of action lead to nonspecific killing of rapidly dividing cells, traditional cytotoxic agents have a very narrow therapeutic index. The dose needed to treat disease does not differ greatly from a dose that could cause potentially dangerous or even lethal damage to normal tissues. The normal cells most frequently affected are those that regularly replenish themselves, such as the bone marrow, mucosal epithelium, hair, and detoxifying organs, including the liver and kidney. The most common side effects include:

- Myelosuppression: Critical depression of bone marrow production leading to reduced peripheral blood counts. Because of the short lifespan of granulocytes, neutropenia is the most significant, increasing the risk for severe

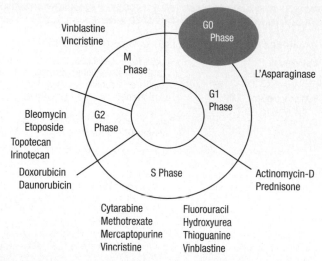

Figure 12.1 Cell-cycle dependent cytotoxic agents and the phase in which they are predominantly active. Go, resting phase: nonproliferation; G1, Gap1 or pre-DNA synthetic phase (12 hrs to days): DNA repair, no net DNA synthesis, diploid, RNA and protein synthesis; G2, Gap2 or post-DNA synthesis (2–4 hrs): Two copies of each chromosome, tetraploid, RNA and protein synthesis; M, mitosis (1–2 hrs); S, DNA synthesis (2–4 hrs).

infection. Thrombocytopenia and anemia may often precipitate the need for transfusion. The lowest counts (nadir) usually occur at 7 to 14 days after the initiation of chemotherapy, with complete recovery by 21 to 28 days.

- Mucositis: Inflammation, ulceration, and potential sloughing of the gastrointestinal (GI) mucosa. May occur anywhere from mouth to anus, impairing one's ability to eat, drink, swallow, or absorb nutrients. Also represents breakdown of an important barrier to infection. Most commonly occurs with the use of the antimetabolites, anthracyclines, and the topoisomerase inhibitors.
- Nausea and vomiting: Rarely dose-limiting but significantly impacting quality of life. Can often be managed quite effectively with antiemetics. The most emetogenic agents include the platinum analogs, nitrogen mustards, dactinomycin, irinotecan, cyclophosphamide, cytarabine, doxorubicin, and methotrexate in higher doses.
- Alopecia: Total body hair loss. Predominantly caused by the alkylating agents, anthracyclines, dactinomycin, and frequently dosed tubulin inhibitors.
- Nephrotoxicity: Most often manifested as renal tubular damage. Dose-limiting with cisplatin and, to a lesser extent, carboplatin. Can also be a significant toxicity of ifosfamide and high-dose methotrexate. Managed with vigorous hydration and electrolyte supplementation.
- Syndrome of inappropriate antidiuretic hormone secretion (SIADH): Leads to water retention and hyponatremia. Seen with high-dose cyclophosphamide and vincristine.
- Hepatotoxicity: Direct hepatocyte toxicity leading to elevation of transaminases, fibrosis, cholestasis, or hepatic venous outflow obstruction. Can be dose-limiting. Most common with methotrexate, 6MP, 6TG, and the alkylating agents in myeloablative doses.
- Cardiotoxicity: Acute toxicity, including arrhythmias, conduction abnormalities, and myopathy, may be seen with the anthracyclines and cyclophosphamide or ifosfamide in high doses. Chronic, late cardiomyopathy is peculiar to the anthracyclines. Risk appears to increase with cumulative exposure (hence, doxorubicin is generally capped at 450 mg/m^2), young age at exposure, and female sex. Dexrazoxane has been shown to be protective.
- Neurotoxicity: Most commonly manifested as reversible peripheral sensory/motor neuropathy and ileus that accompanies the use of vincristine. Outside of cytarabine-induced fever, central nervous system effects are rare and include leukoencephalopathy with frequent intrathecal or high-dose methotrexate and cerebellar toxicity with high-dose cytarabine. Irreversible sensorineural hearing loss can be associated with cisplatin and, to a lesser extent, carboplatin.
- Hypersensitivity: Anaphylactic response may limit use of asparaginase, paclitaxel, and, rarely, cisplatin or bleomycin.
- Infertility: Predominantly associated with the use of alkylating agents with risk based on cumulative exposure. In females, this may be manifested as premature menopause. In males, cisplatin has also been associated with infertility.

13. What can be done to minimize the risks of dose-intensive chemotherapy?

The best defense against toxicity includes aggressive supportive care with antiemetics, fluids, good hygiene, nutrition, blood component transfusions, and antibiotics. Specific chemoprotectants such as mesna and dexrazoxane and rescue agents such as leucovorin can be used. Neutrophil and platelet production can be supported with cytokines, including granulocyte colony–stimulating factor and thrombopoietin or with stem cell rescue. Risks of infertility and the appropriateness of fertility preservation strategies should be addressed before chemotherapy initiation.

14. **Describe the mechanism of hemorrhagic cystitis with ifosfamide and cyclophosphamide and what can be done to prevent it.**
Ifosfamide and cyclophosphamide undergo hepatic transformation to both active and inactive metabolites. One of these metabolites, acrolein, is believed to bind to and irritate the urogenic epithelium and can cause profuse bleeding of the bladder that may be dose-limiting. Mesna (sodium-2-mercaptoethane sulfonate) is rapidly oxidized in plasma to an inert disulfide compound that is resorbed by the kidney and only converted back to its active form in the renal tubules. Therefore it combines and deactivates acrolein and acrolein-precursors by forming nontoxic thioethers only after these metabolites have been excreted in the urine. By giving ifosfamide and cyclophosphamide in conjunction with mesna, vigorous hydration, and frequent voiding, the incidence of hemorrhagic cystitis has been markedly reduced, even in the context of profound dose escalation. (Note: Don't be fooled. Mesna interacts with the colorimetric assay used to detect ketones in urine. A positive dipstick for ketones in a patient receiving mesna usually does not reflect fluid or nutritional status).

15. **How is leucovorin rescue used with methotrexate?**
Methotrexate works by inhibiting dihydrofolate reductase (DHFR), depleting cells of the reduced coenzyme tetrahydrofolate needed for the synthesis of purines, thymidine, and DNA. When high doses of methotrexate are used (usually >100 mg/m^2), leucovorin (folinic acid) supplies normal cells with reduced folate to prevent toxicity (GI, bone marrow, renal, hepatic, and neurologic). Using this "rescue" strategy, doses over 30 g/m^2, previously deemed lethal, may be delivered safely. To prevent rescuing tumor cells, the leucovorin is started 24 hours after the methotrexate is initiated. To prevent toxicity, the leucovorin is not discontinued until serum methotrexate levels fall below 0.1 μmol/L.

16. **What are the most common "druggable" molecular targets in pediatric cancer and some of the targeted agents being used in children?**
See table 12.2 on next page.

17. **Describe some of the most common biochemical mechanisms of drug resistance.**
Drug resistance arises from spontaneous mutation or gene amplification in one generation of tumor cells that is passed on and expanded in subsequent generations under the selective pressure of the drug. Most commonly, the mutation results in increased, decreased, or altered production of a gene product vital to a particular drug mechanism. For example, increased activity of the enzyme glutathione-S-transferase can detoxify the active metabolites of cyclophosphamide. Similarly, increased production of DHFR or an alteration of its affinity for methotrexate can decrease the efficacy of that drug. In the case of targeted agents, the cell may similarly mutate to alter the binding properties to the inhibitor (so-called "gate-keeper mutations" for adenosine triphosphate [ATP]–dependent TKIs), decrease expression of the target (for antibodies), or increase reliance on compensatory or escape pathways.

Traditional "multidrug resistance," first noted in the late 1980s, refers to cross-resistance to a seemingly unrelated, fixed constellation of naturally occurring cytotoxic agents, attributable to a single gene, *MDR-1*, and gene product, the P glycoprotein (Pgp). Pgp is a transmembrane efflux pump capable of ejecting numerous toxins but most notably the vinca alkaloids, anthracyclines, epipodophyllotoxins, taxanes, and dactinomycin. Atypical multidrug resistance occurs when a cell acquires a mutation resulting in increased, decreased, or altered production of a gene product vital to a basic mechanism of cell upkeep. For example, both alkylating agents and topoisomerase inhibitors may be rendered ineffective by the enhanced function or production of DNA repair enzymes or survival signals BCL2 or BCLXL.

18. **What can be done to overcome drug resistance?**
Theoretically, once the biochemical mechanisms of drug resistance can be worked out, new agents can be developed or used in combination with standard agents to counteract or prevent resistance. For example, several agents capable of inhibiting the Pgp efflux pump have been tested in clinical trials, but to date, none have demonstrated significant benefit when given in combination with cytotoxic chemotherapy. For these agents, combination therapy with non–cross-resistant agents still constitutes the best approach. In the case of targeted agents, solving the crystalline protein structure of a kinase that has developed inhibitor resistance by virtue of mutation can allow molecular chemists to rationally develop the next generation of small molecule inhibitors. For example, the T315I point mutation of BCR-ABL, which renders leukemias resistant to imatinib, can be overcome by the novel TKI ponatinib, the use of which is limited to resistant patients because of toxicity.

19. **What is meant by the terms "precision oncology" and "tumor agnostic" indications?**
The hypothesis of precision oncology is that by using molecular diagnostics like next-generation sequencing to identify the key gene or genomic variants driving an individual tumor, one might be better able to select a targeted therapy that is less toxic and more effective for the patient (see Chapter 14). This hypothesis is still under active research with only a few molecularly targeted agents exhibiting extraordinary anticancer activity, particularly in solid tumors. When a molecularly targeted agent is effective based on a specific genetic finding, regardless of tumor histology or location, the Food and Drug Administration (FDA) has granted approval for the agent to be used in adults and children whose

Table 12.2 Molecularly Targeted Agents Used in Childhood Cancers

TARGET CLASS	MOLECULAR TARGET	MECHANISM OF TARGET ACTIVATION/BIOMARKER	RELEVANT PEDIATRIC DISEASE	PROTOTYPIC DRUG EXAMPLES	MECHANISM OF DRUG ACTION
Tyrosine kinase (TK)	ABL1	Translocation (BCR-ABL)	Acute lymphoid leukemia (ALL); chronic myeloid leukemia (CML)	Imatinib[a] Dasatinib[a] Nilotinib[a]	Small molecule adenosine triphosphate (ATP) competitive tyrosine kinase inhibitor (TKI)
	JAK	Activating mutation; pathway upregulation	Leukemias; juvenile myelomonocytic; Graft-versus-host disease	Ruxolitinib[a]	TKI
	FLT3	Internal tandem duplication (ITD)	Acute myeloid leukemia (AML)	Sorafenib Midastaurin Gliteritinib	TKI
	ALK ROS1 NTRK	Translocation; activating mutation (neuroblastoma)	Translocation (+) solid & brain; anaplastic large cell lymphoma (ALCL); neuroblastoma	Crizotinib[a] Lorlatinib Larotrectinib[a] Entrectinib[a]	TKI
	RET	Translocation; activating mutation (thyroid cancer)	Translocation (+) solid & thyroid cancer	Selpercatinib[a] Vandetinib	TKI
	PDGFR KIT MET VEGFR	Translocation; activating mutation; ligand overexpression	Hepatocellular & renal cell carcinoma, sarcoma	Pazopanib Regorafenib Cabozantinib Axitinib	Multi-TKI Antiangiogenesis
Signal transduction protein kinase	mTOR	NF1 loss; TSC1/2 activating mutation; upstream pathway activation	Giant cell astrocytoma; rhabdomyosarcoma	Sirolimus Everolimus[a] Temsirolimus	"Rapalogue" protein kinase inhibitor
	BRAF MEK	BRAF V600E mutation; BRAF translocation; NF1 loss	Biomarker (+), histiocytosis, melanoma, low-grade brain tumors, plexiform neurofibroma	Vemurafenib Dabrafenib[a] Selumetinib[a] Trametinib[a]	Small molecule protein kinase inhibitor

Category	Target	Abnormality	Cancer	Drug	Drug class
Prosurvival/ antiapoptosis regulator	BCL-2	Overexpression; Pathway upregulation	Leukemias, mainly AML	Venetoclax	Small molecule competitive inhibitor
Epigenetic modifier	EZH2	Activating mutation; SMARCB1 (INI1) loss	Epithelioid sarcoma, rhabdoid tumor	Tazemetostat[a]	Small molecule methyltransferase inhibitor
Retinoic acid receptor	PML-RARα	Translocation	APL	Tretinoin	Retinoid induced differentiation
	RAR	Overexpression	Neuroblastoma	Isotretinoin	
Cell lineage marker	CD20	B-cell marker	B non-Hodgkin lymphoma (NHL)	Rituximab[a]	Monoclonal antibody (mAb)
	CD-19	B-cell marker	B-ALL; BNHL	Blinatumomab[a]	Bispecific antibody links blast to activated cytotoxic T-cell
	CD30	Aberrant expression	Hodgkin lymphoma (HL); ALCL	Brentuximab vedotin	Antibody drug conjugate (ADC)
	CD33	Aberrant expression	AML	Gemtuzumab[a] ozogamicin	ADC
	CD22	Aberrant expression	ALL	Inotuzumab ozogamicin	ADC
	GD2	Neuroectodermal marker	Neuroblastoma	Dinutuximab[a] Naxitamab[a]	Chimeric mAb Humanized mAb
Immune regulator	PD1/PDL1	Aberrant expression; increased tumor mutational burden	HL; mismatch repair syndrome	Pembrolizumab[a]	Immune checkpoint mAb

[a]Drugs approved for at least one pediatric indication.

tumors harbor that genetic alteration. Thus far three agents have been given such "tumor agnostic" indications: pembrolizumab for patients with mismatch repair syndrome and high tumor mutational burden and both larotrectinib and entrectinib for neurotrophic TRK (NTRK)–fusion driven cancers.

BIBLIOGRAPHY

1. Fox E, Blaney SM, Moreno L, et al. General principles of chemotherapy. In Blaney SM, Adamson PC, Helman LJ (eds). *Pizzo and Poplack's Pediatric Oncology.* 8th ed. Wolters Kluwer, 2021:239–302.
2. Chabner BA, Longo DL, eds. *Cancer Chemotherapy, Immunotherapy and Biotherapy.* 6th ed. Wolters Kluwer, 2019.
3. Glade Bender J, Sulis ML, Smith MA. General principles of targeted therapy. In Blaney SM, Adamson PC, Helman LJ (eds). *Pizzo and Poplack's Pediatric Oncology.* 8th ed. Wolters Kluwer, 2021:327–361.
4. Wellstein A. General principles in the pharmacotherapy of cancer. In Brunton LL, Hilal-Dandan R, Knollman BC (eds). *Goodman & Gilman's: The Pharmacological Basis of Therapeutics.* 13th ed. McGraw-Hill Education, 2018.

CHAPTER 13

PRINCIPLES OF IMMUNOTHERAPY

Andrew M. Silverman, MD, Hanna E. Minns, and Robyn D. Gartrell, MD, MS

1. **What is immunotherapy?**
   Immunotherapy is a form of cancer therapy that uses the innate or adaptive immune system of a patient to eradicate malignant cells. Although some variations of this therapy directly stimulate or disinhibit the patient's own immune system, other variations of this therapy use immune cells manipulated ex vivo and introduce or reintroduce the cells back to the patient.

2. **How does the immune system interact with a tumor's microenvironment in untreated patients?**
   In addition to unchecked cell division, development of a neovascular network, and accumulation of metastatic potential, a malignant tumor must evade the immune system to grow and thrive. Tumors achieve this immune evasion through a large array of mechanisms, but overcoming the resultant immune privilege within the tumor's microenvironment (TME) is key to treating children with cancer.
   Immune cells interact with cancer via immune surveillance, immune cell infiltration, and tumor cytolysis, allowing for three phases to occur: elimination, equilibrium, and esape. Immune surveillance is the process by which the immune system correctly recognizes cancer cells, leading to their ultimate destruction (elimination). Cancer cells can counteract this response by increasing markers of immune suppression or decreasing expression of surface markers that trigger immune responses (i.e. downregulating human leukocyte antigen [HLA] molecules, etc.). This can lead to an equilibrium where the tumor cells begin to become unrecognizable to the immune cells but there is still some control. Ultimately, escape occurs when the tumor cells overwhelm the immune system and can grow mostly unrestrained.

3. **Describe the lymphocytes in the TME.**
   T Lymphocytes
   There are a variety of T-lymphocyte phenotypes present in normal and tumor microenvironments. These phenotypic subtypes include $CD4^+$ T helper cells (Th cells), $CD8^+$ cytotoxic T cells (CTLs), and regulatory T cells (Tregs). CTLs are activated by interacting with antigens presented by major histocompatibility complex (MHC) class I molecules on antigen-presenting cells (APCs). When this happens, CTLs can recognize infected or cancerous cells and transmit cytotoxic molecules to induce cell death. On the other hand, Th cells and Tregs (which also express CD4 on their surface) are activated by interacting with antigens presented by MHC class II molecules on the surface of APCs. After recognizing specific antigens, these T cells will begin to secrete unique cytokines, stimulating a cytokine-signaling pathway that determines further differentiation of these immune cell subsets.
   For example, interleukin 12 (IL-12) and interferon γ (IFNγ) are the critical cytokines needed to develop a specific subtype of T helper cell called Th1. Th1 cells go on to carry out a variety of functions such as M1 (activating) macrophage and CTL recruitment. The other primary subtype of T helper cells is Th2 cells, which, similar to Tregs, have immunosuppressive functions. These Th2 cells are activated by IL-4 and IL-2 cytokines. IL-2 is also the critical cytokine needed for differentiation into Tregs. Tregs can inhibit an immune response through a variety of mechanisms, including secreting more anti-inflammatory cytokines or modulating APCs so that they do not activate more T cells.
   In cancers, the balance of these immune phenotypes is shifted in favor of immune inhibitory activities. Specifically, $CD4^+$ Th cells and immunosuppressive Tregs tend to be increased, whereas $CD8^+$ CTLs are decreased. This imbalance toward an immunosuppressive TME permits tumor growth and allows cancer cells to evade immune surveillance. Nevertheless, this ratio can also be a predictive indicator of prognosis. For example, a high ratio of $CD8^+$ CTLs to $FOXP3^+$ Treg cells in the ovarian cancer tumor microenvironment has been associated with a favorable clinical outcome.
   B Lymphocytes
   Because relatively few B cells are found in the TME, the role of T cells in cancer progression has been studied more extensively. Nevertheless, over the past few years, several studies have indicated that the presence and functionality of B cells can also be an important prognostic factor. Analysis of RNA sequencing data from The Cancer Genome Atlas demonstrated that high levels of expression of B-cell and plasma cell signature genes correlated with an increased overall survival in some cancer types and with poorer clinical outcomes in others. Moreover, B cells in the TME can elicit both protumor and antitumor responses.
   B cells can concentrate at the tumor edge or form tumor-associated immune aggregates ranging from small unorganized clusters to complex tertiary lymphoid structures (TLS). Although they are found in small numbers, B cells are still able to produce large amounts of cytokines and antibodies that can go on to affect the functions of T cells and various tumorigenic or antitumorigenic processes. The antibodies released by plasma cells can drive antibody-dependent cellular cytotoxicity (ADCC) and phagocytosis, with the class of human immunoglobulin G1 (IgG1) antibodies

especially relevant here. IgG$^+$ memory B cells can produce granzyme B (a CTL activation marker) and tumor necrosis factor-related apoptosis-inducing ligand (TRAIL, which causes apoptosis in tumor cells), while also expressing surface markers characteristic of APCs, secreting IFNγ, and cooperating with CTLs. Thus B cells can actually act similarly to APCs and help maintain the T-cell population intratumorally.

4. Describe Antigen Presenting Cells in the TME.
Macrophages and dendritic cells (DCs) are present in the TME of most cancers and, similar to T lymphocytes, can have inhibitory or stimulatory effects on immune activity. M1 (activating) macrophages are often outnumbered by M2 (inhibitory) macrophages within the TME of growing tumors. Activated M1 macrophages release proinflammatory cytokines like IL-12 and can kill tumor cells themselves, while also recruiting more T cells (IL-12 stimulates the production of Th1 cells, which favor antitumor activities). In comparison, activated M2 macrophages suppress Th1-mediated inflammation and encourage conditions for tumor growth through events like angiogenesis. By secreting cytokines (e.g., IL-4, IL-10, IL-13) favoring this phenotypic selection of M2 macrophages, tumor cells and the regulatory T-cell infiltrate can induce this effect.
   Similarly, DCs are often present within the TME of many tumors and act in an inhibitory manner. These inhibitory phenotypes tend to be favored through similar mechanisms to those seen with macrophage selection but using different cytokines (e.g., IL-1).

5. What are monoclonal antibodies (mAbs) and how are they used in treating cancer?
MAbs are proteins developed in vitro made to have a form and function similar to in vivo immunoglobulins produced by the adaptive immune system. Anticancer mAbs have been developed with intended functions of directly targeting malignant cells, modifying host response to malignant cells, delivering cytotoxic molecules to malignant cells, or retargeting cellular immune activation against malignant cells.

6. How are mAbs used in the clinical setting of pediatric oncology?
"Naked" mAbs are similar in structure and function to native immunoglobulins. They have been used clinically for over 20 years, the first of which to be approved for cancer therapy by the Food and Drug Administration (FDA) was rituximab in 1997. This mAb specifically targets CD20, a cell surface protein present on many malignancies of the B-lymphocyte lineage. It acts via direct mechanisms by signaling induced cell death on the target cell and indirect mechanisms via antibody-directed cell-mediated cytotoxicity (ADCC) and complement-mediated cell death (CDC). Because of its incorporation as monotherapy or as part of a larger multiagent therapeutic approach, rituximab has vastly improved outcomes in cancers expressing CD20 in their TME. In pediatrics, this effect has been most heavily demonstrated in mature B-cell lymphocytic lymphomas.

7. Can mAbs be manipulated to enhance or broaden their efficacy?
Antibody-drug conjugates (ADC) are, as the name suggests, mAbs chemically bound to a cytotoxic chemotherapeutic, allowing for direct delivery of the toxic chemotherapeutic to a patient's TME. This allows for minimal toxicity to the patient without compromising the efficacy of the therapy. Currently FDA-approved in adult patients and refractory pediatric patients with Hodgkin lymphoma, brentuximab vedotin is an ADC that is made up of an anti-CD30 mAb covalently linked by an enzyme-cleavable peptide to monomethylauristatin E (vedotin). This allows for selective delivery of this highly toxic drug (vedotin) to the intracellular compartment of tumor cells expressing CD30 on their cell surfaces via receptor-mediated endocytosis. Once in the cytoplasm of the target cell, the linkage peptide is cleaved and vedotin is released intracellularly in the target Hodgkin cell. Although proven more efficacious than the prior standard of care in adult patients with Hodgkin lymphoma, it is currently under investigation for front-line use in pediatric patients, having demonstrated very promising efficacy in the relapsed setting.
   Bispecific T-cell engagers (BiTEs) are antibody constructs using an anti-CD3 mAb variable region cross-linked to a variable region from a mAb targeting another cell surface protein on the target tumor cell. This induces activation of a T lymphocyte against the target cell, triggering cell death specifically targeted to the tumor cell involved. Blinatumomab is a BiTE therapy that targets CD19, a protein present on the surface of the vast majority of B-lineage leukemia cells. Dosing and efficacy were first demonstrated in pediatric patients in the relapsed or refractory setting, and it is now being used in an upfront trial for newly diagnosed pediatric patients with B-cell acute lymphoblastic leukemia.

8. What are immune checkpoint inhibitors, and how are they used clinically?
Another method of immunotherapy is known as checkpoint inhibition. Tumors learn to trick the immune system into thinking they are self and avoid immune cell killing by displaying "checkpoint" proteins that bind to surface proteins on T cells such as cytotoxic T-lymphocyte-associated protein 4 (CTLA-4) and programmed cell death protein 1 (PD-1). When CTLA-4 or PD-1 binds to its associated ligand, that T cell "turns off" and will not initiate an immune response against cancerous cells. Nevertheless, it has been shown that immune checkpoint inhibitor drugs (ICIs) can reverse this trick that tumor cells play on the immune system and actually realert the immune cells to the tumor. Specifically, CTLA-4 inhibition prevents T-cell inhibition and promotes the activation and proliferation of effector T cells, whereas blockade of the PD-1/PD-L1 pathway leads to the activation of T cells and the reversal of T-cell exhaustion. ICIs such as anti-CTLA-4 (e.g., ipilimumab) and anti-PD-1 (e.g., nivolumab, pembrolizumab) and the combination of ipilimumab and nivolumab have been moderately successful in treating adult

tumors and are currently approved for the treatment of cancer in adults. ICIs have been introduced into pediatrics through phase I/II clinical trials.

Ipilimumab is a monoclonal antibody that binds to CTLA-4 and blocks its interaction with B7-1 and B7-2. When this happens, instead of inhibiting an immune response, B7-1 will preferentially bind to CD28, activating T cells and stimulating the immune system. In 2017, ipilimumab was approved for pediatric patients 12 years and older with unresectable or metastatic melanoma. Similarly, pembrolizumab and nivolumab are highly selective monoclonal antibodies designed to block the binding of PD-1 to its ligands, PD-L1 and PD-L2. If PD-1 cannot bind to its ligands, T cells will remain activated and alert. In 2017, pembrolizumab was approved for children with relapsed/refractory Hodgkin lymphoma and microsatellite instability-high (MSI-H) solid tumors. In 2020, it was approved for children with tumor mutational burdens (TMB) of 10 or higher. Phase I trials have found both anti-PD1 and anti-CTLA-4 agents to be safe for use in pediatric patients. Efficacy has been evaluated in recurrent disease and, unfortunately, no objective tumor regressions were observed with ICIs as the single agent in pediatric recurrent disease outside of Hodgkin lymphoma and melanoma. Because an ICI is unlikely to be successful on its own, combination trials with chemotherapy and/or radiation are underway. The addition of ICIs to these and other therapeutic methods, including targeted therapies, can have astonishing effects on tumor regression and survival compared with single-agent treatment. Lastly, immunotherapy may be more effective when given as part of upfront, initial therapy because the immune system may be depleted and tumor escape more evident at the time of recurrence as immune activation and antitumor response is less likely.

BIBLIOGRAPHY

1. Cole PD, McCarten KM, Pei Q, et al. Brentuximab vedotin with gemcitabine for paediatric and young adult patients with relapsed or refractory Hodgkin's lymphoma (AHOD1221): a Children's Oncology Group, multicentre single-arm, phase 1-2 trial. *Lancet Oncol.* 2018;19:1229–1238.
2. Gajewski TF, Schreiber H, Fu YX. Innate and adaptive immune cells in the tumor microenvironment. *Nat Immunol.* 2013;14:1014–1022.
3. Geoerger B, Kang HJ, Yalon-Oren M, et al. Pembrolizumab in paediatric patients with advanced melanoma or a PD-L1-positive, advanced, relapsed, or refractory solid tumour or lymphoma (KEYNOTE-051): interim analysis of an open-label, single-arm, phase 1-2 trial. *Lancet Oncol.* 2020;21:121–133.
4. Marjanska A, Drogosiewicz M, Dembowska-BagiNska B, et al. Nivolumab for the treatment of advanced pediatric malignancies. *Anticancer Res.* 2020;40:7095–7100.
5. Minard-Colin V, Auperin A, Pillon M, et al. Rituximab for high-risk, mature b-cell non-Hodgkin's lymphoma in children. *N Engl J Med.* 2020;382:2207–2219.
6. Quatromoni JG, Eruslanov E. Tumor-associated macrophages: function, phenotype, and link to prognosis in human lung cancer. *Am J Transl Res.* 2012;4:376–389.
7. Sharonov GV, Serebrovskaya EO, Yuzhakova DV, et al. B cells, plasma cells and antibody repertoires in the tumour microenvironment. *Nat Rev Immunol.* 2020;20:294–307.
8. von Stackelberg A, Locatelli F, Zugmaier G, et al. Phase I/phase II study of blinatumomab in pediatric patients with relapsed/refractory acute lymphoblastic leukemia. *J Clin Oncol.* 2016;34:4381–4389.

CHAPTER 14

PRECISION MEDICINE AND SYSTEMS BIOLOGY

Jovana Pavisic, MD, MA and Jennifer Oberg, EdD, MA

1. **What is precision medicine, and how does it relate to pediatric oncology?**

   Precision medicine refers to approaching the treatment and prevention of disease by tailoring patients' care based on their individual variability in genes, environment, and lifestyle. Oncology has been at the forefront of applying precision medicine principles to the care of patients supported by a rapid expansion in genomic technologies and large-scale databases along with the computational tools for analyzing them. The application of precision medicine is emerging within pediatric oncology as we shift from directing the diagnosis, classification, and management of tumors from the site of tumor origin alone to incorporating individual tumor information at the gene, protein, and environment level. Clinical, histological, and molecular data are integrated with the goal of selecting the most appropriate treatment for an individual patient and the unique biological profile of that patient's tumor. This includes molecularly based classification, use of clinical and molecular features for risk stratification and therapy selection, and the growing use of genomically driven targeted therapies relying on individualized tumor genomic analyses. The goal of precision medicine in pediatric oncology is to select more precise and personalized therapies to cure more patients while minimizing short- and long-term side effects from treatment.

2. **How is the pediatric cancer genome different from that in adults? How does this affect the way precision medicine is applied in pediatric versus adult oncology?**

   Compared with adult cancers, pediatric cancers are much rarer, more often induced by inherited or sporadic errors in development rather than environmental exposures, and typically of mesenchymal rather than epithelial origin. This leads to significant differences in the frequency and spectrum of mutations seen in pediatric cancers compared with adult cancers, including:
   - Lower mutational burden
   - Higher prevalence of structural variations (chromosomal rearrangements, gene fusions)
   - More frequent epigenetic alterations: heritable changes that affect gene expression and activity without underlying nucleotide changes (DNA methylation, histone modifications)
   - Rare occurrence of targetable kinase alterations, such as epidermal growth factor receptor (EGFR) and human epidermal growth factor receptor 2 (HER2)
   - More frequent germline mutations in cancer predisposition genes
       These differences highlight the need for precision medicine in pediatric oncology to:
   - Use more comprehensive sequencing approaches beyond targeted gene panels, including gene expression and DNA methylation analyses.
   - Aggregate clinical and molecular data across institutions to support discovery research and guide clinical decision making in the setting of a rare disease.
   - Focus on inherited cancer susceptibility including the added clinical, computational, and ethical complexity of incorporating routine germline testing into clinical care.

3. **Define next-generation sequencing (NGS). Describe the main NGS methods used clinically in pediatric oncology and their advantages and limitations.**

   NGS, also described as massively parallel or deep sequencing, refers to a newer, fast technology for sequencing of DNA or RNA that is done in a highly parallel, high-throughput, scalable fashion. This has allowed for the sequencing of the entire human genome within a single day and greatly reduced the cost so that routine genomic analysis in the clinical setting to direct patient care is now possible. The main NGS methods used in pediatric oncology clinical practice, along with their advantages and limitations, are detailed in Table 14.1 and Figure 14.1. In addition to the detection of point mutations, these NGS methodologies can identify insertions, deletions, copy number changes, novel gene fusions, and relative gene expression. Compared with older sequencing technologies, NGS can also identify subclonal mutations (present in a low proportion of tumor cells) that can be responsible for therapy resistance and relapse in certain tumors.

4. **What are somatic versus germline mutations?**

   In cancer, the analysis of genetic variation is to identify the origin of the mutations (i.e., whether they are inherited or occur early in the embryogenesis process, referred to as germline, or acquired only in the cancer cells, referred to as somatic). Most mutations in cancer are somatically acquired, meaning that they are not present in normal tissue within the same patient. Unlike adult cancers, underlying germline mutations in cancer predisposition genes are relatively common in pediatric malignancies and can occur in up to 10% of cases. Examples of such germline mutations associated with a

Table 14.1 Next-Generation Sequencing (NGS) Methods Used in Pediatric Oncology

NGS METHOD	DESCRIPTION	ADVANTAGES	LIMITATIONS
Targeted gene/ fusion panel sequencing	• Deep sequencing of a panel of preselected genes or regions associated with cancer	• High sequencing depth to identify rare variants or those at low allele frequency • Commercially available • Cost-effective • Faster, easier, more reliable data analysis	• Often designed for adult cancers (miss important pediatric tumor gene regions) • Limit detection of novel cancer-associated genes not included in the panel
Whole-exome sequencing (WES)	• Sequencing of the protein-coding region of the genome (<2% of entire genome but contains the majority of disease-related variants)	• Can identify novel cancer-associated genes and variants • Relatively cost-effective with smaller, more manageable data compared with whole-genome sequencing (WGS)	• May miss some rare or subclonal variants because of lower depth • Complex interpretation (i.e., variants of unknown significance) • Requires paired sequencing of normal tissue to determine which changes are tumor-related
Whole-genome sequencing (WGS)	• Sequencing of the entire genome, including chromosomal and mitochondrial DNA	• Increased yield for identifying pathogenic variants, including noncoding regions • Higher coverage better identifies copy number changes, structural variants, high focal amplifications, and deletions that can be missed using fragmented data	• Costly • Large amounts of complex data, difficult interpretation (noncoding regions less conserved) • Requires sequencing and data storage systems that are not readily available for everyday clinical practice
Whole transcriptome sequencing (RNAseq)	• Sequencing of coding and multiple forms of noncoding RNA	• Whole transcriptome-based biomarkers have prognostic or therapeutic significance • Important for discovery of novel fusions, allele-specific expression • Relatively cost-effective	• Complicated interpretation and high potential for bias: results are tissue-and time-specific and can vary significantly with the exact sequencing platform

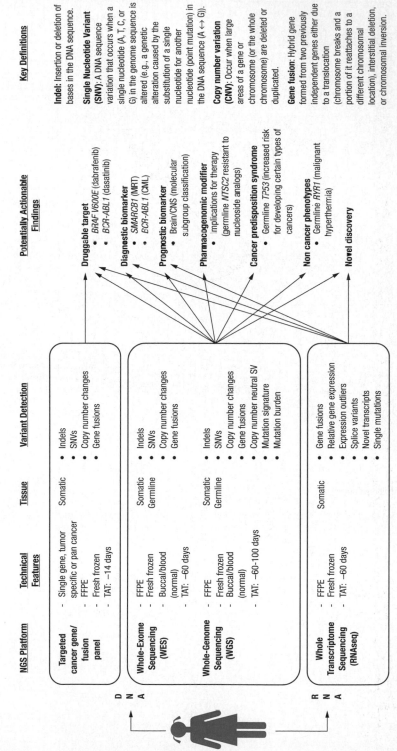

Figure 14.1 Clinical applications of next-generation sequencing (NGS) in pediatric oncology. Different molecular assays can be used to detect relevant somatic and germline alterations of clinical importance. The choice of assay depends on several factors, such as the type of material to be sequenced, performance metrics of the different sequencing platforms, and cost (Table 14.1). *CML*, Chronic myeloid leukemia; *CNS*, central nervous system; *FFPE*, formalin-fixed, paraffin embedded; *MRT*, malignant rhabdoid tumor; *SNV*, single nucleotide variant; *SV*, structural variant; *TAT*, turnaround time.

significant risk for developing certain types of cancer include mutations in the tumor suppressor gene, *TP53*, which is associated with Li-Fraumeni (LFS) syndrome. Patients diagnosed with LFS are at higher risk for developing multiple cancers, notably soft-tissue and bone sarcomas, breast cancer, brain tumors, adrenocortical carcinoma, and acute leukemia, among others. Somatic mutations in *TP53* are also common in pediatric cancers, but these mutations alone are not associated with LFS or increased cancer susceptibility. Another example are germline mutations in tumor suppressor genes, *BRCA1/2*, which are associated with increased susceptibility to developing breast and ovarian cancer.

5. What are actionable variants? In what ways can a molecular finding be actionable?
There are a range of definitions found in the literature to describe actionable molecular findings (alterations). The most restrictive definition refers to identifying a genomic alteration through sequencing analysis that represents a potential therapeutic target (e.g., targeting *BRAF* mutant positive pediatric low-grade gliomas with dabrafenib). More broadly, "potentially actionable" refers to any genomic finding discovered during sequencing analysis that could inform patient care by identifying a targetable (druggable) molecular aberration (e.g., gene variant or fusion), lead to a change in diagnosis or risk stratification, have pharmacogenomic implications (e.g., indicate an ineffectual therapy), or lead to genetic counseling for the patient or other at-risk family members (see Figure 14.1). For example, transcriptome analysis (RNAseq) can identify clinically actionable gene fusions in pediatric leukemias and sarcomas and provide tumor expression subgroup analysis (e.g., medulloblastoma and Ph-like acute lymphoblastic leukemia) and cell-of-origin gene expression analyses for tumors of unknown primary. In addition, rare mutations in actionable genes in unexpected tumor types have been found. Lastly, tumor-germline whole-exome sequencing can detect pathogenic germline mutations in pediatric cancers, even among patients without a family history of cancer.

6. When is comprehensive tumor sequencing indicated?
Given the high efficacy of standardized treatment protocols for the majority of pediatric cancer patients, clinical sequencing efforts typically focus on characterizing patients diagnosed with high-risk malignancies, outlier phenotypes, rare cancers lacking standard therapies, cancer predisposition syndromes, and relapsed/refractory disease to inform patient care. For example, comprehensive sequencing that includes transcriptome analysis can be used to identify targetable fusions, such as *BCR-ABL1* fusions in pediatric CML, which has diagnostic significance and is potentially targetable with a tyrosine kinase inhibitor. Molecular analysis can help refine classification schemas for rare aggressive tumors and lead to a change in diagnosis. For example, identifying loss of *SMARCB1* on chromosome 22q11.2 via copy number analysis is a better diagnostic tool for identifying aggressive malignant rhabdoid tumors of the liver compared with morphology, which often leads to the misclassification of these tumors as small cell variant of hepatoblastoma.[1] Analysis of patient-matched tumor-normal samples can identify pathogenic or likely pathogenic germline mutations in pediatric and adult-onset cancer predisposition genes in 8% to 10% of childhood cancer patients and detect mutations in other noncancer phenotypes. This knowledge may impact clinical management by directing cancer care, prompting further genetic counseling and testing for the patient and other at-risk family members, guide family-planning, and facilitate cancer prevention and surveillance protocols.

7. What is the difference between discovery sequencing and clinical sequencing? What are the major clinical precision medicine initiatives that have advanced the field in pediatric oncology?
Completed discovery sequencing studies typically used banked and archival tissue samples from many patients to identify important insights into the molecular pathology of pediatric cancer. These research/discovery endeavors are not considered precision medicine because their data do not affect the care of the patient from whom the samples were collected. To be considered a precision medicine program, workflows that allow data to impact the care of the patient from whom samples were collected must be in place. This includes having established sample collection and banking procedures, CLIA (Clinical Laboratory Improvement Amendments of 1988)–compliant sample processing, real-time analysis, expert interpretation, and an interface for making results available to clinicians (e.g., instituting a molecular tumor board and transmitting results to the electronic health record). In the United States, clinical sequencing can only be performed by a commercial or academic laboratory that is certified by CLIA. Any results found through sequencing that was not performed in a CLIA-certified laboratory that may impact the care of a patient must be validated in a CLIA-certified laboratory before those results can be acted on in a clinical setting.

Table 14.2 describes the pilot initiatives that demonstrated the feasibility of clinical sequencing for patients with childhood cancers and established a basis for subsequent precision medicine trials that prospectively assess the real-time impact of molecularly targeted therapies in pediatric oncology.

8. What is a precision medicine trial? Discuss and provide examples of precision medicine trial designs used in pediatric oncology. Specifically contrast basket versus umbrella trials.
A precision medicine trial is a clinical trial in which patient eligibility to receive a targeted therapy is determined by the presence or absence of a specific biomarker. Three precision medicine clinical trial designs are commonly used in pediatric oncology with key differences in how patient eligibility is defined: basket trials, umbrella trials, and single-agent targeted therapy trials.[2] Table 14.3 describes and compares these trial designs and lists examples of ongoing trials in pediatric oncology under each category. They are typically seen in the setting of advanced disease, although they are now expanding to the time of initial diagnosis as our knowledge of pediatric cancer genetics grows, especially for the more common childhood cancers such as leukemias, medulloblastoma, and neuroblastoma.

Table 14.2 Selected Published Clinical Sequencing Initiatives in Pediatric Oncology

INITIATIVE [PMID]	TUMOR TYPES	PATIENT POPULATION	PLATFORM	TISSUE EVALUATED	NUMBER OF PATIENTS SEQUENCED (AGE)	POTENTIALLY ACTIONABLE N, %	TARGETABLE ALTERATIONS N, %	DIAGNOSTIC, PROGNOSTIC, RISK STRATIFICATION N, %	GERMLINE N, %
Peds-MiOncoseq[2,6] (University of Michigan) [26325560]	Solid tumors (including CNS); hematological malignancies	Relapsed/refractory, newly diagnosed high-risk or rare cancer types	WES, RNAseq (Non CLIA-certified)[b]	Somatic, germline	91 (<25 years old)	42, 46%	43, 46%	Not evaluated	9, 10%
iCat[2,6,7] (Dana-Farber Cancer Institute)[a] [26822149]	Extracranial solid tumors	Relapsed/refractory, newly diagnosed high-risk	Targeted gene panel sequencing; aCGH (CLIA-certified); RNAseq (non CLIA-certified)[b]	Somatic only	89 (</=30 years old)	43, 48%	31, 35%	3, 3%	11, 12%[c]
BASIC3[2,6,7] (Baylor College of Medicine) [26822237]	Solid tumors including CNS	Newly diagnosed	WES (CLIA-certified)	Somatic, germline	150 (<18 years old)	59, 39%	Diagnostic, prognostic, and/or predictive of treatment in specific tumor type (n = 4, 3%); mutations in members of targetable cancer pathways, gene families or functional groups, regardless of tumor type (n = 29, 27%)	15, 10%	
INFORM[2,6,7] (German Research Center)[a] [27479119]	Solid tumors including CNS and hematological malignancies	Relapsed/refractory, newly diagnosed high-risk	WES, low coverage WGS, RNAseq, methylation, expression microarray (CLIA equivalent)	Somatic, germline	52 (<41 years old)	26, 50%	26, 50%	Note evaluated	2, 4%
MBB Program[2,6] (Institute Curie, France) [27896933]	Solid tumors including CNS	Relapsed/refractory, newly diagnosed high-risk	Targeted gene panel sequencing; aCGH (CLIA equivalent)	Somatic only	58 (<22 years old)	23, 40%	23, 40%	Not evaluated	Not evaluated
PIPseq[2,6] (Columbia University) [28007021]	Solid tumors including CNS and hematological malignancies	Relapsed/refractory, newly diagnosed high-risk	Targeted gene panel, WES, CNV, RNAseq (CLIA-certified, NYS DOH approved)	Somatic, germline	101 (<27 years old)	67, 66%	38, 38%	38, 38%	20% (18/90)

Study	Tumor type	Disease status	Methods	Analysis	No. (age)				
MOSCATO–01[2,6] (Gustave Roussy, France) [28733441]	Solid tumors including CNS	Relapsed, refractory	Targeted gene panel sequencing, aCGH, WES, RNAseq (CLIA equivalent)	Somatic, germline	69 (<25 years old)	42, 61%	42, 61%	15, 22% detected or confirmed disease-defining gene fusions in 12 patients (3pts dx change)	10% (5/48)
Zero Childhood Cancer Program[8] (Australia)[a] [33020650]	Solid tumors including CNS and hematological malignancies	Initial diagnosis, relapse/refractory disease, secondary cancer	WGS, CNV, methylation, RNAseq (CLIA equivalent)	Somatic, germline	247 (0–31 years old)	231 (94%)	134, 67%	67, 27%	40, 16%

[a]Multicenter study.

[b]Clinically significant results were required to be validated through a CLIA (Clinical Laboratory Improvement Amendments of 1988)-certified lab before being used in patient care.

[c]Somatic alterations indicating the possible presence of a cancer predisposition syndrome and patients were referred for genetic counseling for further evaluation.

Table 14.3 Precision Medicine Clinical Trial Designs and Examples in Pediatric Oncology

	BASKET TRIAL	UMBRELLA TRIAL	SINGLE-AGENT TARGETED THERAPY TRIAL
Descriptior / Settings Used	• Tumor agnostic (multiple diagnoses) • Eligibility for different arms of targeted therapies based on results of tumor sequencing • Ideal when genomic variants that could predict targeted therapy response occur at low or unknown frequency across diseases → very important in pediatric oncology given rarity of tumor types and low mutational burden • Currently used only for relapsed/refractory disease	• Tumor specific (single diagnosis) • Eligibility for different arms of targeted therapies based on results of tumor sequencing • Requires significant discovery sequencing information in the specific tumor type to understand potentially actionable mutations and ensure frequency is sufficient for the study to be feasible • Used at diagnosis for common tumor types and for relapsed/refractory disease	• Primarily tumor agnostic in pediatric oncology given low patient numbers but can be tumor specific • Eligibility for the single-study arm includes a genomic biomarker • Often industry sponsored using drugs primarily developed for gene variants present in the more common adult cancers • Typically used for relapsed/refractory disease

Examples in Pediatric Oncology:

Basket Trial	• **National Cancer Institute (NCI)–Children's Oncology Group (COG) Pediatric MATCH** (Molecular Analysis for Therapeutic Choice): Uses a targeted gene panel to assign patients to different single-agent targeted therapy arms across relapsed/refractory hematologic, solid, and central nervous system (CNS) tumors (NCT03155620) • **AcSe-ESMART**: Similar trial in Europe (NCT02813135)
Umbrella Trial	Relapsed/refractory disease: • **NEPENTHE (Next-Generation Personalized Neuroblastoma [NBL] Therapy):** uses a targeted gene panel to assign patients with relapsed NBL to different arms of combinations of targeted therapies (NCT02780128) Newly diagnosed disease: • **Total Therapy XVII for Newly Diagnosed Patients with ALL (acute lymphoblastic leukemia):** separate arms based on genomic features, including use of tyrosine kinase inhibitors (dasatinib) or Janus kinase (JAK) inhibitors (ruxolitinib) with chemotherapy for newly diagnosed patients with Ph+ or Ph-like ALL or CRLF2/JAK/STAT mutations, respectively (NCT03117751) • **St. Jude Clinical and Molecular Risk-Directed Therapy for Newly Diagnosed Medulloblastoma:** tumor molecular subtype (WNT, SHH, Non-WNT Non-SHH) incorporated into risk stratification and therapy selection including addition of vismodegib-targeted therapy for participants with SHH+ tumors (NCT01878617)
Single-Agent Targeted Therapy Trial	• **Larotrectinib** in pediatric advanced solid or CNS NTRK fusion–positive tumors (NCT02637687) • **Crizotinib** for adult or pediatric tumors with an anaplastic lymphoma kinase (ALK), hepatocyte growth factor receptor (MET), or ROS1 alteration (NCT02034981) • **Dabrafenib with trametinib** for BRAF V600–mutated pediatric low-grade glioma or relapsed/refractory high-grade glioma (NCT02684058) • EZH2 inhibitor **tazemetostat** in pediatric relapsed/refractory integrase interactor 1 (INI-1)–negative tumors (NCT02601937)

9. **Provide three examples of precision medicine–targeted therapies developed for pediatric hematologic, solid, and central nervous system malignancies.**

   The treatment of Philadelphia chromosome-positive acute lymphoblastic leukemia (ALL; Ph+ ALL) is a classic early example of applying precision medicine to pediatric oncology. Targeting the canonical BCR-ABL1 translocation by an ABL1 kinase targeting drug—initially imatinib and now the second-generation dasatinib—in combination with chemotherapy has transformed the dismal outcomes for this group of patients such that they no longer require bone marrow transplantation in first remission. Furthermore, genomic profiling has identified a new subtype of high-risk ALL that is Philadelphia chromosome-like (Ph-like ALL, ~15% of patients). These patients are defined by gene expression signatures similar to Ph+ ALL but lack the hallmark BCR-ABL1 fusion. A diverse set of mutations contribute to this molecular subtype, activating three common, targetable pathways: Janus kinase (JAK)-signal transducer and activator of transcription proteins (STAT), ABL, and PI3K/AKT/mammalian target of rapamycin (mTOR). Groups are now studying the upfront efficacy of combining dasatinib or ruxolitinib with chemotherapy for patients with Ph-like ALL with ABLI class fusions or JAK/STAT pathway alterations, respectively.[3]

   Another example is the use of crizotinib, a hepatocyte growth factor receptor (HGFR, c-MET) and anaplastic lymphoma kinase (ALK) inhibitor, initially developed for ALK-mutated lung cancer, in a phase 1/2 trial for pediatric patients with refractory solid tumors or anaplastic large-cell lymphoma (ALCL). Significant responses were seen in ALCL and inflammatory myofibroblastic tumors harboring ALK fusions, eventually leading to the Food and Drug Administration (FDA)-approval of crizotinib for ALK-positive ALCL in children and young adults.[4] Responses were also seen in neuroblastoma patients with ALK mutations; however, these were mixed because ALK mutations in neuroblastoma differ from those seen in lung cancer. Newer drugs targeting ALK, such as ceritinib, are being explored in neuroblastoma (NCT02780128). The Trk inhibitor, larotrectinib, is also showing significant efficacy in a phase 1/2 study for treatment of pediatric patients with advanced solid or primary CNS tumors harboring NTRK fusions (NCT02637687).

   For pediatric CNS malignancies, the use of BRAF inhibitors (vemurafenib, dabrafenib) is emerging from the application of precision medicine principles. Genomic analyses showed that a proportion of pediatric gliomas harbor somatic alterations in BRAF, most commonly translocations resulting in the loss of BRAF regulation and activation of the mitogen-activated protein (MAP) kinase pathway but also the BRAFV600E point mutations that leads to constitutive activation of BRAF. BRAF inhibitors have since been effectively used in several clinical trials for pediatric gliomas harboring the V600E mutation. They are contraindicated in patients with BRAF fusions because they result in feedback-loop-mediated upregulation of the pathway and accelerated tumor growth. Alternatively, MAP kinase inhibitors are under investigation in this cohort of patients.

10. **What are the persistent challenges and barriers to implementing pediatric precision cancer medicine?**

    Precision medicine has the potential to change the paradigm for diagnosing and treating pediatric cancer. Yet precision medicine still faces challenges to broad clinical implementation. These challenges are highlighted in the following bullet points:

    - Logistical challenges related to NGS:
      - Reagent and equipment costs have declined but infrastructure and personnel costs related to bioinformatics, computational pipeline generation, data processing time, and data storage through cloud computing are still high.
      - Turnaround time for results from comprehensive sequencing can exceed 100 days.
      - Clinical NGS is poorly reimbursed or not reimbursed by most healthcare payers, restricting to whom NGS can be offered.
      - Interpreting pathogenic or likely pathogenic variants of uncertain significance identified by comprehensive sequencing remains a challenge.
      - Returning incidental germline pathogenic variants (i.e., variants unrelated to cancer or other known patient phenotype) may have ethical implications for patients and families, including the potential for genetic discrimination in the future.
    - Drug access challenges:
      - Few Food and Drug Administration (FDA)-approved drugs for adult cancer indications include pediatric labeling information because of a paucity of efficacy or safety data in pediatric tumors.
      - Lack of pediatric-friendly formulations.
      - Process for obtaining non-FDA approved experimental drugs through compassionate use/access programs for pediatric patients is lengthy and access to drugs is rarely granted for younger patients.
      - Insurance carriers are not obliged to provide coverage for off-label use of newer, high-cost agents.
      - Lack of available clinical trials and, when a clinical trial is available, access may be limited by geography, availability of treatment slots, or strict eligibility criteria.
    - Challenges to precision medicine clinical trials:
      - Treatment regimens are tailored to small subsets of genomically defined patients and use a single-arm design rather than a randomized design (the impact of the intervention is compared with a historical control).
      - Single-arm studies are intended to detect a signal in a histology agnostic cohort of patients based on a specific genetic marker and do not assess agent activity for a prespecified tumor type.

11. **What is systems biology? How is it used to study cancer, and what are its potential applications in pediatric oncology?**

Systems biology is an approach to biomedical research that uses sophisticated computational models and large amounts of data at the molecular, cellular, tissue, organism, or environmental level to understand how the different components interact together. Its goal is to model and discover properties of complex biological systems that cannot be inferred by studying its individual pieces (i.e., engineering metabolic, cell signaling, or gene regulatory networks). Cancer systems biology specifically focuses on studying tumorigenesis and treatments using multiomic data (e.g., genomics, proteomics, metabolomics, phenomics), advanced computational tools, and in vitro and in vivo tumor models to integrate in silico modeling of cancer development, growth, and therapy response with experimental validation.[5] It provides an opportunity to:

- Better understand the regulatory mechanisms contributing to the tumor cell state and their association with underlying genetic changes;
- Model targeted therapy response at the molecular and cellular level;
- Optimize classification of tumors; and
- Generate more robust predictive models of therapy response and outcomes.

In pediatric oncology, systems biology principles can be applied to generate and interrogate comprehensive molecular data sets such as that developed by the Therapeutically Applicable Research to Generate Effective Therapies (TARGET) study, infer novel targetable tumor dependencies and effective therapeutic strategies based on in silico tumor modeling, and integrate the growing body of multiomic data to optimize tumor classification, risk stratification, and therapy selection.

BIBLIOGRAPHY

1. Faratian D, Bown JL, Smith VA, Langdon SP, Harrison DJ. Cancer systems biology. *Methods Mol Biol.* 2010;662:245–263.
2. Fazlollahi L, Hsiao SJ, Kochhar M, Mansukhani MM, Yamashiro DJ, Remotti HE. Malignant rhabdoid tumor, an aggressive tumor often misclassified as small cell variant of hepatoblastoma. *Cancers (Basel).* 2019;11(12):1992.
3. Forrest SJ, Geoerger B, Janeway KA. Precision medicine in pediatric oncology. *Current Opinion in Pediatrics.* 2018;30(1):17–24.
4. Glade Bender J, Verma A, Schiffman JD. Translating genomic discoveries to the clinic in pediatric oncology. *Curr Opin Pediatr.* 2015;27(1):34–43.
5. Mody RJ, Prensner JR, Everett J, Parsons DW, Chinnaiyan AM. Precision medicine in pediatric oncology: lessons learned and next steps. *Pediatr Blood Cancer.* 2017;64(3), e26288.
6. Tran TH, Shah AT, Loh ML. Precision medicine in pediatric oncology: translating genomic discoveries into optimized therapies. *Clinical Cancer Research.* 2017;23(18):5329–5338.
7. Vo KT, Parsons DW, Seibel NL. Precision medicine in pediatric oncology. *Surg Oncol Clin N Am.* 2020;29(1):63–72.
8. Wong M, Mayoh C, Lau LMS, et al. Whole genome, transcriptome and methylome profiling enhances actionable target discovery in high-risk pediatric cancer. *Nat Med.* 2020;26(11):1742–1753.

CHAPTER 15

PREDISPOSITION SYNDROMES

Manuela Orjuela-Grimm, MD, ScM and Lianna J. Marks, MD

1. **What percent of childhood cancer is attributable to inherited mutations?**
   In a recent study of 1120 children and adolescents with cancer, germline mutations in cancer-predisposing genes were identified in 8.5% of the cases. With the exception of this small percentage of cases attributable to hereditary cancer syndromes or genetic syndromes such as Down syndrome, the etiology of most childhood cancers is unknown. Importantly family history does not appear to predict presence of cancer predisposition in the majority of hereditable pediatric cancers.

2. **Discuss the importance of rare cancers attributable to inherited mutations to the practice of pediatric oncology.**
   Despite their rarity, these syndromes and their underlying genetics permit a greater understanding of the processes underlying the development of malignancy. In addition, by identifying children at risk because of inheritance of a genetic defect, we can screen these children for the tumors for which they are at risk and potentially decrease the morbidity and mortality from their malignancy.

3. **A child referred to your service with presumed Wilms tumor is found to have tumor present in both of her kidneys. Describe the underlying genetic changes present when patients have bilateral Wilms tumor.**
   Wilms tumor is thought to originate from pluripotent embryonic renal precursors. Five to ten percent of children diagnosed with Wilms tumors present with bilateral disease and develop tumors at an earlier age (circa 2 years) than children with unilateral disease (average age at diagnosis, 5 years). Tumors of children with bilateral disease contain persistent nephrogenic rests (undifferentiated blast cells), which normally disappear shortly after birth. Their persistence in Wilms tumor suggests a constitutional abnormality in renal differentiation.

   Most children with bilateral Wilms tumor have de novo germline mutations in *WT1*. *WT1* is a tumor suppressor gene located on chromosome 11p13, which encodes a zinc finger transcription factor and is inactivated in the germline of children with genetic predisposition to Wilms tumor and in 15% of sporadic Wilms. *WT1* is a critical regulator of organ-specific differentiation; its inactivation or disruption triggers malignant transformation in embryonic cell types. *WT1* is expressed in glomerular precursors of the developing kidney, and mice who lack both copies of *WT1* do not develop kidneys.

4. **Name the genetic syndromes associated with Wilms tumor. How should children with these syndromes be followed?**
   The WAGR (Wilms tumor, aniridia, genitourinary defects, and mental retardation) and Beckwith-Wiedemann syndromes (BWS) are both associated with a predisposition to the development of Wilms tumor, and both are associated with developmental abnormalities, as well as with germline abnormalities involving gene loci on chromosome 11.

   Patients with WAGR have gross cytogenetic deletions at 11p13. This locus includes the *WT1* gene, and *PAX6*, a gene responsible for directing eye development. Loss of one copy of *WT1* in nephrogenic cells leads to genitourinary malformations, whereas Wilms tumor, which occurs in 40% of these children, results from acquired point mutations occurring in the remaining WT1 allele in renal precursor cells. Loss of one allele for *PAX6* leads to aniridia. Children with WAGR should be followed closely for abdominal masses and should have renal ultrasonograms every 3 months until they turn 7 years old.

   Children with BWS can present with asymmetric organomegaly, hypoglycemia, and umbilical hernias; in addition, they are predisposed to developing adrenocortical carcinoma, hepatoblastoma, and Wilms tumor. BWS is associated with abnormalities at the 11p15 gene locus. Fifteen percent of cases are familial. Some cases of BWS have a duplication of paternal 11p15 with no maternal contribution (uniparental isodisomy). These cases appear to have increased expression of *IGF2,* the insulin dependent growth factor 2 gene, which is also located in this chromosomal region. Other cases of BWS with demonstrated maternal imprinting (where the paternal gene is not expressed) have inactivating mutations in p57, a cyclin-dependent kinase inhibitor, identified as a cell cycle regulator, which is also located on 11p15. These children should also be followed with abdominal ultrasonograms every 3 months until the age of 7, and serum alpha fetoprotein (AFP) levels should be taken every 3 months until age 4 years.

5. **What genetic lesion characterizes desmoplastic small round cell tumors?**
   Desmoplastic small round cell tumor (DSRCT) is an embryonic neoplasm that occurs primarily in adolescent males and typically has an aggressive clinical course. These tumors normally arise within the abdomen, usually from the

peritoneal lining. Their cells express markers of epithelial, muscle, and neural lineages, suggesting that they derive from pluripotent progenitor cells. DSRCTs are characterized by the t(11;22) (p13;q12) chromosomal translocation, which fuses the N-terminal domain of the Ewing sarcoma gene *EWS* to the three C-terminal zinc fingers of *WT1*. *WT1* is normally expressed at high levels in the mesothelial cells that line visceral organs and the pleural, peritoneal, and pericardial surfaces. *WT1* is thought to play a role in regulating the mesenchymal-to-epithelial cell conversion, which is normally seen in these mesothelial cells. DSCRT is thought to arise in these mesothelial cells lacking normal *WT1* function because of the translocation.

6. A school-age child in your care is diagnosed with juvenile chronic myeloid leukemia. On examination, you notice that she has multiple café-au-lait spots greater than 5 mm. Her parents report that these spots have been present since infancy. She also has freckles in her axillae. What underlying genetic defect is this child likely to have? What other tumors is she at risk to develop?

This child likely has neurofibromatosis type 1 (NF1) or von Recklinghausen disease. NF1 is an autosomal dominant inherited disorder that affects 1 in 4000 individuals and is caused by mutations in the *NF1* gene located on 17q11.2. In newly diagnosed patients with NF1, approximately 50% of the germline mutations are de novo, not present in their parents, and occur preferentially in the paternally inherited allele. *NF1* encodes several alternatively spliced transcripts. Its product is neurofibromin, a cytoplasmic protein belonging to the *Ras* guanosine triphosphatase (GTPase) activating group of proteins, which acts as a tumor suppressor. Neurofibromin is expressed in most tissues, but it is found at highest levels in the central nervous system (CNS) and peripheral nervous system and in the adrenal gland, which is consistent with the distribution of organs most frequently affected by this disease.

Diagnostic criteria for NF1 include the presence of at least two of the following:
- Six café-au-lait spots of at least 5 mm in diameter if prepubertal (or >15 mm if postpubertal)
- Axillary or inguinal freckling
- Two or more neurofibromas (originating from Schwann progenitor cells)
- One plexiform neurofibroma
  - An optic nerve glioma
  - A distinctive osseous lesion (such as sphenoid wing dysplasia)
- A first degree relative with NF1.

Children with NF1 are at increased risk for developing benign and malignant solid tumors, which include iris hamartomas (Lisch nodules), glioblastoma multiforme, rhabdomyosarcomas, pheochromocytomas, and carcinoid tumors, as well as hematologic malignancies, including de novo juvenile chronic myelogenous leukemia, monosomy 7 syndrome, and acute myelogenous leukemia. In addition, 5% of plexiform neurofibromas progress to malignant peripheral nerve sheath tumors. The majority of gliomas found in patients with NF1 are pilocytic astrocytomas arising within the optic nerve.

7. A teenage boy is found to have a thyroid nodule on routine examination. Endocrinologic studies reveal that his serum calcitonin levels are elevated. His younger brother has Hirschsprung disease. They are foster children, and the foster parents have been told that the biological mother had a "kidney" tumor. Which genetic syndrome might this family have? What genetic test would you do for this child and his sibling? What would you recommend as follow-up for the younger brother if the test were positive?

This family history suggests that the older brother may have medullary thyroid carcinoma, a malignant tumor derived from parafollicular C cells in the thyroid. These brothers may be affected by one of the multiple endocrine neoplasia type 2 (MEN2) syndromes, MEN2A or MEN2B, which are autosomal dominant genetic syndromes associated with specific germline mutations in the *RET* proto-oncogene. *RET*, located at chromosome 10q11.2, encodes a receptor functioning as a tyrosine kinase. Germline mutations in this gene are observed in 95% of patients with MEN2B and in 98% of those with MEN2A. The nature and location of these mutations correlates closely with the syndrome type.

Most familial cases (60%) are MEN2A. In addition to medullary thyroid carcinoma, the most frequently associated diseases in MEN2A are pheochromocytomas (in 50% of patients) and hyperparathyroidism, which can occur before or after the diagnosis of thyroid disease. In some families with MEN2A, children are at increased risk for Hirschsprung disease in their first years of life.

MEN2B is an aggressive and rare disorder representing 5% of inherited medullary thyroid cancers that occur early in life. The syndrome involves locally invasive thyroid tumors that can cause compressive symptoms and frequently have early mediastinal and lung metastases. MEN2B is associated with developmental abnormalities including marfanoid habitus; overgrowth of neural tissue of the lips, tongue, and conjunctivae; and ganglioneuromatosis of the intestinal tract. Pheochromocytomas are also present, usually bilaterally, and are usually diagnosed after the thyroid disease. This form is not associated with primary hyperparathyroidism.

Familial screening for MEN2 is now offered to detect thyroid disease before clinical manifestations so that curative presymptomatic thyroidectomies can be performed. Screening is based on *RET* mutation detection in genomic DNA extracted from peripheral blood leukocytes. This genetic testing should be performed at birth in children suspected of having the MEN2B syndrome and before the age of 1 year in those with possible MEN2A. If specific *RET* gene mutations are noted, total thyroidectomy is recommended as soon as the diagnosis is established. For MEN2A patients, thyroidectomy should be performed before 5 years of age, whereas patients with MEN2B may need surgery during the first 6 months to 1 year of life. Given this family history, the younger brother is most likely to have a genetic defect consistent with MEN2A; if so, then prophylactic thyroidectomy should be performed before he turns 5 years.

8. A 12-year-old girl presents with knee pain and is found to have an osteogenic sarcoma arising in the distal femur. She is brought by her father because her mother is undergoing treatment for breast cancer. Her brother died at age 6 of a brain tumor. On further questioning, you discover that two maternal aunts also had breast cancer in their 30s. The patient's 10-year-old sister is clinically well. What genetic syndrome do you suspect? What tumor suppressor protein is associated with this syndrome? How would you follow her and her sister?
This family appears to have Li-Fraumeni Syndrome (LFS), an autosomal dominant disorder characterized by germline mutations in the *P53* tumor suppressor gene, which is located on chromosome 17p13. Patients with LFS are at increased risk for early onset of bone and soft tissue sarcomas, breast and adrenal cortex carcinomas, brain tumors, especially primitive neuroectodermal tumors and astrocytomas, and acute leukemia. The *P53* gene was first described as a result of studying families with this syndrome. It encodes a protein, p53, which is expressed at low levels in many cell types. This tumor suppressor protein plays a key role in controlling cell cycle progression and providing DNA repair after oxidative damage or mutagenic DNA damage. Hypoxic and mutagenic DNA damage leads to nuclear accumulation and activation of p53. In addition, p53 transcriptionally activates genes that induce cell cycle arrest and apoptosis. Mutant p53, such as that found in patients with LFS, is unable to suppress tumor development and can inhibit wild-type P53. Somatic *P53* mutations are also found in tumor cells in sporadically occurring tumors. The most common types of *P53* mutations in both LFS and in sporadically occurring tumors are point mutations causing cytosine-to-adenine transitions at CpG sites (G:C changes to A:T) and arise from deamination of 5-methylcytosine. Although these types of mutations can occur spontaneously, they are usually corrected by DNA repair mechanisms.

DNA from this child can be examined to look for mutations in *P53*. These would be expected to be present both in her tumor DNA and in her genomic DNA (and thus in her leukocytes). Once a *P53* mutation is found, her sister's leukocytes could be examined to probe for the mutation. If her sister is found to have mutant *P53,* she can be counseled and followed closely to detect potential cancers at earlier stages. This patient will also need to be followed closely for early development of breast cancer. It is unknown whether avoidance of risk factors associated with development of sporadic breast cancer will decrease her probability of developing this disease.

9. A teenager presents in the emergency department with a history of severe headaches and sudden loss of consciousness. He is found on magnetic resonance imaging (MRI) to have multiple cystic lesions in his cerebellum. His hemoglobin is 16 mg/dL. His father reports that the boy's grandfather died of a kidney tumor and that he himself was also recently diagnosed with a kidney tumor. The boy's 8-year-old sister is completely well. What genetic syndrome do you suspect in this family, and what do you expect these cystic lesions contain? How should this boy and his younger sister be followed?
This family probably has von Hippel-Lindau (VHL) disease, which is transmitted through autosomal dominant inheritance of a germline mutation of the *VHL* tumor suppressor gene located on chromosome 3p5-26. The VHL protein (pVHL) is involved in cell cycle regulation (with the transition from G2 into G0, the quiescent phase) and angiogenesis (deficiency of pVHL is associated with overexpression of vascular endothelial growth factor). The *VHL* gene is expressed in epithelial cells in skin; gastrointestinal, respiratory, and urogenital tracts; and endocrine and exocrine organs. In the CNS, pVHL is found primarily in the Purkinje cells of the cerebellum.

The characteristic clinical findings in VHL disease include multiple capillary hemangioblastomas in the CNS (primarily in the cerebellum, brainstem, and spinal cord and usually accompanied by cysts or syrinxes), retinal hemangioblastomas, renal cell carcinoma, pheochromocytomas, clear cell renal carcinoma, and pancreatic and inner ear tumors. This youth has a typical presentation that likely consists of multiple hemangioblastomas and adjacent cysts. The cysts can cause impaired cerebrospinal fluid flow and increased intracranial pressure, which can lead to the presenting symptoms. The hemangioblastomas themselves are often present in the walls of the large cysts. Because these tumors can produce erythropoietin, patients can present with secondary polycythemia.

Mortality in patients with VHL is primarily caused by effects secondary to the cranial hemangioblastomas. Affected individuals should undergo periodic MRI to detect presymptomatic cranial lesions. Treatment is usually surgical or with gamma-knife radiation, although tyrosine kinase inhibitors and monoclonal antibodies targeting the VEG-F pathway are currently in experimental trials. Patients should also have regular ophthalmologic examinations to detect and remove retinal hemangioblastomas before they cause significant retinal damage. This boy and his sister (and his father and other paternal family members) should have genetic testing done to look for *VHL* mutations.

10. **A child presents with newly diagnosed Wilms tumor. You notice that the child is smaller than expected for her age and that she has malar hypoplasia and a telangiectatic rash on her cheeks. Her parents report that the rash worsens with sun exposure and that she has been small since birth. Describe the genetic defect this child might have**

This child may have Bloom syndrome, a rare autosomal recessive disorder involving a mutation in the *BLM* gene, which is located at 15q26.1. The *BLM* gene encodes a DNA helicase, and functional mutations in this gene lead to defective DNA repair characterized by increased sister chromatid exchanges. Bloom syndrome is characterized by prenatal and postnatal growth retardation, photosensitivity (causing a facial telangiectatic rash), and malar hypoplasia. Twenty-five percent of persons with Bloom's syndrome develop some form of malignancy including leukemia, lymphoma or Wilms tumor as children and breast, stomach, or colon adenocarcinomas as adults, often with an early age of onset.

11. **An infant presents with hepatoblastoma. His maternal grandmother was diagnosed with colon cancer before she was 40, and his mother and maternal aunts have undergone prophylactic colectomies. Name the genetic syndrome this family is likely to have. What is the underlying genetic defect? What follow-up should this child and his siblings receive?**

This family probably suffers from familial adenomatous polyposis (FAP), an autosomal dominant inherited syndrome characterized by the presence of adenomatous polyps in the colon and rectum and development of colorectal cancer. Children in these families are also at an increased risk for hepatoblastoma. FAP is caused by germline mutations in the adenomatous polyposis coli (*APC*) gene. The *APC* gene, located on chromosome 5q21-22, encodes a large multidomain protein that plays an integral role in the Wnt-signaling pathway, intercellular adhesion, stabilization of the cytoskeleton, and possibly regulation of the cell cycle and apoptosis. *APC* mutations almost always result in a truncated protein product with abnormal function. Inheritance of *APC* germline mutations has a penetrance of almost 100%, but phenotypic expression is quite variable. Persons affected by FAP develop thousands of adenomatous polyps in their colon and rectum usually by adolescence or by age 30. Colorectal cancer invariably develops by age 40. Colorectal tumors from FAP patients carry additional somatic APC mutations or loss of heterozygosity at this locus in addition to the original germline mutation.

One variant of FAP, Gardner's syndrome, is characterized by the presence of innumerable colonic polyps, in addition to epidermoid skin cysts and benign osteoid tumors of the mandible and long bones. Follow-up for this child should follow the recommended screening for children with APC, which includes colonoscopy starting at age 10 years and prophylactic colectomy. The value of screening for hepatoblastoma is controversial but includes serum AFP levels and abdominal ultrasound every 3 months until age 7 years.

This chapter does not include discussion of retinoblastoma, which is also a cancer predisposition syndrome. Please see the chapter on retinoblastoma for discussion of this entity.

BIBLIOGRAPHY

1. Achatz M, Porter CC, Brugières L, et al. Cancer screening recommendations and clinical management of inherited gastrointestinal cancer syndromes in childhood. *Clin Cancer Res.* 2017;23(13):e107–e114. PMID: 28674119.
2. Evans DGR, Salvador H, Chang VY, et al. Cancer and central nervous system tumor surveillance in pediatric neurofibromatosis 1. *Clin Cancer Res.* 2017;23(12):e46–e53. PMID: 28620004.
3. Glasker S. Von Hippel-Lindau disease: current challenges and future prospects. *Onco Targets Ther.* 2020;13:5669–5690. PMID: 32606780.
4. Kalish JM, Doros L, Helman LJ, et al. Surveillance recommendations for children with overgrowth syndromes and predisposition to Wilms tumors and hepatoblastoma. *Clin Cancer Res.* 2017;23(13):e115–e122. PMID: 28674120.
5. Valdez JM, Nichols KE, Kesserwan C. Li-Fraumeni syndrome: a paradigm for the understanding of hereditary cancer predisposition. *Br J Haematol.* 2017;176(4):539–552. PMID: 27984644.
6. Wasserman JD, Tomlinson GE, Druker H, et al. Multiple endocrine neoplasia and hyperparathyroid-jaw tumor syndromes: clinical features, genetics, and surveillance recommendations in childhood. *Clin Cancer Res.* 2017;23(13):e123–e132. PMID: 28674121.
7. Zhang J, Walsh MF, Wu G, et al. Germline mutations in predisposition genes in pediatric cancer. *N Eng J Med.* 2015;373(24):2336–2346. PMID: 26580448.

⊕ Additional references available online.

CHAPTER 16

HEALTH EQUITY AND DISPARITIES IN PEDIATRIC AND ADOLESCENT/ YOUNG ADULT ONCOLOGY

Melissa P. Beauchemin, PhD, RN, CPNP and Justine M. Kahn, MD, MS

1. **What are health disparities?**
   In discussions about cancer-related outcomes, the word "disparity" is often used interchangeably with other words like "difference" or "inequity." But disparities are not simply "any" differences in health. Rather, disparities, as defined by the World Health Organization (WHO), are *avoidable* differences in health arising from the social and economic conditions that determine an individual's risk of illness, and the actions taken to prevent or treat said illness.

2. **What are *cancer* health disparities?**
   The National Cancer Institute (NCI) defines cancer health disparities as adverse differences in cancer incidence, prevalence, cancer-related mortality, survivorship, and burden of cancer or related health conditions that exist among disadvantaged or minority populations in the United States.

3. **What is a vulnerable population?**
   The Health and Human Services (HHS) Office of Minority Health defines a health disparity as a particular type of difference in health in which socially disadvantaged groups, including poor patients, racial/ethnic minorities, women, LGBTQIA, and any other people who face persistent disadvantage and discrimination systematically experience worse health or greater risk than more advantaged social groups. These groups who systematically experience worse health outcomes are known collectively as vulnerable populations.

4. **What factors contribute to cancer health disparities?**
   Factors contributing to differential outcomes among diverse groups can be biologic or non-biologic in etiology. In general, when speaking about health disparities, the emphasis is on non-biologic factors, specifically, the social determinants of people's lives that impact their ability to achieve good health. Factors contributing to cancer outcome disparities – and health inequities – operate at many levels. These range from policy factors, like insurance coverage and Medicaid/Medicare, to system-levels, like access to transportation and high-quality medical care, to individual level factors at both the patient and provider levels, including bias, discrimination, mistrust, or health beliefs.

5. **What are social determinants of health?**
   The underlying social and structural factors that drive disparities in risk and outcome are referred to as social determinants of health (SDOH). Broadly, SDOH are defined as the upstream social and economic conditions in which people are born, grow, live, work, and age that shape both individual and population differences in health status. These determinants include five domains:
   - Economic stability
   - Education access and quality
   - Neighborhood and built environment
   - Social and community context
   - Health care access and quality.

6. **Explain the difference between "genetic ancestry" and "race/ethnicity."**
   Both biologic and socioeconomic mechanisms have been proposed as causes of cancer disparities. Underlying genetic variations associated with ancestry may lead to differences in tumor biology and pharmacogenetics for some childhood cancers. However, race and ethnicity are not the same as genetic ancestry. Race is highly correlated with socioeconomic status (SES), particularly in the United States, where institutionalized racism continues to place Black and Hispanic patients at risk of living in underresourced neighborhoods with high rates of poverty.

7. **How does the NCI define the adolescent/young adult (AYA) age group?**
   The NCI definition of AYA includes patients ages 15 to 39 years old.

8. **Why is the AYA population of concern in terms of cancer-related outcomes?**
   Improving the quality of cancer treatment and survivorship care for AYAs with cancer is a priority area in the United States because this group has not experienced the survival gains enjoyed by other age groups over the past two decades. This is an important public health need: Cancer is the leading cause of nonaccidental death in AYAs. Progress

in AYA outcomes has been hampered by their underrecognized cancer risk, the lack of knowledge about the most effective treatment settings and survivorship care for this population, and the poorer access to health and supportive care because this age group has historically been the most highly uninsured in the United States. Inferior outcomes among AYAs vs. children are compounded in patients from vulnerable populations like, non-White race/ethnicity, or those from low-income groups.

9. **How does cancer care delivery influence outcomes?**
   In the context of disparities, cancer care delivery research examines how inequities (meaning avoidable differences in cancer care) can be evaluated and addressed to reduce disparities in vulnerable populations.

10. **What are some examples of observed disparities in pediatric oncology?**
    Compared with White children, Black and Hispanic children experience lower survival from many cancers, including leukemias, lymphomas, central nervous system (CNS) tumors, and extracranial solid tumors. The underlying causes of racial/ethnic survival differences are not well understood and may vary by cancer type; examples include the following:
    - Acute lymphoblastic leukemia (ALL): Several studies have reported racial/ethnic survival differences in children with ALL. One analysis of Children's Cancer Group studies found that Black and Hispanic patients were significantly more likely than White patients to have relapsed disease. In another analysis from the Dana-Farber Cancer Institute ALL Consortium, Hispanic patients treated on the clinical trial were significantly more likely than White patients to have disease recurrence.
    - Acute myeloid leukemia (AML): Black children with AML are more likely than White children to present with high acuity disease and to require admission to the Intensive care unit. As a result, studies have shown that the rates of death during the first cycle of AML therapy is significantly increased in Black versus White patients.
      In a separate analysis of phase 3 clinical trials in children with AML, Hispanic and Black patients treated with chemotherapy had significantly worse overall survival compared with White children, even within the context of a cooperative group clinical trial, suggesting the possibility of differences in leukemia biology across groups.
    - Hodgkin lymphoma: Both population-based and cooperative group analyses have reported significantly worse outcomes for children and AYAs with newly diagnosed Hodgkin lymphoma. In those with relapsed disease, Black and Hispanic patients are up to three times more likely to die than White patients.
    - CNS tumors: Population-based studies have reported racial/ethnic differences in the histologic subtypes of certain CNS tumors. A recent study using population-based data reported higher risk of death in Black and Hispanic children (versus White) children with CNS tumors.
    - Neuroblastoma: Cooperative group analyses have reported higher prevalence of high-risk disease among Black and Native American patients (versus White). This accounts for the reported worse event-free survival observed in these patients.

11. **Discuss inequities in cancer supportive care.**
    There is a wide variability in clinical settings, and evidence-based supportive care clinical practice guidelines are not consistently implemented in practice. For example, prevention of chemotherapy-induced nausea and vomiting, common treatment-related adverse effects for children and adolescents with cancer, are not consistently managed according to published clinical practice guidelines. Racial and socioeconomic disparities in receipt of guideline concordant care for antiemetic prophylaxis have been reported. Similarly, studies have shown that those with commercial insurance are significantly more likely to receive GCC compared with those with public insurance. Disparities in provision of high-quality GCC may not only affect tolerability of treatment regimens but also negatively impact long-term health-related quality of life.

12. **Describe ongoing efforts to address cancer health disparities.**
    Just as the drivers of cancer disparities happen at multiple levels from the society to the patient, interventions are happening at all levels. The clearest example of this at the federal level was the Affordable Care Act, and many states are implementing policies to ensure even more insurance coverage for their poorest citizens. At the cancer research level, much attention is being paid to clinical trial participation in under-represented populations. Clinical trials are considered essential for the discovery and development of better drugs and treatments for cancer. For example, the NCI's Community Oncology Research Program aims to reduce cancer disparities by offering patient's access to cancer clinical trials in community practices.

13. **What is financial toxicity?**
    Financial toxicity is broadly defined as the "harmful personal financial burden (i.e., demands on household income) faced by patients receiving cancer treatment." Financial toxicity is a potentially devastating adverse effect of cancer therapy. In adult cancer patients, three domains of financial toxicity have been described: material hardship (loss of income, high out of pocket costs), psychological responses (distress or anxiety related to the costs of cancer care), and coping behaviors (skipping or modifying medications or treatments because of costs and modifying spending or financial savings behavior). In adults with cancer, financial toxicity has been associated with poorer health outcomes and earlier mortality. Currently, much research is ongoing to better understand financial toxicity in pediatric oncology to ultimately intervene and improve cancer outcomes, particularly among vulnerable populations.

14. **How are children and adolescents with cancer, and their families, impacted by financial toxicity?**

Although the full scope of financial toxicity is not well understood in pediatric oncology, with 80% of children and adolescents expected to become long-term survivors of cancer at diagnosis, the effect is likely significant and potentially lifelong for the patient and their family. Because successful treatment of pediatric cancer requires a commitment to intensive therapy, often including hospitalizations, oral chemotherapy, and other components of care that have additional costs, current research to understand and develop strategies to mitigate financial toxicity is imperative. Finally, with the extensive impact of the COVID-19 pandemic on financial status and psychological burden, we must be cognizant to develop feasible, acceptable, and sustainable interventions because financial hardships may be protracted.

BIBLIOGRAPHY

1. Altice CK, Banegas MP, Tucker-Seeley RD, et al. Financial hardships experienced by cancer survivors: a systematic review. *J Natl Cancer Inst.* 2016;109(2):djw205.
2. Aristizabal P. Diverse populations and enrollment in pediatric cancer clinical trials: challenges and opportunities. *Pediatr Blood Cancer.* 2020. e28296.
3. Beauchemin M, Sung L, Hershman DL, et al. Guideline concordant care for prevention of acute chemotherapy-induced nausea and vomiting in children, adolescents, and young adults. *Support Care Cancer.* 2020;28(10):4761–4769.
4. Beauchemin, M, Santacroce, SJ, Bona, K, et al. Rationale and design of Children's Oncology Group (COG) study ACCL20N1CD: financial distress during treatment of acute lymphoblastic leukemia in the United States. *BMC Health Serv Rcs.* 2022;22,832.
5. Kahn JM, Cole PD, Blonquist TM, et al. An investigation of toxicities and survival in Hispanic children and adolescents with ALL: Results from the Dana-Farber Cancer Institute ALL Consortium protocol 05-001. *Pediatr Blood Cancer.* 2018;65(3):10.1002/pbc.26871.
6. Kahn JM, Keegan TH, Tao L, et al. Racial disparities in the survival of American children, adolescents, and young adults with acute lymphoblastic leukemia, acute myelogenous leukemia, and Hodgkin lymphoma. *Cancer.* 2016;122(17):2723–30.
7. Kahn JM, Kelly KM, Pei Q, et al. Survival by race and ethnicity in pediatric and adolescent patients with Hodgkin lymphoma: a children's oncology group study. *J Clin Oncol.* 2019;37(32):3009–3017.
8. Koh HK, Piotrowski JJ, Kumanyika S, Fielding JE. Healthy people: a 2020 vision for the social determinants approach. *Health Educ Behav.* 2011;38(6):551–557.
9. Marmot MG, Bell R. Action on health disparities in the United States: commission on social determinants of health. *JAMA.* 2009;301(11):1169–1171.
10. Santacroce SJ, Kneipp SM. A conceptual model of financial toxicity in pediatric oncology. *J Pediatr Oncol Nurs.* 2019;36:6–16.
11. Venkatapuram S, Marmot M. Epidemiology and social justice in light of social determinants of health research. *Bioethics.* 2009;23(2):79–89.
12. Warner EL, Kirchhoff AC, Nam GE, et al. Financial burden of pediatric cancer for patients and their families. *J Oncol Pract.* 2015;11:12–18.
13. Winestone LE, Getz KD, Miller TP, et al. The role of acuity of illness at presentation in early mortality in black children with acute myeloid leukemia. *Am J Hematol.* 2017;92(2):141–148.
14. Yousuf Zafar S. Financial toxicity of cancer care: it's time to intervene. *JNCI.* 2015;108(5):djv370.

CHAPTER 17

CLINICAL EMERGENCIES IN CHILDREN WITH CANCER

Andrea Webster Carrion, MD and Michael Weiner, MD

1. **What is tumor lysis syndrome?**

   Tumor lysis syndrome (TLS) is defined by the metabolic derangements that result from massive release of intracellular contents into the systemic circulation secondary to the initiation of cytotoxic therapy. The laboratory findings of TLS include hyperuricemia, hyperkalemia, hyperphosphatemia, hypocalcemia, and an increasing serum creatinine; clinically, TLS may cause renal failure, cardiac arrhythmias, seizures, or sudden death. Serum lactate dehydrogenase (LDH) is not a component of the syndrome; however, it can be used as a risk assessment surrogate for rapid cell turnover. Occasionally, in situations where the initial tumor burden is extremely high, such as in Burkitt lymphoma, acute lymphoblastic leukemia (ALL) with white blood cell (WBC) count greater than 100,000/mm^3, and acute myelogenous leukemia (AML) with WBC greater than 50,000/mm^3, a phenomenon referred to as hyperleukocytosis, TLS may occur spontaneously.

2. **Describe the management of TLS.**

   It is imperative to perform a tumor lysis risk assessment at the time of initial presentation and disease diagnosis. Risk should be assessed based on patient comorbidities, laboratory criteria, tumor type, cell burden, cell lysis potential, rate of proliferation, and degree of renal impairment. Continuous monitoring, a high index of suspicion, and preparation for early intervention are mandatory. The most important measures are ensuring adequate urine output and the use of hypouricemic agents. Allopurinol, a xanthine analog, works as a competitive xanthine oxidase inhibitor, slowing the production of uric acid and decreasing the risk of acid crystallization in kidney tubules. Rasburicase is the preferred prophylactic agent in cases of high-risk TLS and as treatment in patients with hyperuricemia. Rasburicase is a recombinant urate oxidase that catalyzes the oxidation of uric acid to allantoin, which is 5 to 10 times more urine soluble than uric acid. G6PD screening should always be performed to prevent methemoglobinemia or severe hemolytic anemia. Allopurinol should be stopped if rasburicase is started.

3. **What are hyperleukocytosis and leukostasis?**

   Hyperleukocytosis is defined as a WBC greater than 100,000/mm^3. Leukostasis is the term used to describe the tissue hypoperfusion associated with hyperleukocytosis. Hyperleukocytosis is usually seen in T-cell ALL, infant ALL, monocytic or monoblastic subtypes of AML, acute promyelocytic leukemia (APL), and chronic myelogenous leukemia. Leukostasis, however, is more commonly seen in AML because myeloid blasts are relatively larger in size, less deformable, and more adherent to the vasculature than lymphoblasts.

   The intracerebral and pulmonary circulations are most vulnerable to the effects of leukostasis; the most common pulmonary symptoms include dyspnea, tachypnea, hypoxemia, and right-sided heart failure. Chest radiographs can reveal varying degrees of diffuse interstitial or alveolar infiltrates. Life-threatening cardiorespiratory failure may result. Neurologic involvement can present with frontal headaches, seizures, mental status changes, weakness, papilledema, or retinal venous distention. Hemorrhagic stroke is a feared complication that can be seen in acute promyelocytic leukemia. Other organ systems are less frequently involved but can present as oliguria, anuria, priapism, disseminated intravascular coagulopathy (DIC), renal vein thrombosis, and retinal hemorrhage, among others.

   The management should include emergent cytoreductive therapy and hyperhydration for reduction of blood viscosity and prevention of TLS. Rasburicase is recommended. Additionally, monitoring for DIC and ensuring a platelet count greater than 20×10^9/L in nonbleeding patients is beneficial. To date, leukapheresis has failed to show evidence of mortality reduction and its use remains controversial because of potential complications.

4. **Describe the spectrum of cytokine release syndrome.**

   Cytokine release syndrome (CRS) is the term used to describe a spectrum of reactions seen after administration of targeted therapies, such as chimeric antigen receptor (CAR) T-cell therapies and bispecific T-cell engaging antibodies, that cause significant activation of the immune system. In contrast to cytokine storm, the term CRS is usually used to describe a delayed onset of clinical symptoms as a result of T-cell activation and proliferation. Nevertheless, no single definition of cytokine storm or the cytokine release syndrome is widely accepted. The cytokines that are consistently found to be elevated are interleukin (IL)-6, IL-10, and interferon (IFN)-γ. CRS may occur 1 to 14 days after CAR T-cell infusion and rarely develops more than 17 days after infusion. Initial presentation can mimic a flu-like illness and sepsis. It can progress to vasodilatory shock, acute respiratory distress syndrome, multiorgan failure, and DIC. Laboratory abnormalities commonly include cytopenias, elevated creatinine, heightened liver enzymes, deranged coagulation parameters, and a high C-reactive protein (CRP).

If CRS is suspected, a severity scoring system should be used to better assess the need to start treatment. The most widely used grading scheme for the severity of CRS was developed by the National Cancer Institute (NCI). Consider early intensive care unit (ICU) referral. Patients that develop grade 3 or 4 CRS toxicity should immediately receive treatment with tocilizumab. This is an approved monoclonal antibody against the IL-6 receptor that has been found to be effective in CRS, without affecting the CAR T-cell therapy function. Corticosteroids should generally be avoided as first-line treatment of CRS in patients receiving CAR T cells and should be reserved for refractory cases or in severe neurotoxicity.

5. **Describe superior vena cava syndrome.**
Superior vena cava (SVC) syndrome is a clinical phenomenon that develops when a mass lesion obstructs the blood flow through the SVC. The obstruction can be because of external compression, invasion of an adjacent tumor into the SVC, or thrombosis. Collateral veins of the thorax, neck, and head engorge and produce the classic symptoms that include dyspnea; fullness and plethora of the face, head, and upper extremities; periorbital edema; dysphagia; cough; and chest pain. The more acute the onset of the SVC obstruction, the more significant the signs and symptoms present and the more imperative it is to initiate lifesaving therapy. It is crucial to identify patients with life-threatening symptoms such as cerebral edema, severe laryngeal edema, and hemodynamic compromise.

Malignant tumors are the most common cause of SVC syndrome in pediatric patients. The "terrible Ts"—T-cell non-Hodgkin lymphoma (lymphoblastic lymphoma or large cell lymphoma), T-cell acute lymphoblastic leukemia, malignant teratomas, thyroid cancer, and thymomas—may all cause this syndrome. Hodgkin disease is not infrequently associated with SVC syndrome, whereas neuroblastoma, rhabdomyosarcoma, and Ewing sarcoma are rare causes. Occlusion of a central venous catheter, as in the case of thrombus, in a child with cancer may cause a secondary form of SVC syndrome.

On initial imaging, a chest radiograph can reveal mediastinal widening or pleural effusion. The imaging modality of choice is a contrast-enhanced computed tomography (CT) venogram. In severe cases, it may be necessary to initiate empiric therapy with high-dose glucocorticoids and/or directed, targeted radiotherapy. The biopsy to confirm the diagnosis should be delayed until it can be performed safely. Airway management should be decided by a multidisciplinary team and should include determination of anesthesia risk because of high risk of tracheal collapse, inability to ventilate, and worsening hypotension with the use of sedatives and paralytics.

6. **Describe the signs and symptoms of spinal cord compression.**
Back pain and localized tenderness occur in most children with spinal cord compression at presentation. In children with a history of cancer, the presence of these signs and symptoms should cause concern for spinal cord compromise until proven otherwise. Additional neurologic findings, if present, will depend on the spinal level involvement and degree of compression. Weakness that may lead to partial or complete paralysis and incontinence tend to develop later in the course if the symptoms persist. Sensory deficits may also occur but are difficult to elicit, especially in younger children.

Spinal cord compression is present in 3% to 5% of children with cancer at diagnosis and can also be seen in metastatic, relapsed, or disease progression cases. The most common pathologies associated with spinal cord compression are neuroblastoma and sarcomas, such as Ewing sarcoma and rhabdomyosarcoma. Less frequent causes are metastatic central nervous tumors, lymphomas, meningiomas, AML, and osteosarcomas.

Early diagnosis and proactive treatment are vital to improving prognosis and survival. When spinal cord dysfunction is suspected based on history and physical examination findings, dexamethasone should be given immediately. Plain films have low sensitivity and are usually unhelpful. Magnetic resonance imaging (MRI) is the ideal modality and should include the entire neural-axis (brain and whole spine). Sedation and analgesia may be required to allow for adequate patient positioning. Additional therapeutic options should be considered by a multidisciplinary team depending on the etiology. Interventions include surgical decompression, radiation, and chemotherapy.

7. **What is the differential diagnosis of a child with right lower quadrant abdominal pain and neutropenia?**
Necrotizing colitis of the cecum, also known as typhlitis, is a major concern in a child with prolonged, severe neutropenia who presents with localized right lower-quadrant abdominal pain. Bacterial invasion of the mucosa may progress from inflammation to infarction and perforation. *Clostridium septicum* and *Pseudomonas aeruginosa* are most often involved. Children with AML are at higher risk because of the prolonged neutropenic phase and the common use of chemotherapeutic regimens that are toxic to the gastrointestinal tract. CT scan may reveal thickening of the cecal wall or, in advanced cases, pneumatosis intestinalis. Treatment is primarily supportive with antibiotic coverage for gram-negative and anaerobic organisms; however, a surgical consult should be requested because some patients may require surgical intervention.

8. **Which chemotherapeutic agents are associated with a risk of acute cerebral infarctions?**
L-asparaginase can cause either cerebral vascular hemorrhage or thrombosis as a result of its inhibition of synthesis of coagulation factors. Cisplatin can lead to cerebral ischemia from renal wasting of magnesium inducing arterial spasm or direct thrombotic endothelial injury. Methotrexate, after either high-dose intravenous or intrathecal administration, may also lead to cerebral infarction, either from direct vascular injury or from an embolic effect. In a series of pediatric patients with acute cerebral infarctions, 30% were directly related to chemotherapy.

BIBLIOGRAPHY

1. Henry M, Sung L. Supportive care in pediatric oncology: oncologic emergencies and management of fever and neutropenia. *Pediatr Clin North Am.* 2015;62(1):27–46.
2. Freedman Jason L, Rheingold Susan R, Fisher Michael J. Chapter 38: oncologic emergencies. In: Poplack Pizzo Philip A, David G (eds). *Principles and Oractice of Pediatric Oncology. 7th ed.* Lippincott Williams & Wilkins, 2016:967–991.
3. Mullen EA, Gratias E. Oncologic emergencies. In: Orkin SH, Fisher DE, Ginsburg D, Look AT, Lux SE, Nathan DG (eds). *Nathan and Oski's Hematology and Oncology of Infancy and Childhood.* 8th ed. Elsevier Saunders, 2015:2267–2291.
4. Shimabukuro-Vornhagen A, Gödel P, Subklewe M, et al. Cytokine release syndrome. *J Immunother. Cancer.* 2018;6(1):56.
5. Williams SM, Killeen AA. Tumor lysis syndrome. *Arch Pathol Lab Med.* 2019;143:386–393.

CHAPTER 18

TRANSFUSION MEDICINE

Chinwe Madubata, Maha Al-Ghafry, and Stuart P. Weisberg

1. Describe the collection processes, storage conditions, clinical indications, and pediatric dosing for red blood cells, fresh frozen plasma, platelets, and cryoprecipitate (see Table 18.1).
   Red blood cells (RBCs):
   - Indication: Increase oxygen-carrying capacity
   - Collection: Apheresis or centrifugation of whole blood
   - Storage: 1°C to 6°C
   - Dosing: 10 to 15 mL/kg
   Fresh frozen plasma (FFP):
   - Indication: Broad coagulation factor replacement
   - Collection: Apheresis from single donors, centrifugation of whole blood, or pooled and solvent detergent treated from multiple donors
   - Storage: -18°C
   - Dosing: 10 to 15 mL/kg
   Platelets:
   - Indication: To prevent or treat bleeding because of thrombocytopenia or qualitative platelet defect
   - Collection: Apheresis from single donors but also may be separated from units of whole blood
   - One "unit" of single donor apheresis platelet product is roughly equivalent to 6 "units" of whole blood–derived platelets
   - Storage: 20°C to 24°C with gentle agitation
   - Dosing: 5 to 10 mL/kg
   Cryoprecipitate:
   - Indication: To prevent or treat bleeding because of hypofibrinogenemia or factor XIII deficiency
   - Collection: Cold-insoluble precipitate of FFP during thawing

2. Describe transfusion reactions that frequently present with dyspnea and the clinical testing needed to evaluate new dyspnea during transfusions (see Table 18.2).
   Transfusion-associated acute lung injury (TRALI) is an inflammation mediated acute lung injury caused by donor antibodies targeting recipient white blood cell (WBC) human leukocyte antigens (HLA) or human neutrophil antigens (HNA). Symptoms include dyspnea and hypoxemia with or without fever within 6 hours of transfusion. Chest imaging is indicated, and the blood supplier must be notified to identify anti-HLA and anti-HNA antibodies in the donor with specificity for antigens in the recipient. The presence of donor antibodies affirms the diagnosis of TRALI.

   Transfusion-associated circulatory overload (TACO), cardiogenic pulmonary edema, is caused by fluid overload from excessive transfusion volumes or rate. Symptoms include dyspnea and hypoxemia with signs of elevated central venous pressure within 6 hours of transfusion. Evaluation with chest imaging and the assessment of N-terminal pro–B-type natriuretic peptide (BNP) levels, a biomarker for heart failure, are indicated. TACO usually responds well to diuresis.

   Allergen-induced airway compromise results from allergic reaction to an immunoglobulin (Ig) caused by E and histamine-mediated reaction to allergens in donor plasma. Symptoms of wheezing and/or bronchospasm along with other allergic symptoms (e.g., hives, itching, angioedema, flushing, hypotension) with spectrum of severity from mild to severe anaphylaxis may occur. Patients with history of severe allergic transfusion reaction should be tested for IgA deficiency and haptoglobin deficiency.

3. When is performing a direct antiglobulin test clinically indicated?
   A direct antiglobulin test (DAT) is clinically indicated for conditions in which antibody-mediated RBC destruction is suspected:
   - Newborns with elevated bilirubin or jaundice to assess for hemolytic disease of the fetus and newborn (HDFN)
   - Transfusion recipients with suspected acute or delayed hemolytic transfusion reaction
   - Patients with suspected autoimmune hemolysis
   - Hematopoietic stem cell transplant (HSCT)-related alloimmune hemolysis during early engraftment. In major ABO incompatibility transplant, the recipient harbors antibodies and antibody-producing plasma cells against donor RBC. In minor ABO incompatibility transplant, donor lymphocytes cause formation of antibodies against recipient RBC (passenger lymphocyte syndrome).

Table 18.1 Blood Products With their Pediatric Dosing, Indications, Processing, and Storage

COMPONENT DOSAGE FOR PATIENTS <50 KG	INDICATIONS	COLLECTION PROCESS	STORAGE TEMPERATURE
Red blood cells (RBCs) 10–15 mL/kg for 2–3 g/dL increase in hemoglobin (Hb)	Anemia (symptomatic or severe)	Sedimentation or centrifugation of whole blood Apheresis	1°C–6°C
Platelets (plts) 5–10 mL/kg for platelet count rise of 50,000–100,000/µL	Massive hemorrhage Bleeding because of thrombocytopenia or platelet dysfunction (e.g., uremia, aspirin, extracorporeal membrane oxygenation [ECMO], bypass)	Separation from whole blood Apheresis	20°C–24°C
Plasma 10–15 mL/kg for 15%–20% increase in factor levels	Replacement of multiple plasma coagulation factors to prevent or manage bleeding (e.g., diffuse intravascular coagulation, warfarin reversal, liver disease, massive hemorrhage) Management of factor or plasma protein deficiencies when factor concentrates or recombinant proteins are unavailable Thrombotic thrombocytopenic purpura	Separation from whole blood Apheresis	≤-18°C
Cryoprecipitated antihemolytic factor (Cryoprecipitate) 1–2 units/10 kg for 60–100 mg/dL increase in fibrinogen	Prevention/management of bleeding because of fibrinogen deficiency or factor XIII deficiency Management of von Willebrand disease or hemophilia A (factor VIII deficiency) when factor concentrate or recombinant factor is unavailable.	Isolation of the cold-insoluble precipitate by centrifugation during thawing of fresh frozen plasma	≤-18°C

Table 18.2 Transfusion Reactions Causing Respiratory Distress

TRANSFUSION COMPLICATION[a]	PATHOGENESIS	CLINICAL PRESENTATION
Transfusion-associated acute lung injury (TRALI)	Donor anti-human leukocyte antigen (HLA) and/or anti-human neutrophil antigens (HNA) antibodies targeting recipient white blood cells. This is most likely to occur with donors who were previously sensitized by pregnancy.	Hypoxemia and noncardiogenic pulmonary edema within 6 hours of transfusion. Identification of donor antibodies targeting recipient HLA or anti-HNA supports the diagnosis.
Transfusion-associated circulatory overload (TACO)	Cardiogenic pulmonary edema caused by transfusion of large fluid volumes or rapid transfusions.	Dyspnea, distended neck veins, S_3 on cardiac auscultation, hypoxemia that improves with diuresis. Newly elevated B-type natriuretic peptide supports the diagnosis.
Allergic reaction	Donor allergens trigger immunoglobulin (Ig) E–mediated histamine release in sensitized recipient.	Spectrum from mild to severe (anaphylaxis) including wheezing and bronchospasm with associated hives, itching, angioedema, hypotension, and flushing.

[a]These diagnoses may only be made in the absence of other causes of the presenting symptoms.

DAT

Add anti-human globulin (AHG)

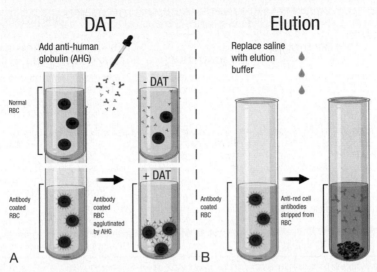

Normal
RBC

- DAT

Antibody
coated
RBC

Antibody
coated
RBC
agglutinated
by AHG

+ DAT

A

Elution

Replace saline
with elution
buffer

Antibody
coated
RBC

Anti-red cell
antibodies
stripped from
RBC

B

Figure 18.1 Schematic of the direct antiglobulin test (DAT) and elution. (A) Red blood cells (RBC) from a patient with suspected antibody-mediated hemolysis are washed, resuspended in saline, and treated with anti-human globulin, which binds to human antibodies, thus cross-linking antibody-coated RBC together. Formation of visible agglutinates indicates a positive DAT and lack of agglutinates indicates a negative DAT. (B) If the DAT is positive, an elution is performed where antibodies coating the RBC are removed into elution buffer. Antibody identification is then performed on the eluate. (Created with BioRender.com).

4. **How is the DAT performed, and how should positive and negative results be interpreted?**
   The DAT informs the presence of antibodies bound to the patient's circulating RBC with or without complement fixation. Anti-human globulin (AHG) is added to washed patient RBC. AHG binds human antibodies, thus cross-linking together antibody-coated RBC to form visible agglutinates. Lack of agglutinates indicates a negative DAT (Figure 18.1A). In parallel, the RBC may be reacted with anti-human complement component C3 to detect complement fixation. In severe hemolysis because of ABO incompatibility, the DAT can be falsely negative because of rapid destruction of antibody-coated RBC.

5. **What blood bank testing should follow-up a positive DAT, and how can this testing elucidate the cause of hemolysis?**
   Follow-up testing of a positive DAT involves an elution procedure where antibodies coating the patient RBC are removed using an elution buffer (see Figure 18.1B). This "eluate" is then assessed for antigen specificity using reagent "panel" RBC. In HDFN, antibodies in the newborn's eluate will show specificity for the antigen(s) expressed by the newborn to which the mother is sensitized. These may include antibodies to major ABO (e.g., the mother is group O and newborn group A) or minor blood group antigens (e.g., Rh[D] and Kell). In hemolytic transfusion reactions, the transfusion recipient's RBC eluate will show specificity for the mismatched RBC alloantigen to which they are sensitized. In patients with autoimmune hemolysis, the patient's RBC eluate is panreactive and typically shows reactivity to most panel RBC with no apparent specificity. In HSCT-related alloimmune hemolysis, the patient's RBC eluate will show specificity for major or minor blood group antigens for which there is donor-recipient mismatch. If the eluate is nonreactive with panel RBC, then it may contain antibodies against RBC antigens not represented on the reagent RBC (e.g., a drug-induced antigen). Also, if ABO incompatibility is suspected, ensure that the lab tests the eluate against A+ and/or B+ reagent RBC.

6. **Describe the transfusion reactions that frequently cause fever, the blood products implicated, and the clinical testing needed to evaluate fever during transfusions.**
   Hemolytic transfusion reaction (Table 18.3) may be a life-threatening reaction caused by antibody- and complement-mediated lysis of incompatible blood. It is most often associated with transfusion of incompatible RBC. In pediatric patients, however, transfusion of ABO-incompatible plasma can cause hemolysis of patient RBC, a process called "reverse hemolysis." Presenting symptoms include fever, back pain, chest pain, hemoglobinuria, hypotension, and diffuse intravascular coagulation (DIC). Delayed hemolytic reactions (2–12 days after transfusion) occur in sensitized recipients, when transfused cells trigger production of alloantibodies by memory cells. Increased antibody levels lead to destruction of circulating donor RBC. Clinical evaluation includes DAT, hemolysis markers, a recheck of patient blood group and antibody screen results, and a clerical check to ensure correct product was given.

Table 18.3 Transfusion Reactions Causing Fever

TRANSFUSION COMPLICATION[a] (IMPLICATED PRODUCTS)	PATHOGENESIS	CLINICAL PRESENTATION (LABORATORY FINDINGS)
Febrile nonhemolytic transfusion reaction (RBC > Plts >> FFP)	Pyrogens associated with white blood cells	Fever ($\geq$38°C) with temperature increase of at least 1°C during transfusion or within 4 hours after a transfusion (No evidence for hemolysis, DAT negative)
Hemolytic transfusion reaction (acute and delayed) (RBC >> Plts, FFP)	Antibody-mediated destruction of incompatible donor or recipient RBCs	Fever, tachycardia, back pain, chest pain, dyspnea, hypotension, DIC, hemoglobinuria (DAT positive, positive hemolysis indices - hemoglobinemia, low haptoglobin, increased indirect bilirubin)
Transfusion transmitted bacterial infection (Plts >> RBC, FFP)	Bacterial contamination of blood product leading to systemic inflammation	Temperature increase of $\geq$2°C, chills, and hypotension during or shortly after transfusion (Positive blood and product culture)

[a]These diagnoses may only be made in the absence of other causes of the presenting symptoms.

DAT, Direct antiglobulin test; *DIC*, disseminated intravascular coagulation; *FFP*, fresh frozen plasma; *Plts*; platelets; *RBC*, red blood cells.

Transfusion-transmitted bacterial infections are life-threatening infections caused by bacterial contamination of blood products, most often platelets. Symptoms overlap with those of sepsis, including fever, chills, rigors, hypotension, and DIC. The clinical evaluation includes blood culture, product culture, and visual assessment of product for signs of contamination, such as increased opacity, clotting, and gas bubbles. Febrile nonhemolytic reaction is the most common and least severe of the febrile transfusion reactions and a diagnosis of exclusion. It is caused by pyrogens associated with WBCs in cellular blood components. Hemolytic transfusion reaction, sepsis, and TRALI must be adequately ruled out.

7. **What are the most common causes of hemolytic transfusion reactions, and how can they be prevented and mitigated?**
   The Food and Drug Administration (FDA) and AABB (formerly the American Association of Blood Banks) specify strict protocols to address the most common causes of hemolytic transfusion reactions, which are because of incorrect pretransfusion sampling—wrong blood in tube—or incorrect transfusion recipient. The recipient sample must be labeled with two unique identifiers (e.g., name plus date of birth or medical record number) with date/time of collection and the initials of the phlebotomist. Samples not appropriately labeled must be rejected by the blood bank. In addition, at least one other independently collected sample, or the historical record, must provide confirmation of the recipient's ABO group and Rh(D) type. Another cautionary procedure is to repeat a type and screen every 3 days for those who have been transfused in the prior 3 months or who are pregnant.
   Administration protocols to ensure the correct recipient and rapidly identify signs of severe transfusion reaction must be in place, and the transfusionist must identify the correct recipient by two unique identifiers of the assigned blood product unit, ideally with confirmation of another person. The recipient should have vital signs assessed before transfusion, 15 minutes after beginning transfusion, periodically during transfusion as needed, and at the end.

8. **What causes allergic transfusion reactions, how can these be prevented, and how do these mitigation strategies affect the blood products?**
   Allergic transfusion reactions are among the most common transfusion reactions seen in children, with platelets most commonly implicated. Modifications in blood component manufacturing can mitigate allergic transfusion reactions caused by allergens in donor plasma to which recipients are sensitized. Plasma mitigation techniques include the following:
   - Platelet and RBC washing prevent allergic transfusion reactions but reduce component shelf life and functionality and are cumbersome.
   - Prestorage replacement of platelet plasma with platelet additive solution (PAS) has little impact on shelf life or function and, in large retrospective studies, PAS platelets are associated with reduced allergic reactions in adults and children.
   - Solvent detergent–treated pooled plasma products are associated with reduced rates of allergic reactions.

To prevent severe allergic reactions in patients with absolute IgA deficiency and sensitization to IgA, washed cellular blood products and/or components from IgA deficient donors is recommended. There is little evidence for efficacy of diphenhydramine premedication in patients with no history of allergic reactions.

9. **What causes febrile nonhemolytic transfusion reactions, and how can these be prevented?**

Febrile nonhemolytic reactions are among the most common transfusion reactions seen in children, with RBC with platelets most commonly implicated. Although typically harmless, they usually cause transfusions to be stopped to rule out more serious transfusion reactions (see question #6). They are caused by recipient responses to donor WBC antigens and pyrogens. Prestorage leukoreduction markedly reduces febrile nonhemolytic transfusion reactions without having a significant effect on the blood product function. There is no evidence that premedication with acetaminophen is useful for preventing these reactions.

10. **How are patients with sickle cell disease uniquely susceptible to hemolytic transfusion reactions, and how can this risk be mitigated?**

Individuals with sickle cell disease (SCD) are exposed to many units of donor RBC over time to prevent or manage complications of the disease, and minor RBC antigens vary widely between individuals. Estimated rates of alloimmunization range from 18% to 47% and circulating alloantibody levels may fluctuate over time. If alloantibody levels are low at the time of antibody screening and cross-matching, these tests may not reflect previous sensitization to RBC antigens. Transfusion of mismatched RBC may then trigger memory cell production of alloantibodies, resulting in a delayed hemolytic transfusion reaction (DHTR). DHTRs may be complicated by hyperhemolysis, in which hemoglobin falls below pretransfusion levels because of lysis of native RBC in addition to antigen-positive donor RBC. Hyperhemolysis may be lethal.

The risk of hemolytic transfusion reactions in SCD patients may be reduced by careful documentation of patient alloantibody profiles from all institutions where the patient receives care. In addition, prospective phenotype matching may help prevent alloimmunization. In this process, a laboratory identifies the antigens to which the patient may become sensitized by documenting their RBC antigen profile and avoids transfusing RBC expressing those antigens.

11. **What causes hemolytic disease of the fetus and newborn? Describe the testing needed to evaluate and mitigate HDFN.**

In HDFN caused by ABO incompatibility, naturally occurring IgG antibodies from the maternal circulation cross the placenta and destroy incompatible fetal RBC. This is most commonly seen in a mother with type O blood (with anti-A and anti-B antibodies) against a fetus that is type A.

In HDFN caused by alloantibodies, maternal exposure to fetal RBC antigens that she does not express causes formation of IgG alloantibodies that can cross the placenta to destroy fetal RBC. This is most commonly seen in D-negative mothers with D-positive pregnancies. HDFN because of anti-D is dramatically reduced in areas with widespread use of Rho(D) immunoglobulin (RHIg). Pregnant women with clinically significant anti-RBC alloantibodies should have serial antibody titers to monitor for increasing sensitization and fetal middle cerebral artery Doppler velocity to monitor for fetal anemia. In mothers with known anti-RBC alloantibodies or if HDFN is suspected, evaluation of the cord blood should include DAT and, if positive, elution with antibody identification and assessment of hemoglobin and bilirubin levels.

12. **What is an appropriate blood component composition for neonates undergoing manual RBC exchange for HDFN and hyperbilirubinemia?**

The units should be antigen negative and selected to avoid the clinically significant anti-RBC antibodies from the mother (e.g., Kell negative if the mother has anti-Kell). Use fresh units, less than 14 days old. Older units have increased risk of lysis with elevated levels of potassium, which could cause arrhythmias and metabolic complications. Irradiation to destroy lymphocytes should be performed, thus preventing graft versus host disease and leukoreduction to remove WBCs, which decreases risk of febrile reactions and also removes cells with intracellular cytomegalovirus (CMV), leading to a CMV-safe product. The blood component should be hemoglobin-S negative to prevent sickling. Washing the product to remove the anticoagulant, preservative solution, and excess potassium and reconstitution with ABO-compatible plasma to the desired final hematocrit, typically 50%, is recommended.

13. **For fetal and neonatal alloimmune thrombocytopenia, what are the recommended blood component strategies?**

The most common implicated antibodies are maternal anti-HPA-1a and anti-HPA-5b; thus for neonates requiring platelet transfusion (typically a platelet count $< 30 \times 10^9$/L or for bleeding), the following procedures should be employed:

- Maternal platelets (because they lack the incompatible platelet antigen), washed to remove antibodies
- HPA-selected platelets negative for the incompatible platelet antigen
- Random-donor platelets
- All platelets should be leuko-reduced and irradiated

BIBLIOGRAPHY

1. Association for the Advancement of Blood & Biotherapies. Circular of Information for the Use of Human Blood and Blood Components. October 2017.
2. Delaney M, Matthews DC. Hemolytic disease of the fetus and newborn: managing the mother, fetus, and newborn. *Hematology. American Society of Hematology Education Program.* 2015;2015:146–151.
3. Goel R, Tobian AAR, Shaz BH. Noninfectious transfusion-associated adverse events and their mitigation strategies. *Blood.* 2019; 133(17):1831–1839.
4. Jorgenson M. Administration of blood components. In Cohn CS, Delaney M, Johnson ST, Katz LM (eds). *Technical Manual.* AABB; 2020:537–551.
5. Parker V, Tormey CA. The direct antiglobulin test: indications, interpretation, and pitfalls. *Arch Pathol Lab Med.* 2017;141(2):305–310.
6. Vossoughi S, Perez G, Whitaker BI, Fung MK, Stotler B. Analysis of pediatric adverse reactions to transfusions. *Transfusion.* 2018;58 (1):60–69.
7. Zerra PE, Hendrickson JE, Josephson CD. Neonatal and pediatric transfusion medicine. In Shaz BH, Hillyer CD, Gil MR (eds). *Transfusion Medicine and Hemostasis.* 3rd ed. Elsevier; 2019:295–299.

CHAPTER 19

PEDIATRIC RADIATION ONCOLOGY

Matthew Gallitto, MD, Eileen Connolly, MD, PhD, and Cheng-Chia Wu, MD, PhD

1. **How does radiation therapy work?**
   In the realm of external beam radiation (the most commonly used radiotherapy), a linear accelerator produces a beam of high-energy electrons, which hits a metal target at the head of the machine. Upon striking the target, electron energies are subsequently converted to x-ray (photon) energies. Filters and multileaf collimators (MLCs) are placed distal to the target in the head of the machine to selectively block and shape the x-ray radiation as it exits the linear accelerator and enters the patient. When these uncharged photons collide with a charged electron in the body, this excited electron can cause damage either directly or indirectly:

   Direct Action: The ionizing event leads to DNA damage and triggers cell death.
   Indirect Action: The ionizing event forms free radicals (most commonly hydroxyl) that can then cause DNA damage and cell death.

2. **Describe the simulation process.**
   The simulation session allows the radiation therapist to place patients in a reproducible position that is used each day during treatment. A variety of immobilization devices are available to minimize patient motion and maximize reproducibility for the duration of treatment. Sometimes permanent tattoos are placed to help align the patient for a reproducible setup. Once the computed tomography (CT) scan is complete with the customized immobilization devices, other imaging modalities such as positron emission tomography (PET) and magnetic resonance imaging (MRI) can be used to help identify the tumor target and normal organs at risk (OARs).

3. **Which structures are contoured and how?**
   The most common target volumes used for radiation planning are gross tumor volume (GTV), clinical target volume (CTV), and planning target volume (PTV):
   - *GTV:* Represents tumor that is visible on CT scan (MRI or PET information can be used).
   - *CTV:* Represents GTV + microscopic disease. This typically includes a margin around the GTV plus any regions concerning for lymphatic spread.
   - *PTV:* Represents an expansion around the CTV that takes into account patient motion and setup variation.
     Additionally, OARs near the target volumes are delineated to generate a plan that maximizes dose to the tumor while minimizing toxicity to nearby structures.

4. **What are the different techniques used to deliver external beam radiation?**
   There are several factors that influence radiation technique:
   - The type and frequency of imaging of the patient before radiation delivery
   - The complexity of the type of radiation to be delivered (i.e., physicians manually placing the beams versus using computer-based algorithms to customize radiation beam delivery to spare OARs)
   - How quickly the radiation is delivered
     The different techniques include three-dimensional conformal radiotherapy (3D-CRT), intensity-modulated radiotherapy (IMRT), standard fractionated radiotherapy, stereotactic radiotherapy, and hypofractionated radiotherapy:

   3D-CRT: This technique is for simple palliative treatments, such as for Wilms tumors. Using CT scans to visualize the tumor, the radiation oncologist and planners can design the radiation plan without software algorithm assistance.
   IMRT: This is a more advanced form of CT-based radiation planning. Radiation delivery is customized with different intensities of radiation coming at different angles to target the tumor and avoid normal tissue. By using a computer algorithm, the tumor target volume, and the OARs, the computer generates a customized plan for treatment.
   Standard Fractionated Radiotherapy: The treatment is typically 1.5 to 2 Gy per treatment delivered over several weeks. One can have standard fractionated 3D-CRT or standard fractionated IMRT.
   Stereotactic Radiotherapy: Using the same techniques as in IMRT, stereotactic radiotherapy refers to the delivery of high doses of radiation (6 Gy or more) in five or fewer fractions. Stereotactic radiosurgery (SRS) refers to treatment of intracranial lesions, whereas extracranial stereotactic radiation therapy is referred to as stereotactic body radiotherapy (SBRT).
   Hypofractionated Radiotherapy: Treatment courses that are shorter than the standard fractionated treatments but do not fit criteria for stereotactic radiotherapy are considered hypofractionated radiotherapy. One can be treated with 3D-CRT or IMRT with hypofractionation.

5. **Is total dose simply additive?**
   No. Dose alone fails to represent the effect of radiation on biological tissue if it is delivered in 1 versus 10 daily fractions. Biologically effective dose (BED) is a measure of the true biological dose delivered by a particular combination of dose per fraction and total dose to a particular tissue. There are modeling formulas to calculate the BED of a treatment. In general, for the same overall dose, if the treatment is given in shorter treatments at a higher dose per fraction, the overall effect is stronger. For example, 20 Gy given in 1 treatment is significantly stronger than 20 Gy given over 10 treatments.

6. **Can other modalities and/or sources be used aside from photons?**
   Yes, in addition to the use of photon beams to deliver external beam radiotherapy, several other radiotherapy options exist. Electron beam therapy can also be used for superficial tumors and scars because they have a finite range and dose falls off rapidly once reaching the skin surface. Protons and electrons have a finite entrance and exit dose upon entering and leaving the body. Given the unique molecular composition of protons, however, they deposit nearly all of their energy at the end of their path and there is virtually no exit dose from the body. Thus proton beam therapy is being extensively studied as a way to further minimize toxicity to normal tissues.
   In contrast to external beam radiotherapy, brachytherapy treats cancer tissue from the inside, and the radiation does not travel through healthy tissue to reach its target. This requires the implantation of radioactive sources (i.e., cobalt, iridium, palladium) into the patient through intracavitary, intraluminal, or interstitial applicators.

7. **When is stereotactic body radiotherapy used in pediatric patients?**
   In patients with metastatic Ewing or rhabdomyosarcoma, radiation is frequently used for consolidation to treat all metastatic disease. Historically, standard fractionated radiotherapy was used. This can be time consuming and limit quality of life for patients. SBRT is being investigated with the Children's Oncology Group (COG) as a method to treat all metastatic sites. Typically, 30 to 40 Gy in 5 fractions is used.

8. **What is the role for craniospinal irradiation?**
   Craniospinal irradiation (CSI) is used for malignancies with high risk of spread to the craniospinal axis or for patients with metastatic disease in the spine. Historically, CSI is delivered with 3D-CRT planning; however, more recently, patients have been treated with protons to prevent normal tissue toxicity anterior to the vertebral body. IMRT techniques are also being explored for photon-based CSI. CSI is largely used for medulloblastoma, nongerminomatous germ cell tumors of the central nervous system (CNS), and pineoblastoma, to name a few. Patients with atypical teratoid rhabdoid tumor (ATRT) were historically treated with CSI; however, with results from COG ACNS0333, focal radiotherapy is used.

9. **When is total lung irradiation used?**
   Total lung irradiation is commonly used for patients with metastatic Wilms tumors, Ewing sarcoma, and rhabdomyosarcoma with lung involvement. Historically, 3D-CRT was used to treat the entire lung using one beam from the front and one from the back. More recently, IMRT has been used for more focused lung irradiation while sparing the heart. Typically 12 Gy is used for Wilms and 15 Gy for Ewing/rhabdomyosarcoma.

10. **When is whole ventricular irradiation used?**
    Historically, pure germ cell tumors/seminomas of the CNS were treated with CSI with excellent outcomes. To further decrease toxicities, efforts have been made to decrease the radiation field size. It was found that whole ventricular irradiation (WVI) with a boost to the gross disease achieved similar outcomes to CSI. Furthermore, neoadjuvant chemotherapy with carboplatin and etoposide allowed further radiation dose reduction. Of note, WVI was examined in patients with nongerminomatous germ cell tumor (NGGCT) in COG ACNS1123 and increased failure was reported in the spine.[3] CSI thus remains the standard of care for NGGCT.

11. **When is involved-field radiation therapy used?**
    Historically, lymphoma has been treated with involved-field radiation therapy (IFRT). This involves treating larger volumes defined on anatomical boundaries, including an entire lymphatic region. In adult lymphoma, standard treatment has transitioned toward involved-site radiation therapy (ISRT). This factors in prechemotherapy extent and postchemotherapy response to target a smaller treatment area. ISRT for high-risk Hodgkin lymphoma in children is being tested in COG AHOD1331.

12. **What is the purpose of lung blocks, and when are they indicated for use in total body irradiation?**
    Total body irradiation (TBI) using photon beams is used to treat several diseases, including multiple myeloma, leukemias, lymphomas, and certain solid tumors. TBI is also used commonly as a conditioning regimen before stem cell transplantation to accomplish the following:
    - Deplete the bone marrow
    - Eliminate residual malignant cells
    - Prevent rejection via immunosuppression

    The most common TBI schedules include a total dose of 12 Gy delivered in 1.8 to 2 Gy fractions. Most facilities use customized lung blocks for shielding to keep the median lung doses to 8 Gy to decrease the risk of pneumonitis/pulmonary fibrosis. In select patients that have to be treated supine, other blocking techniques can be used.

In patients who cannot tolerate standard TBI regimens or those undergoing TBI for nonmalignant hematologic diseases, there are reduced-intensity regimens consisting of 2 to 4 Gy delivered in 1 to 2 fractions. Lung blocks are not needed in these reduced-intensity regimens. Some newer techniques are currently under investigation, including total lymphoid and marrow irradiation.

BIBLIOGRAPHY

1. Kalapurakal JA, Gopalakrishnan M, Walterhouse DO, et al. Cardiac-sparing whole lung IMRT in patients with pediatric tumors and lung metastasis: final report of a prospective multicenter clinical trial. *Int J Radiat Oncol Biol Phys.* 2019;103(1):28–37.
2. Fangusaro J, Wu S, MacDonald S, et al. Phase II trial of response-based radiation therapy for patients with localized CNS nongerminomatous germ cell tumors: a children's oncology group study. *J Clin Oncol.* 2019;37(34):3283–3290.
3. Reddy AT, Strother DR, Judkins AR, et al. Efficacy of high-dose chemotherapy and three-dimensional conformal radiation for atypical teratoid/rhabdoid tumor: a report from the Children's Oncology Group Trial ACNS0333. *J Clin Oncol.* 2020;38(11):1175–1185.
4. Specht L, Yahalom J, Illidge T, et al. Modern radiation therapy for Hodgkin lymphoma: field and dose guidelines from the international lymphoma radiation oncology group (ILROG). *Int J Radiat Oncol Biol Phys.* 2014;89(4):854–862.
5. Wong JYC, Filippi AR, Dabaja BS, Yahalom J, Specht L. Total body irradiation: guidelines from the International Lymphoma Radiation Oncology Group (ILROG). *Int J Radiat Oncol Biol Phys.* 2018;101(3):521–529.
6. Wong JYC, Filippi AR, Scorsetti M, Hui S, Muren LP, Mancosu P. Total marrow and total lymphoid irradiation in bone marrow transplantation for acute leukaemia. *Lancet Oncol.* 2020;21(10):e477–e487.

CHAPTER 20

PRINCIPLES OF INFECTIOUS DISEASE AND MANAGEMENT OF FEBRILE NEUTROPENIA

Marc D. Foca, MD

1. **What are typical infectious complications in pediatric oncology patients?**
   Typical infectious complications include bacterial sepsis, systemic or organ-specific infections caused by either primary or reactivated viruses (e.g., cytomegalovirus [CMV], Epstein-Barr virus [EBV]), respiratory viruses (e.g., influenza, respiratory syncytial virus [RSV]), and invasive fungal infections (e.g., *Candida*, *Aspergillus* sp.)

2. **How does bacterial infectious risk vary across the spectrum of oncology patients?**
   The risk of infection coincides with the intensity of chemotherapy, leading to profound myelosuppression, mucositis, and nutritional deficiencies. Bacteremia is most common in relapsed acute lymphocytic leukemia (ALL) and acute myelocytic leukemia (AML) followed by allogeneic hematopoietic stem cell transplantation (HSCT). Estimates of bacterial infections vary by study and year published but can approach 50% in relapsed ALL and AML. Embryonal central nervous system (CNS) tumors and high-risk neuroblastoma are other high-risk diagnoses. Across all conditions, indwelling foreign devices such as central venous catheters and ventriculoperitoneal shunts increase infection risk.

3. **What is the recommended empiric antibiotic coverage for febrile neutropenia?**
   Antibiotic coverage should be based on the local hospital antibiogram and should offer combined coverage for:
   - *Pseudomonas* and related gram-negative organisms
   - The majority of typical gram-positive organisms, including *Staphylococcus aureus* and Viridans group *Streptococci.*
   Therefore antibiotics should include an antipseudomonal agent, which has additional gram-positive coverage, typically a penicillin (piperacillin-tazobactam) or cephalosporin (cefepime). Vancomycin is not routinely indicated as empiric coverage for stable febrile children with neutropenia unless there is a high probability of a resistant gram-positive pathogen (e.g., signs of catheter site infection, skin and soft tissue infection, and/or a previous history of methicillin-resistant *Staphylococcus aureus* [MRSA] or resistant viridans group *Streptococci*).

4. **What is the role of antibiotic prophylaxis for limiting bacterial infections in oncology patients?**
   Evidence suggests that the use of preemptive systemic antibacterial therapy (e.g., levofloxacin) can decrease bacteremia rates in a select group of patients at the highest infectious risk. In a randomized clinical trial, bacteremia in patients with ALL receiving levofloxacin prophylaxis was significantly lower (21.9% vs 43.4% for patients with acute leukemia [a significant difference]) and lower but not statistically different (11.0% vs 17.3%) in those who underwent HSCT. Current guidelines suggest consideration of systemic antibacterial prophylaxis for children receiving intensive chemotherapy for acute AML and relapsed ALL. Routine use of systemic antibacterial prophylaxis is not currently recommended during induction chemotherapy for ALL, autologous HSCT, and allogeneic HSCT. Antibacterial prophylaxis should be reserved for instances where prolonged neutropenia is anticipated and balanced against the evolution of antibacterial resistance.

5. **What are investigations that are useful in the neutropenic patient with persistent fever?**
   Management of persistent fever of a greater than 96-hour duration in the neutropenic patient despite appropriate antibacterial coverage should be addressed with institutional protocols. Radiology investigations including computed tomography (CT) with contrast of chest and/or ultrasound of the abdomen can be done to look for abscesses, infectious foci (which may need drainage), or evidence of pulmonary nodules that may indicate the presence of fungal disease. Sinus imaging could be performed if suggestive symptoms are present. Choice of antibacterial therapy could be revisited in the setting of local antibiograms to cover for resistant organisms. Routine serum fungal markers, such as galactomannan, beta-D-glucan, or fungal polymerase chain reaction (PCR), are not recommended, although consideration of galactomannan as a marker for invasive aspergillosis in the setting of radiographic evidence can be entertained. Serum beta D-glucan can be used as a marker for *Pneumocystis jiroveci* pneumonia. Drug fever and *Clostridium difficile* infections are also important to rule out.

6. **What is an important resistance mechanism, and what are some novel beta-lactam antibiotics available for treatment of resistant gram-negative bacterial infections?**
   An important resistance mechanism is the production of enzymes (beta-lactamases), which degrade the beta-lactam class of antibiotics, such as penicillins, cephalosporins, and carbapenems. These include extended spectrum beta-lactamases (ESBLs), which hydrolyze third-generation cephalosporins (in *Escherichia*, *Klebsiella* sp. commonly), chromosomally mediated beta-lactamases that can be expressed on exposure to antibiotics (amp-C beta lactamases in *Enterobacter* species), and carbapenemases, which degrade carbapenems (e.g., *Klebsiella pneumoniae* carbapenemase). Antibiotic options for ESBL-producing organisms include piperacillin-tazobactam (for urinary sources) and carbapenems (noting the absence of *Pseudomonal* coverage for ertapenem). Cefepime, or carbapenems, are options for organisms that produce AmpC beta-lactamases. Novel combinations of beta-lactam/beta-lactamase inhibitors now available to treat carbapenem-resistant *Enterobacteriaceae* (CREs) include ceftazidime/avibactam, meropenem/vaborbactam, and imipenem/relebactam. Ceftolozane/tazobactam is another agent that is typically used to treat multidrug-resistant *Pseudomonas*. Dosing for the agents have not been fully defined in younger age groups.

7. **Define an approach to evaluate antibiotic allergies in pediatric oncology patients.**
   Antibiotic allergies should be carefully evaluated before modifying therapy. A nonsevere, nontype-1 hypersensitivity (e.g., a rash that develops later in antibiotic course) is not a contraindication to using an alternate beta-lactam antibiotic. True cross-reactivity rates between different classes of beta lactams are low (1%–3%) and within the same class are determined by the side chain attached to the beta-lactam ring. Serious systemic reactions are rare and usually present with mucosal involvement (Steven-Johnson syndrome) or organ failure/lymphadenopathy (drug reaction with eosinophilia and systemic symptoms [DRESS]). Alternatives to antibiotic coverage for patients with serious beta-lactam allergies include aztreonam, a monobactam that does not provide gram-positive coverage, or an alternate antibiotic class (e.g., fluoroquinolones).

8. **What are risk factors for and common pathogens that cause invasive fungal disease in pediatric oncology patients?**
   Risk factors for invasive fungal disease include older age, prolonged neutropenia, high-dose steroid exposure, intensive-timing chemotherapy for acute myeloid leukemia, and acute and chronic graft versus host. *Candida* and *Aspergillus* spp. are the predominant pathogens that cause this in children with cancer, but there is increasing prevalence of other non-*Aspergillus* molds (*Fusarium*, *Scedosporium*, and *Mucorales*).

9. **What is the spectrum of activity of currently available antifungal agents?**
   All available azole agents (e.g., fluconazole, voriconazole) are active against *Candida* sp. Some species (*C. glabrata*, *C. krusei*) demonstrate decreased fluconazole susceptibility. Most *Candida* species are susceptible to echinocandins (e.g., caspofungin, micafungin). *C. auris* can be resistant to multiple antifungal agents and can be rapidly transmitted in healthcare settings. Voriconazole is commonly used as an anti-*Aspergillus* agent and requires monitoring of drug levels and can be associated with adverse events (hepatitis, QT prolongation, and interactions with vincristine through the CYP hepatic pathway). Newer-generation azoles (posaconazole and isavuconazole) offer expanded coverage against non-*Aspergillus* molds and currently are most often used for prophylaxis but can be used as salvage therapy in pediatrics. Echinocandins (e.g., micafungin) have some mold activity but are not ideal coverage. Amphotericin B is active against a broad range of yeasts and molds (including *Mucorales*), but use is limited by significant toxicity (acute kidney injury, electrolyte disturbances).

10. **What are common viral infections in pediatric oncology patients and some strategies to decrease their impact?**
    Viral infections can include both primary infections (typically respiratory viruses) and secondary reactivations (e.g., CMV, EBV). Common respiratory viral infections (e.g., RSV, parainfluenza) show increased shedding, more involvement of the lower respiratory tract, and increased morbidity, particularly in patients post-HSCT.
    Therapy is mostly supportive. Antiviral agents for influenza include oseltamivir, inhaled zanamivir, and, in the United States, intravenous peramivir (single dose). Ribavirin in oral formulation can be considered for RSV, although evidence is sparse for its use for parainfluenza infections. Cidofovir is an available agent for severe adenoviral infections.
    Risk factors for CMV infection/reactivation include HSCT patients with discordant serostatus (specifically R+/D-), pre-HSCT CMV DNAemia, unrelated/mismatched donors, and graft versus host disease. Valganciclovir prophylaxis can be used to decrease the risk of CMV reactivation, although it is less likely to be used in patients who have not yet engrafted. Letermovir is a new antiviral, with a different mechanism of action (terminase complex inhibitor), less toxicity, and which can be used for CMV prophylaxis in older adolescents. It does not cause myelosuppression, so it can be used as immediate prophylaxis in high-risk patients who are CMV negative by PCR at the time of initiation. First-line therapy for CMV is ganciclovir. Alternate agents (foscarnet and/or cidofovir) are considered in patients with antiviral resistance (typically mediated by mutations in DNA polymerase and/or thymidine kinase), ganciclovir-related toxicity (e.g., myelosuppression), or those not yet engrafted. Oncology patients are at lower risk of CMV disease, and as such, routine screening for CMV is not recommended. In certain high-risk patients (i.e., younger age, high-risk ALL, and relapsed ALL), it can be considered.

Two main strategies are used to prevent CMV reactivation and disease. Prophylaxis is the provision of antiviral therapy to either all patients or high-risk patients only for a defined period of time after transplant. Preemptive therapy is the provision of antiviral therapy only after the detection of CMV at scheduled screening intervals, usually by PCR assay, in asymptomatic or symptomatic patients. A combination of these strategies can also be employed on an individualized basis. Preemptive therapy is most often used after HSCT.

11. **What are some special aspects of COVID-19 in pediatric oncology patients?**
Children with COVID-19 are less likely to develop severe disease or require hospitalization compared with adults. Although other respiratory viral infections (e.g., influenza) are more severe in immunocompromised patients, the role of immunosuppression as a specific risk factor in pediatric COVID-19 is not established and the overall morbidity and mortality in published case series is low. Immune compromise has not been described as a risk factor for multisystem inflammatory disease. Immunosuppressed patients are likely to have prolonged PCR positivity, and although evidence suggests that this is usually prolonged shedding of nonviable nucleic acid fragments, studies have also recovered viable virus. A therapeutic agent of particular relevance for immunocompromised adolescents are anti SARS-CoV-2 monoclonal antibodies, which are authorized for children 12 or older with mild to moderate disease who are not hospitalized for COVID-19.

BIBLIOGRAPHY

1. Alexander S, Fisher BT, Gaur AH, et al. Effect of levofloxacin prophylaxis on bacteremia in children with acute leukemia or undergoing hematopoietic stem cell transplantation: a randomized clinical trial. *JAMA.* 2018;320(10):995–1004.
2. Blumenthal KG, Peter JG, Trubiano JA, Phillips EJ. Antibiotic allergy. *Lancet.* 2019;393(10167):183–198.
3. Fisher BT, Robinson PD, Lehrnbecher T, et al. Risk factors for invasive fungal disease in pediatric cancer and hematopoietic stem cell transplantation: a systematic review. *J Pediatric Infect Dis Soc.* 2018;7(3):191–198.
4. Lehrnbecher T, Fisher BT, Phillips B, et al. Guideline for antibacterial prophylaxis administration in pediatric cancer and hematopoietic stem cell transplantation. *Clin Infect Dis.* 2020;71(1):226–236.
5. Lehrnbecher T, Robinson P, Fisher B, et al. Guideline for the management of fever and neutropenia in children with cancer and hematopoietic stem-xell transplantation recipients: 2017 update. *J Clin Oncol.* 2017;35(18):2082–2094.
6. Madhusoodhan PP, Pierro J, Musante J, et al. Characterization of COVID-19 disease in pediatric oncology patients: the New York-New Jersey regional experience. *Pediatr Blood Cancer.* 2020;18:e28843.
7. Meesing A, Razonable RR. New developments in the management of cytomegalovirus infection after transplantation. *Drugs.* 2018;78 (11):1085–1103.
8. Tamma PD, Aitken SL, Bonomo RA, Mathers AJ, van Duin D, Clancy CJ. Infectious Diseases Society of America guidance on the treatment of extended-spectrum β-lactamase producing Enterobacterales (ESBL-E), carbapenem-resistant Enterobacterales (CRE), and *Pseudomonas aeruginosa* with difficult-to-treat resistance (DTR-P. aeruginosa). *Clin Infect Dis.* 2021;72(7):1109–1116.

CHAPTER 21

NEOPLASTIC HEMATOPATHOLOGY

Bachir Alobeid, MD and Andrew Myles Parrott, MD

1. **What is B-cell acute lymphoblastic leukemia, and how is it diagnosed?**

   B-cell acute lymphoblastic leukemia (B-ALL) is a neoplasm of B lineage lymphoid progenitors (B lymphoblasts). It includes multiple distinct subtypes characterized by constellations of genetic alterations, including aneuploidy, chromosomal rearrangements, DNA copy number alterations, and sequence mutations. The bone marrow (BM) usually shows extensive involvement by lymphoblasts at initial presentation. Rarely the marrow can show less than 20% involvement. The peripheral blood (PB) can be variably involved, ranging from minimal involvement, detectable only by flow cytometry (FC), to extensive involvement with hyperleukocytosis. Diagnostic work-up involves morphologic evaluation, immunophenotypic analysis by FC and immunohistochemistry (IHC), cytogenetics including conventional karyotype and fluorescence in situ hybridization (FISH), and molecular studies including next-generation sequencing (NGS).

2. **What is the role of flow cytometry in B-ALL at diagnosis and follow-up?**

   Because different leukemias have different therapy regimens and prognosis but can look similar on routine morphology, the phenotype of blasts needs to be established at diagnosis. FC analysis plays a crucial role in the diagnostic work-up and subsequent detection of measurable (formerly minimal) residual disease (MRD), critical in the follow-up and management of B-ALL. Leukemic cells are positive for the B-cell associated markers CD19 and CD79a, whereas CD20 expression is variable. In addition, leukemic cells show variable expression of the immaturity markers CD34, CD10, and terminal deoxynucleotidyl transferase (TdT).

3. **What is the role of cytogenetics in B-ALL diagnosis and classification?**

   B-ALL involves many subtypes associated with distinct gene expression profiles that have variable age-related prevalence, driven by three main types of initiating genetic alteration:
   - Chromosomal aneuploidy
   - Rearrangements that deregulate oncogenes or encode chimeric transcription factors
   - Point mutations

   High hyperdiploidy (>50 chromosomes) is present in up to 30% of childhood B-ALL and is associated with mutations in the Ras pathway, chromatin modifiers such as CREBBP, and favorable outcomes. Low hypodiploidy (31–39 chromosomes) is present in approximately 1% of children and in more than 10% of adults with B-ALL. It is characterized by the deletion of IKZF2 and by near-universal TP53 mutations, which are inherited in approximately half the cases. Near-haploidy (24–30 chromosomes) is present in approximately 2% of childhood B-ALL and is associated with Ras pathway mutations (particularly NF1) and deletions of IKZF3. Both low-hypodiploid and near-haploid B-ALL are associated with unfavorable outcomes. B-ALL with intrachromosomal amplification of chromosome 21 (iAMP21) is most common in older children and has poor prognosis, but outcomes have improved with intensive treatment.

   Of B-ALL subtypes characterized by translocations, the most common in childhood is t(12;21)(p13;q22) encoding ETV6-RUNX1, which is typically cryptic on cytogenetic analysis and associated with favorable prognosis. The t(1;19)(q23;p13) translocation and variants encode TCF3-PBX1, which is more common in African Americans and associated with frequent central nervous system (CNS) relapse and inferior outcomes with older, but not contemporary, treatment regimens. The t(9;22)(q34;q11.2) translocation results in the formation of the Philadelphia chromosome encoding BCR-ABL1 and is found in a subset of childhood B-ALL associated with unfavorable outcomes, although prognosis has improved with combined chemotherapy and tyrosine kinase inhibition. Rearrangement of KMT2A (MLL) at 11q23 to more than 80 partners, most commonly t(4;11) (q21;q23) encoding KMT2AAFF1, is common in infant B-ALL and is associated with a dismal prognosis.

4. **What is T-cell acute lymphoblastic leukemia and T lymphoblastic lymphoma?**

   T lymphoblastic lymphoma (T-LBL) is the second most common type of non-Hodgkin lymphoma (NHL) in childhood and adolescence, accounting for 25% to 35% of all cases. T-LBL often affects older males with a median age of onset around 9 years old and involves mediastinal and cervical lymph nodes in the vast majority of patients. Patients commonly present with an anterior mediastinal mass arising from the thymus that can cause airway compression or superior vena cava syndrome and is frequently accompanied with pleural or pericardial effusions. About 15% to 20% of patients exhibit BM infiltration. Peripheral blood and/or BM involvement by more than 25% T lymphoblast cells is required for the diagnosis of the leukemic phase of disease, acute T-cell lymphoblastic leukemia (T-ALL). Although debate exists whether T-ALL and T-LBL are distinct entities or a spectrum of the same disease, they do share many similar molecular alterations.

5. **What are the pathologic features of T-LBL?**
   Histologically, T-LBL shows an infiltrate of small- to medium-sized blast cells. Further evaluation either by FC (of malignant effusions and/or fresh tissue) or IHC analysis of biopsies is needed to confirm the diagnosis. T-LBL cells express cytoplasmic (or less frequently membrane-bound) CD3, with consistent expression of CD7. In addition, the majority of cases are positive for TdT and variably positive for CD1a, CD34, CD10, CD2, CD4, CD5, and CD8. They are further subclassified by the differentiation stage of T lymphoblasts on their passage through the thymus (pro, pre-, cortical and medullary).

   More recently, a T-ALL phenotype of very early differentiation, termed early T-precursor acute lymphoblastic leukemia (ETP-ALL), has been recognized. It occurs in 10% to 15% of patients with T-ALL and is defined by expression of CD7 and low level CD5 and absence of CD1a, CD4, and CD8 expression. ETP-ALL is associated with increased incidence of acute myeloid leukemia (AML)-type mutations rather than T-ALL/LBL-associated *NOTCH1* mutations. ETP-ALL was associated with an increased rate of induction failures, but with current treatment protocols there is no significant difference in prognosis.

6. **What is Classic Hodgkin lymphoma and nodular lymphocyte predominance Hodgkin lymphoma?**
   Hodgkin lymphoma (HL) is composed of two distinct disease entities: classic HL (cHL) and nodular lymphocyte predominance HL (NLPHL). In contrast with most other lymphomas, in which the neoplastic cells are a major population of the tumor cell constituents, the neoplastic cells in both HL entities usually account for less than 10% of the tumor bulk against a predominant reactive background. cHL is a nodal disease with virtually all cases arising in lymph nodes, commonly in the mediastinum, and, when the disease advances, infiltration into the spleen, liver, and other extranodal locations.

   There are four major types of cHL:
   - Nodular sclerosis (NOS), the most common subtype, tends to affect adolescents and young adults and usually presents with localized disease involving cervical, supraclavicular, and mediastinal regions.
   - Mixed cellularity (MC) is more prevalent in the pediatric and older age groups and commonly is associated with a more advanced stage of disease with poorer prognosis.
   - Lymphocyte-depleted is a rare form occurring mainly in older age patients and in patients with acquired immune deficiency syndrome.
   - Lymphocyte-rich is a subtype recognized more recently and morphologically can closely mimic NLPHL (see later).

7. **What are the pathologic features of cHL?**
   The presence of multinucleated giant Hodgkin/Reed-Sternberg (HRS) or variant (lacunar or mummified) cells within a mixed reactive cellular background (small lymphocytes, histiocytes, plasma cells, and granulocytes) is the pathologic hallmark of cHL. The RS cells of cHL are unique in their abundant cytoplasm and characteristic bilobed nuclei with eosinophilic prominent nucleoli, imparting an "owl-eye" appearance. HRS cells are of B-cell derivation; they stain positively for CD30, CD15, and Pax5 but typically lack expression of CD45 and other B-cell markers. Epstein-Barr virus (EBV)–positive cHL is observed more frequently in childhood (<10 years) and in older adults (>60 years) and is highest in MC type.

8. **What is NLPHL, and how it is different from cHL?**
   NLPHL is a unique clinicopathologic entity that is more prevalent in males, usually presents with limited nodal disease that typically affects the neck region and spares the mediastinum, and rarely presents with constitutional symptoms or extranodal disease. Thus NLPHL has a more indolent clinical course compared with cHL, with a tendency for late recurrences.

9. **What are the pathologic features of NLPHL?**
   NLPHL lacks typical HRS cells and instead is characterized by a neoplastic population of large cells with folded/lobulated nuclei known as lymphocyte-predominant (LP) cells. Unlike HRS cells, LP cells are CD20+ and typically negative for CD30 and CD15. LP cells comprise a minority of cells, most commonly seen in large, abnormal follicular structures made up predominantly of small lymphocytes. They are typically rimmed by rosettes of follicular helper T-cells (CD4+, PDL1+, and CD57+).

10. **What are the most common hematopoietic neoplasms in patients with Down syndrome?**
    Children with Down syndrome (DS) manifest three main hematologic disorders:
    - Transient abnormal myelopoiesis (TAM) at birth.
    - Myeloid leukemia associated with DS (ML-DS).
    - B-ALL.

11. **What is TAM?**
    TAM is a unique condition closely associated with DS and found exclusively in neonates. It is characterized by increased circulating blast cells that harbor germline trisomy 21 and prenatally acquired *GATA1* mutations that cooperatively contribute to the disease. TAM has a variable clinical presentation ranging from asymptomatic with incidental detection to symptomatic with fatal outcome. Accordingly, TAM affects at least 5% to 10% of neonates with

DS; however, the incidence could be much higher. The majority of cases resolve spontaneously, but approximately 20% of patients die and 20% to 30% of survivors subsequently develop ML-DS (see later).

12. **What is ML-DS?**
After the clinical resolution of TAM with normalization of blood counts, up to 30% of neonates will subsequently develop ML-DS, typically before 4 years of age. In some patients the progression to leukemia is heralded by a period of falling blood counts and dysplasia, a myelodysplastic phase frequently preceding the development of AML. Therefore the spectrum of both myelodysplastic syndrome (MDS) and AML are known collectively as ML-DS. Compared with AML in children without DS, ML-DS has a disproportionately high proportion of cases with megakaryoblastic morphology and phenotype (formerly FAB-M7). *GATA1* mutations are identified in all cases of ML-DS with other additional somatic mutations; therefore monitoring *GATA1* in DS patients may assist with an earlier diagnosis of ML-DS.

13. **What are the features of B-ALL in DS patients?**
There is an estimated 10- to 20-fold increased risk of B-ALL in DS children, with the majority of cases occurring before 15 years of age and older than 1 year of age. There are no phenotypic features unique to DS B-ALL. However, frequencies of B-ALL subtypes with poor prognosis (hypodiploidy, t(9;22), and 11q23 translocations) and those with good prognosis (ETV6-RUNX1 fusion transcripts and high hyperdiploidy) are lower in DS B-ALL compared with non-DS B-ALL.

14. **What are the post-transplant lymphoproliferative disorders?**
Post-transplant lymphoproliferative disorders (PTLDs) are a major complication of solid organ and allogeneic hematopoietic stem cell transplantation that develop as a consequence of immunosuppression. They encompass a wide spectrum of hematolymphoid and/or plasmacytic proliferations. PTLDs are currently classified into two major categories: nondestructive and destructive lesions. The nondestructive lesions include plasma cell hyperplasia, infectious mononucleosis-like PTLD, and florid follicular hyperplasia. The destructive lesions include two major categories: polymorphic and monomorphic PTLDs; the latter include diffuse large B-cell lymphoma (DLBCL), Burkitt lymphoma (BL), plasma cell myeloma, plasmacytoma, and other B-cell neoplasms. The monomorphic lesions also include T-cell neoplasms, such as hepatosplenic T-cell lymphoma (HSTCL, see later).

15. **What are the features and pathogenesis of PTLDs?**
PTLDs occur more commonly in intestine, heart, and lung transplant recipients, likely because of the greater degree of immunosuppression and the amount of lymphoid tissue in the transplant. They can involve different organs including lymph nodes, gastrointestinal (GI) tract, and CNS and can be disseminated. The oncogenic EBV plays a major role in the pathogenesis of many PTLDs, especially those arising earlier in the post-transplant period (first 1–2 years). Subsequently, EBV sero-mismatch between a sero-positive donor and sero-negative recipient, younger age at transplant, and intensity of immunosuppression are all recognized risk factors.

16. **What types of B-cell non-Hodgkin lymphomas can be encountered in children?**
Most B-cell NHLs (B-NHLs) encountered in the pediatric age group are of large cell type (LBCLs). Although they have morphological and phenotypic features similar to those observed in their adult counterparts, the more favorable outcome of most pediatric patients after high-dose chemotherapy hints at different underlying biology. Aggressive mature B-NHL in children and young adults include BL, primary mediastinal large B-cell lymphoma (PMBL), DLBCL, and DLBCL, NOS. Pediatric LBCLs and BL are treated with intensive chemotherapy protocols, and although curable, approximately 10% of cases relapse. Certain types of indolent B-cell lymphomas can also be encountered in children:
- *Pediatric-type follicular lymphoma* is a distinct clinicopathologic entity that makes up 1% to 2% of all pediatric NHL cases. It is regarded as a nodal disease, commonly involving the cervical lymph nodes. Most patients present with localized disease and after local excision show complete remission with excellent prognosis. A "watch and wait" approach and follow-up is currently recommended.
- *LBCL with IRF4 rearrangement* is a newly recognized provisional entity, which usually presents in the Waldeyer ring and/or cervical lymph nodes but can also arise in the GI tract. It may be exclusively follicular, follicular and diffuse, or diffuse. This lymphoma predominates in the pediatric population, has a favorable outcome after therapy, and consistently overexpresses IRF4 because of genetic translocation.
- *Pediatric nodal marginal zone lymphoma (NMZL)* is a variant of NMZL with male predominance that commonly occurs in adolescents and has excellent prognosis. This variant presents as asymptomatic localized disease involving lymph nodes of the head and neck area.

17. **What types of peripheral T-cell lymphomas can be encountered in children?**
ALK-1 positive anaplastic lymphoma (ALCL) is the most common type of peripheral T-cell lymphoma (PTCL) in children and accounts for approximately 10% to 15% of all pediatric NHL; however, other PTCL can be seen:
- *ALCL* is an aggressive CD30$^+$ PTCL, showing aberrant ALK activity, most commonly because of the t(2;5)(p23;q35) translocation. Patients often present at advanced clinical stage with peripheral, intra-abdominal, or mediastinal lymph node involvement, frequently associated with B symptoms and extranodal spread to skin, liver, lung, soft tissue, and bone. Because of loss of several pan T-cell antigens, some cases may have an apparent "null" phenotype but show evidence of a T-cell lineage at the molecular level. Tumors associated with the t(2;5)

(75%–80% of cases) express NPM1-ALK fusion protein and show a characteristic cytoplasmic, nuclear, and nucleolar staining pattern. Nevertheless, variant translocations involving ALK and other partner genes can occur and result in different distributions of ALK staining depending on the translocation partner.

- *Hepatosplenic* T-cell lymphoma (HSTCL) preferentially affects teenagers and young adults with male predominance and is associated with long-term immunosuppression, in particular after solid organ transplantation and in patients with Crohn disease. HSTCL is characterized by hepatosplenomegaly, lack of lymphadenopathy, frequent B-symptoms, BM involvement, and elevated serum lactate dehydrogenase (LDH) levels. Histologically, the tumor constitutes small- to intermediate-sized cells that infiltrate the splenic red pulp cords and sinuses, hepatic sinusoids, and BM sinuses. The disease is aggressive, and most patients die within 2 years, even after initial remission.

- *Subcutaneous panniculitis-like T-cell lymphoma* (SPTCL) is defined as a T-cell receptor α/β-positive T-cell lymphoma of CD8$^+$ cytotoxic T-cells, exclusively involving the subcutaneous tissue, which can have overlapping features with lupus panniculitis. It is rare but has been shown to affect all age groups including infants and children. SPTCL is associated with autoimmune disorders such as systemic lupus erythematosus and immunodeficiency syndromes. Histology shows infiltration by irregular lymphoid cells, adipocytic rimming, nuclear debris, lipophages, and macrophages with hemophagocytosis and fat necrosis. Overall, SPTCL has a good prognosis, and its clinical course depends on the presence or absence of a frank hemophagocytic syndrome, which develops in approximately 20% of cases.

BIBLIOGRAPHY

1. Agostinelli C, Akarca AU, Ramsay A, et al. Novel markers in pediatric-type follicular lymphoma. *Virchows Arch.* 2019;475(6):771–779.
2. Attarbaschi A, Abla O, Padilla LA, et al. Rare non-Hodgkin lymphoma of childhood and adolescence: a consensus diagnostic and therapeutic approach to pediatric-type follicular lymphoma, marginal zone lymphoma, and nonanaplastic peripheral T-cell lymphoma. *Pediatr Blood Cancer.* 2020;67(8), e28416.
3. Burkhardt B, Hermiston ML. Lymphoblastic lymphoma in children and adolescents: review of current challenges and future opportunities. *Br J Haematol.* 2019;185(6):1158–1170.
4. Inaba H, Mullighan CG. Pediatric acute lymphoblastic leukemia. *Haematologica.* 2020;11:247031. Online ahead of print.
5. Maloney KW, Taub JW, Ravindranath Y, et al. Down syndrome preleukemia and leukemia. *Pediatr Clin North Am.* 2015;62(1):121–137.
6. Piris MA, Medeiros LJ, Chang K-C. Hodgkin lymphoma: a review of pathological features and recent advances in pathogenesis. *Pathology.* 2020;52(1):154–165.
7. Robinson CH, Coughlin CC, Chanchlani R, Dharnidharka VR. Post-transplant malignancies in pediatric organ transplant recipients. *Pediatr Transplant.* 2021;25(1), e13884.
8. Swerdlow SH, International Agency for Research on Cancer, & World Health Organization. *WHO classification of tumours of haematopoietic and lymphoid tissues.* 4th ed. International Agency for Research on Cancer, 2020.
9. Ramis-Zaldivar JE, Gonzalez-Farré B, Balagué O, et al. Distinct molecular profile of IRF4-rearranged large B-cell lymphoma. *Blood.* 2020;135(4):274–286.
10. Turner SD, Lamant L, Kenner L, Brugières L. Anaplastic large cell lymphoma in paediatric and young adult patients. *Br J Haematol.* 2016;173(4):560–572.

PEDIATRIC SOLID TUMORS PATHOLOGY

Larisa Debelenko, MD, PhD

1. **Histology is one of the most important factors that play a role in risk stratification of neuroblastomas. What features differentiate between favorable and unfavorable histology, and how do they relate to patient age?**

   Neuroblastoma (NB) is the most prevalent pediatric sarcoma characterized by a significant heterogeneity affecting the tumor behavior and prognosis. The tumor originates from a subset of nerve crest cells programmed to differentiate toward sympathetic ganglia and adrenal medulla. NB belongs to the group of neuroblastic tumors that show a spectrum of differentiation reflected by variable proportions of its cellular and stromal components, which include:
   - Immature neurons (neuroblasts) at different stages of their differentiation
   - A specific fibrillary matrix (neuropil) produced by differentiating neuroblasts
   - A specialized glial tissue (Schwannian stroma), which supports growing neuroblasts

   NBs are Schwannian-stroma poor tumors composed of more than 50% of neuroblasts and less than 50% of Schwannian stroma. The International Histology Neuroblastoma Classification (the Shimada system) provides criteria distinguishing favorable and unfavorable histology and is based on three factors:
   - Degree of neuroblastic differentiation accompanied by accumulation of neuropil
   - Mitotic activity and tumor apoptosis reflected by mitotic-karyorrhectic index (MKI)
   - Patient's age at diagnosis

   Accordingly, NB is subclassified into three categories:
   - Undifferentiated (tumors composed of undifferentiated neuroblasts and lacking neuropil)
   - Poorly differentiated (tumors containing no more than 5% of differentiating neuroblasts producing neuropil)
   - Differentiating (tumors containing more than 5% of differentiating neuroblasts, differentiated ganglion cells, and abundant neuropil)

   MKI is defined as a cumulative number of mitotic and apoptotic figures counted in 5000 tumor cells under the microscope. MKI of less than 100 per 5000 cells (or 2%) is low, 100 to 200 per 5000 cells (or 2%–4 %) is intermediate, and more than 200 per 5000 cells (or 4%) is high.

   Favorable histology NBs are diagnosed in patients younger than 5 years if they show signs of neuroblastic differentiation and low or intermediate MKI. Thus all differentiating tumors with low or intermediate MKI are favorable and all undifferentiated tumors with high MKI are unfavorable. However, in patients younger than 18 months at diagnosis, undifferentiated and poorly differentiating tumors with low or intermediate MKI are also favorable. In patients older than 18 months at diagnosis, undifferentiated and poorly differentiated tumors are unfavorable regardless of MKI.

   Histology of all NBs (Schwannian-stroma poor tumors) is unfavorable in patients older than 5 years. All Schwannian-stroma rich or dominant neuroblastic tumors called ganglioneuroblastoma and ganglioneuroma, respectively, are favorable regardless of age.

   Examples of favorable and unfavorable histology in neuroblastoma are presented in Figure 22.1.

2. **What separates favorable from unfavorable histology in Wilms tumor?**

   Wilms tumor (nephroblastoma) recapitulates renal development and consists of different proportions of epithelial and stromal elements and undifferentiated blastema (Figure 22.2A–C). Diffuse anaplasia is the key feature that distinguishes favorable and unfavorable histology (see Figure 22.2D).

   Generally, the term "anaplasia" implies an extreme de-differentiation of tumor cells and is used arbitrarily; however, because of its prognostic significance, it is strictly defined in nephroblastoma. This definition includes cellular gigantism (cells 3-to-4 times larger than their neighbors) and, most importantly, atypical (asymmetrical) mitotic figures.

   Biologically, anaplasia reflects extreme polyploidy and aneuploidy of tumor cells resulting from chromosomal instability because of genetic alterations of important cell cycle check points, such as *TP53*. Anaplasia is usually seen in the blastemal component; however, stromal anaplasia is also known.

   Originally, anaplasia in Wilms tumor was described as focal and diffuse and both types were considered unfavorable in the early treatment protocols. Further analysis, however, showed that some isolated stage 1 Wilms tumors with anaplasia behaved similarly to their favorable counterparts without anaplasia, which led to reevaluation of the criteria and significance of focal anaplasia. Currently, focal anaplasia is defined, using both quantitative and topographical parameters, as anaplastic nuclear changes confined to one or several discrete foci of primary tumor

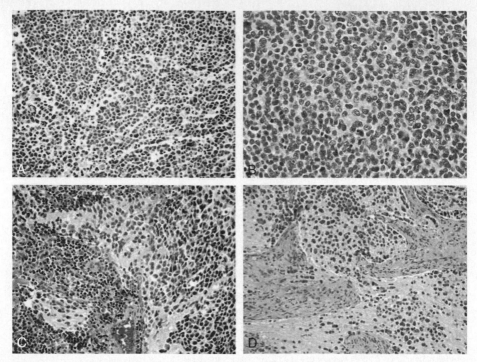

Figure 22.1 Histology of neuroblastoma (NB). (A) Undifferentiated NB with high mitotic-karyorrhectic index (MKI). Note sheets of undifferentiated "small round blue cells" and numerous mitotic and apoptotic figures. (B) Undifferentiated NB with low MKI. The tumor cells show primitive round cell morphology without signs of differentiation. The cumulative number of mitoses and apoptosis (karyorrhectic nuclei) is less than 2%. (C) Poorly differentiated NB with low MKI. Note fine fibrillary extracellular matrix (neuropil) and scatted within the matrix enlarged cells with signs of differentiation toward ganglion cells. (D) Differentiating NB with low MKI. Note abundant neuropil and tumor cells on variable stages of differentiation. Tongues of spindle cell proliferation (Schwannian stroma) are also present but occupy less than 50%.

located within boundaries of a tumor section on a slide without anaplasia or cellular unrest in the surrounding tumor and, most importantly, extrarenal sites (renal sinus, vessels, renal/tumor capsule, or metastases).

Focal anaplasia does not mean unfavorable histology; however, histological evaluation of the entire primary tumor and metastases (if any) are necessary to confirm that the observed anaplasia is focal. Thus anaplasia observed in a random tumor biopsy does not meet definitions of focal and is considered diffuse.

It is thought that anaplasia is the predictor of tumor responsiveness to therapy rather than the marker of innate tumor aggressiveness and Wilms tumors with diffuse anaplasia are characterized by poor therapeutic response and, thus, poor prognosis.

3. How may tumor and lymph nodes sampling affect staging of pediatric renal tumors?
   Staging of renal tumors is different in children and in adults. The Pediatric Oncology Group (POG) identifies 5 stages of Wilms tumor:
   Stage 1: Tumor limited to kidney and completely resected
   Stage 2: Tumor extending outside the kidney (penetrating renal capsule, extensively involving soft tissue or vessels of renal sinus) but completely resected
   Stage 3: Residual tumor confined to abdomen (nonhematogenous metastases to regional lymph nodes, penetration of peritoneum, peritoneal implants, positive resection margins, pre- or intraoperative tumor spillage, tumor removed in more than one piece)
   Stage 4: Hematogenous (liver, lung, bone, brain) and/or lymph node metastases outside abdominal cavity
   Stage 5: Bilateral renal involvement at diagnosis (each side should be staged separately according to the aforementioned criteria)
   To properly assign the stage, It is mandatory to sample and microscopically examine regional lymph nodes (hilar, periaortic, or inguinal). In many cases of low-grade tumors, the hilar lymph nodes are small and difficult to identify during surgery; therefore sampling of periaortic or inguinal lymph nodes should be planned. It is also important to take proper sections of the tumor for microscopic examination to examine the renal capsule and sinus. Renal sinus is the

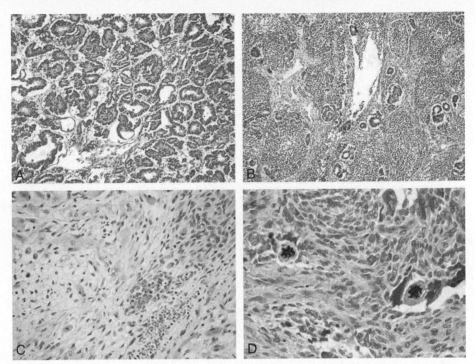

Figure 22.2 Histology of Wilms tumor (WT). (A) Predominantly epithelial WT composed of gland-like proliferation, recapitulating renal tubular development, with intervening stroma. (B) Predominantly blastemal WT with lobular proliferation of primitive round small cells (blastema) with admixed scattered epithelial (tubular) and nephrogenic elements and spindle cell tumor stroma. (C) Predominantly stromal (rhabdomyoblastic) WT. Note spindle tumor cells with focal sings of rhabdomyoblastic differentiation (eccentric eosinophilic cytoplasm with rare striations). A small amount of undifferentiated round cells (blastema) is also seen on the right. (D) Anaplastic WT. The tumor composed of undifferentiated blastema showing hyperchromasia and polymorphism with scatted giant cells with atypical mitotic figures.

concave region on the medial aspect of the kidney that contains most of the pelvicalyceal system and vessels and nerves passing to and from the kidney.

Failure of the sampling of renal sinus, renal capsule, and regional lymph nodes may result in an unnecessary upstaging of the tumor, preventing some patients from eligibility for Stage 1 management, which includes minimal or no postsurgical therapy, because to qualify for Stage 1, the tumor should have an intact capsule and documented absence of involvement of renal sinus and regional lymph nodes.

4. **How important is histological subtyping of rhabdomyosarcoma onto alveolar, embryonal, and other variants?**

Rhabdomyosarcoma (RMS) is a malignant soft tissue neoplasm originating from immature precursors of striated muscle cells. The tumor cells, rhabdomyoblasts, are arrested in early stages of differentiation and have a predominantly primitive morphology with indiscernible striations (Figure 22.3A–C). Nevertheless, rhabdomyoblasts express transcriptional factors, which normally govern muscular differentiation but are silenced in mature myocytes. Some of these transcriptional factors, such as MyoD-1 and myogenin, detected by immunohistochemistry (see Figure 22.3D), are used to differentiate RMS from other sarcomas.

RMSs have divergent morphologies: thus tumors resembling developing limbs seen in embryos have been called embryonal; tumors resembling primitive alveoli have been called alveolar; tumors growing under mucosal surfaces and grossly resembling a bunch of grapes have been called botryoid; and tumors showing extreme pleomorphism and anaplasia have been called pleomorphic (the latter subtype is very rare in children). In a subset, RMS cases show overlapping morphologic features, complicating the precise subclassification.

Chromosomal translocations resulting in fusions of *FOXO1* (located on chromosome 13) and *PAX2* (located on chromosome 2) or, alternatively, *PAX7* (located on chromosome 1), have been discovered in a majority of alveolar, but not in embryonal, RMS cases. Subsequently, gene expression analysis demonstrated a sharply demarcated signature defining a distinct biology of fusion-positive RMSs. Additionally, Children's Oncology Group (COG) studies revealed unfavorable outcomes associated with *PAX* fusions. The current COG protocol uses the fusion status rather than histology to define RMS risks.

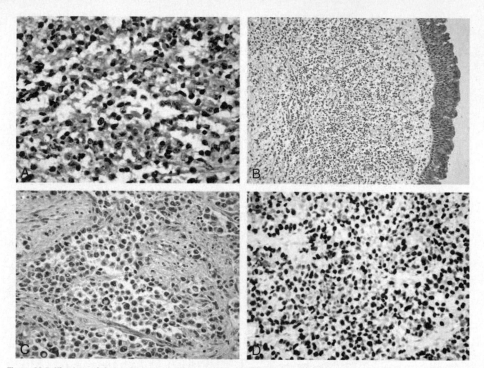

Figure 22.3 Histology of rhabdomyosarcoma (RS). (A) Embryonal RS showing round-to-oval tumor cells scattered in a "patternless" pattern. Note cells with eccentric eosinophilic cytoplasm showing morphologic signs of rhabdomyoblastic differentiation. (B) Botryoid RS. Pleomorphic tumor proliferation, admixed with chronic inflammatory infiltrate, is located under the intact bladder lining (urothelium). (C) Alveolar RS. Large undifferentiated predominantly round tumor cells are characterized by poor adhesion with formation of nascent "alveoli" separated by stromal septa. (D) Positive myogenin nuclear staining in alveolar RS.

Unlike alveolar RMS cases featuring translocations t(2;23) and t(1;13), most embryonal RMS cases are characterized by numerical chromosomal abnormalities with near triploid chromosomal content, including trisomies 2, 7, 8, 19, and 20. Recent studies also proposed a spindle cell/sclerosing variant of rhabdomyosarcoma, which includes (1) highly aggressive tumors with activating mutations of *MYOD1;* (2) less aggressive and sometimes congenital tumors with recurrent gene fusions involving *VGLL2* and *NCOA2* genes; and (3) mutation/translocation negative spindle-cell RMS cases characterized by predominantly abdominal and paratesticular locations.

Thus RMS histology has been useful in identifying distinct tumor groups; however, in cases of mixed and overlapping morphologies, the underlying molecular mechanisms appear to be more accurate in predicting the tumor behavior.

5. Describe the differences between Ewing and Ewing-like sarcomas.
Ewing sarcoma (ES) was first described as a bone tumor by James Ewing of Cornell University in the early 1920s. In 1983 the reciprocal translocation t(11;22) was identified in tumor cell lines and primary tumor tissue, leading to the cloning of the *EWSR1* gene on chromosome 22 named after the tumor. Identical translocations were identified in peripheral neuroepithelioma and Askin tumor, which shared primitive round cell morphology and malignant behavior with ES. These findings led to the understanding that all three neoplasms represented one entity, with primary tumors arising in either bone, soft tissues, or viscera; hence the term ES family tumors was introduced. Interestingly, tumors with t(11;22) are exceedingly rare in the brain.

ES is an archetypical round cell tumor characterized by a diffuse sheet-like growth of primitive monomorphic cells with uniform nuclei with fine chromatin and scant clear cytoplasm (Figure 22.4A). The primitive tumor cells are rich in glycogen. The exact cell of origin is not known, but it is thought that the tumor arises from early mesenchymal cells that reside in bone marrow or even earlier stem cells that retain capacity to differentiate along both mesenchymal and ectodermal/neuroectodermal lines. The most consistent immunohistochemical marker is CD99, which, albeit not specific, has a characteristic strong membranous pattern in ES (see Figure 22.4B).

The classical ES has translocations involving *EWSR1* or, seldom, *FUS* genes (which are closely related) with members of the ETS gene family of transcription factors, most frequently *FLI-1* and *ERG*. However, primitive sarcomas with different translocations have been identified. Called Ewing-like sarcomas by the previous World Health Organization (WHO) classification, they were reclassified in the 2020 edition as round cell sarcomas with *EWSR1*

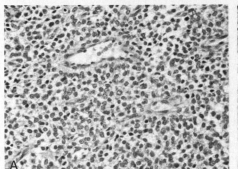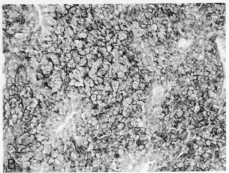

Figure 22.4 Histology of Ewing sarcoma (ES). (A) The tumor is composed of sheet-like proliferation of uniform tumor cells with round nuclei, clear cytoplasm, and indiscernible boundaries. Prominent capillaries with hyperplastic endothelium are characteristic. (B) CD99 stain shows the strong membranous staining pattern, resembling Olympic rings.

(*FUS*)-non ETS fusions. The following non-ETS partners have been reported thus far: *NFATC2*, *PATZ1*, and *VEZF1*. These tumors are characterized by mildly heterogeneous morphology with ovoid and spindled cells, extracellular matrix, and variable immunoreactivity with CD99. Although the number of studied tumors is small, non-ETS fusion partners imply a different biology.

Ewing-like sarcomas in the previous WHO classification also included undifferentiated sarcomas with different translocations, namely, involving *CIC* with *DUX4* or other partners and tumors with *BCOR* alterations, including *BCOR* internal tandem duplications or its fusions with *CCNB3* or other partners. The body of information accumulated in recent years has allowed us to reclassify these tumors as stand-alone entities.

Thus *CIC*-rearranged sarcomas, originally described in children, are now recognized to be more prevalent in young adults. Histologically they are composed of mildly pleomorphic round cells with vesicular nuclei, prominent nucleoli, and amphophilic cytoplasm. The tumors show only patchy CD99 staining but are frequently positive for ETB4 and WT1. The prognosis is poor and worse than in ES.

BCOR-activated sarcomas include tumors with internal tandem duplications, like infantile undifferentiated round cell tumors (and related clear cell sarcoma of kidney) or primitive myxoid mesenchymal tumors of infancy. Tumors with *BCOR-CCNB3* fusions affect predominantly males in the second decade and have a predilection to long bone. The tumors are composed of slightly ovoid primitive cells and express BCOR by immunohistochemistry, although this marker is not specific.

In summary, the classification of primitive sarcomas is a work in progress and currently includes classical ES with *EWSR1-ETS* fusions, Ewing-like sarcomas with *EWSR1-*non *ETS* fusions, and undifferentiated round cell sarcomas with different molecular alterations.

6. Why are some of the pediatric sarcomas called "epithelioid" and "rhabdoid," and what is the biological significance of these morphologic features?
"Epithelioid" and "rhabdoid" are descriptive terms used to designate *undifferentiated* tumors composed of cells that morphologically resemble epithelial cells and rhabdomyoblasts, respectively. Rhabdoid features include large cellular size, eosinophilic (pink) cytoplasm, and centrally or eccentrically located round to ovoid nucleus with prominent nucleolus. Epithelioid features include ovoid cellular shape and relatively abundant, so-called "plump," cytoplasm. This phenotypic resemblance is accompanied by the immunohistochemical mimicry: thus, both rhabdoid and epithelioid tumors frequently express markers of epithelial (cytokeratins), muscular (actin and desmin), and other lines of differentiation.

Both malignant rhabdoid tumor (MRT), located in soft tissues and viscera, and its central nervous system counterpart, atypical rhabdoid-teratoid tumor (ARTT), are composed of sheets of undifferentiated rhabdoid cells (Figure 22.5A). Affecting predominantly very young children, these highly aggressive malignancies are associated with germ-line mutations or deletions of *SMARCB1* gene on chromosome 22 in approximately 30% of cases. The tumors develop according to the two-hit Knudson model, with the second mutation knocking out the *SMARCB1* in somatic tumor cells, which leads to cessation of the constitutive expression of the encoded protein called by its aliases: INI-1 or BAF47. Lack of INI-1 expression in tumor cells by immunohistochemistry is useful in the pathology diagnosis of MRT (see Figure 22.5B).

Epithelioid sarcoma (EpS) is a distinctive soft tissue neoplasm, affecting predominantly young males. The classical type is localized to distal parts of the body (fingers, toes, tongue) and mimics chronic (granulomatous) inflammation both clinically and pathologically, which can sometimes cause a delay in cancer diagnosis. The proximal type has a predilection to pelvic-perineal deep soft tissue but may occur in any location, except the most distal parts of extremities. The tumor cells have epithelioid, histiocytoid, or rhabdoid morphologic features and strongly express cytokeratins and other markers of epithelial differentiation, hence, the name, EpS. Similarly to MRT, loss of function

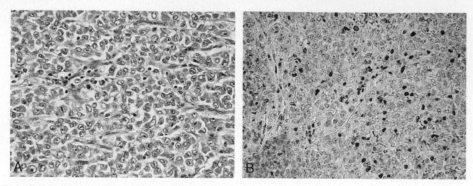

Figure 22.5 Histology of malignant rhabdoid tumor (MRT) (A) The tumor is composed of large cells with focal eccentric eosinophilic cytoplasm, resembling rhabdomyoblasts. Characteristic prominent nucleoli are present. (B) INI-1 staining is absent in the tumor cells, whereas the admixed inflammatory and endothelial cells show normal constitutive expression of the protein in their nuclei.

alterations of *SMARCB1* or other members of the SWI/SNF gene family members underlie the pathogenesis of EpS and the INI-1 is not expressed in 80% to 100% of EpS cases.

Tumors featuring inactivation of *SMARCB1* or other SWI/SNF gene family members are not limited to MRT, ARTT, and EpS. Thus the same mechanism underlies small cell carcinoma of the ovary (hypercalcemic type), epithelioid variant of malignant peripheral nerve sheath tumors, undifferentiated/dedifferentiated carcinomas occurring in gastrointestinal, genitourinary, and respiratory tracts, chordomas, subsets of synovial sarcomas and myoepithelial tumors of soft tissues, and other even more rare tumors. Although in a large proportion of these tumors, epithelioid and rhabdoid morphologies correlate with SWI/SNF gene inactivation, this association is not absolute and there are tumors with epithelioid features but different underlying molecular mechanisms and vice versa.

In summary, tumor histology and genetics combined provide the basis for tumor classification and to accurately predict prognosis and response to therapy they need to be interpreted in appropriate clinical contexts.

BIBLIOGRAPHY

1. Agaimy A. SWI/SNF Complex-deficient soft tissue neoplasms: a pattern-based approach to diagnosis and differential diagnosis. *Surg Pathol Clin.* 2019;12:149–163.
2. Alaggio R, Zhang L, Sung YS, et al. A molecular study of pediatric spindle and sclerosing rhabdomyosarcoma: identification of novel and recurrent VGLL2-related fusions in infantile cases. *Am J Surg Pathol.* 2016;40:224–235.
3. Anderson WJ, Doyle LA. Updates from the 2020 World Health Organization Classification of Soft Tissue and Bone Tumours. *Histopathology.* 2021;78(5):644–657.
4. Beckwith JB, Zuppan CE, Browning NG, Moksness J, Breslow NE. Histological analysis of aggressiveness and responsiveness in Wilms' tumor. *Med Pediatr Oncol.* 1996;27:422-8.
5. Dome JS, Cotton CA, Perlman EJ, et al. Treatment of anaplastic histology Wilms' tumor: results from the fifth National Wilms' Tumor Study. *J Clin Oncol.* 2006;24:2352–2358.
6. Faria P, Beckwith JB, Mishra K, et al. Focal versus diffuse anaplasia in Wilms tumor - new definitions with prognostic significance: a report from the National Wilms Tumor Study Group. *Am J Surg Pathol.* 1996;20:909–920.
7. Green DM, Breslow NE, Beckwith JB, et al. Treatment with nephrectomy only for small, stage I/favorable histology Wilms' tumor: a report from the National Wilms' Tumor Study Group. *J Clin Oncol.* 2001;19:3719–3724.
8. Parham DM, Giannikopoulos P. Rhabdomyosarcoma: from obscurity to clarity in diagnosis … but with ongoing challenges in management: The Farber-Landing Lecture of 2020. *Pediatr Dev Pathol.* 2021;24(2):87–95.
9. Shimada H, Ambros IM, Dehner LP, et al. Terminology and morphologic criteria of neuroblastic tumors: recommendations by the International Neuroblastoma Pathology Committee. *Cancer.* 1999;86:349–363.
10. Shimada H, Ambros IM, Dehner LP, et al. The International Neuroblastoma Pathology Classification (the Shimada system). *Cancer.* 1999;86:364–372.
11. Tsuda Y, Zhang L, Meyers P, Tap WD, Healey JH, Antonescu CR. The clinical heterogeneity of round cell sarcomas with EWSR1/FUS gene fusions: impact of gene fusion type on clinical features and outcome. *Genes Chromosomes Cancer.* 2020;59:525–534.

CHAPTER 23

MOLECULAR PATHOLOGY

Mahesh M. Mansukhani, MD and Justin L. Kurtz, MD

1. Compare and contrast DNA and RNA as targets for molecular testing.

   DNA is double-stranded with A-T and C-G pairs of deoxyribonucleotides; it includes exons, introns, and intergenic regions; all nucleated normal cells have the full DNA complement; and DNA is relatively stable. RNA is usually single stranded using uracil in place of thymine; ubiquitous ribonucleases make RNA unstable outside of living cells requiring rapid/immediate sample processing (warm ischemia during surgical resection should especially be avoided); each cell expresses RNAs from only a subset of genes, with dynamic temporal changes, and variable (often short) half-life; and mature RNA lacks introns. DNA is the preferred target for mutation testing and for chimerism analysis after transplant; RNA is the preferred target for detecting gene fusions and performing gene expression analysis. Translocations that do not result in gene fusions will not be detected by RNA analysis, although they may be suspected by aberrant expression of RNA.

2. What are the different tests for genomic rearrangements (translocations), and their strengths and weaknesses?

   Karyotyping requires growing tumor cells in culture. It will detect most rearrangements that result in visible chromosomal alterations (Figures 23.1A, 23.2A, and 23.3A).; however, the resolution is limited and "interstitial" rearrangements involving only short segments of chromosomes may be missed. Karyotyping will not identify the involved genes, and it requires viable tumor cells.

   In-situ hybridization uses probes with different colors (fluorescent or chromogenic) targeting distant genomic regions brought together by the rearrangement ("fusion probes"; see Figures 23.1B and 23.2B) or probes flanking one of the breakpoints, with colors separating as a result of the translocation ("break-apart probes"; see Figure 23.3B–C). A different probe set is needed for each rearrangement, although break-apart probes will detect all rearrangements of a gene that has multiple partners (e.g., EWSR1) without identifying the fusion partner.

   Reverse-transcriptase polymerase chain reaction (PCR) can identify rearrangements that create chimeric RNA (e.g., BCR-ABL1, the various EWSR1 transcripts), but a different primer set and/or test may be needed for each fusion variant. It requires intact RNA and special handling of samples to preserve RNA. Quantitative and highly sensitive tests (tests with low detection limits) can be designed to monitor response to treatment and minimal residual disease.

   DNA PCR can detect rearrangement with or without RNA fusions, but DNA breakpoints of rearrangements can vary tremendously from case to case, so only a subset of rearrangements will be detected with each assay. Even multiplexed assays will miss some rearrangements, resulting in variable sensitivity for the various rearrangements.

   Targeted next-generation cDNA sequencing using anchored multiplexed PCR can detect RNA fusions of multiple targets at a time and will detect both known and novel partners of targeted genes. It works with partially degraded RNA and with small amounts of RNA. It will only detect fusions involving targeted genes, although modifications allow detection of novel partners.

   Whole transcriptome sequencing has the potential to detect all possible rearrangements that result in RNA fusions but is dependent on the level of expression of the fusion RNA. In addition, many nonspecific "fusions" are seen, necessitating careful analysis and, sometimes, confirmatory tests to report novel rearrangements.

   Whole-genome sequencing can potentially detect any genomic rearrangement but requires a high tumor percentage in the sample, needs infrastructure to analyze massive amounts of data, and may require additional testing to predict the effects of genomic rearrangements.

3. Name the recurrent cytogenetic abnormalities used for classification of B-cell acute lymphoblastic leukemia (B-ALL) and the impact of each on prognosis?

   High risk: Hypodiploid genome (45 or fewer chromosomes); *KMT2A (MLL)* rearrangements, most commonly t(4;11)(q21;q23) *KMT2A-AFF1 (MLL-AF4)*, t(11;19)(q23.3;p13.3) *(KMT2A-MLLT1)* and over forty others; t(9;22)(q34;q11.2) *BCR-ABL1* (standard risk with *ABL1* inhibitor); Ph-like *(IKZF1* deletions); *CRLF2* rearrangements (e.g., t(X;14)(p22;q32)); activating kinase mutations; intrachromosomal amplification of chromosome 21 (iAMP21); *MEF2D* rearrangements.

   Intermediate (standard) risk: t(1;19)(p23;q13.3) *TCF3-PBX1 (E2A-PBX1)* (standard risk with intensive chemotherapy); t(5;14)(p31;q32) *IL3-IGH; ZNF384* rearrangements.

   Low risk: *ETV6-RUNX1* (TEL-AML1)/t(12;21) (p13;q22) (the most common rearrangement in B-ALL); hyperdiploidy (51–65 chromosomes because of whole chromosome gains); *DUX4-IGH* gene rearrangements.

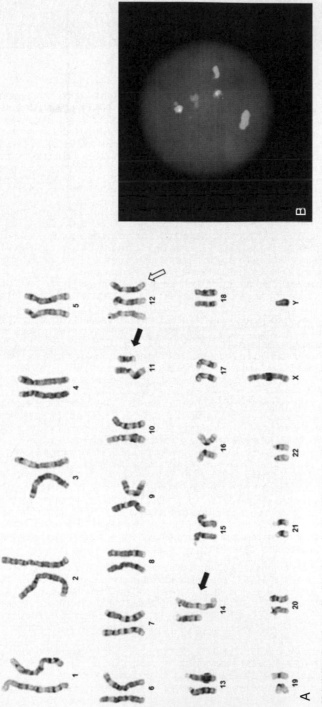

Figure 23.1 (A) Karyotype of a mantle cell lymphoma, showing a t(11;14)(q13;q32) translocation (*black-filled arrows*) and trisomy 12 (*white arrow*). (B) Interphase dual color IGH–CCND1 fusion probe of the same specimen. The two overlapping fused gray and bright white signals (*red and green* fluorescent probes, respectively) represent the translocation, with two bright IGH signals, and one gray CCND1 signal.

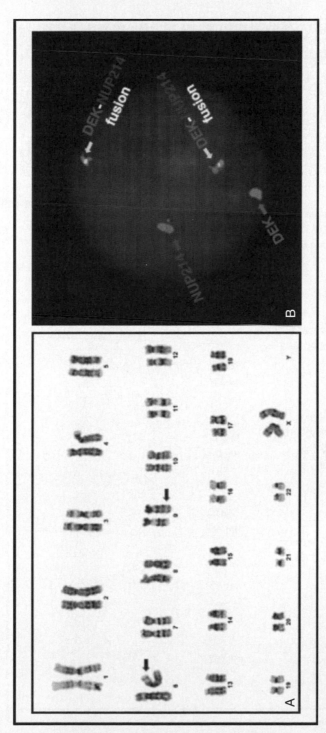

Figure 23.2 (A) Karyotype of an acute myeloid leukemia showing a t(6;9)(p22;q34) translocation (*filled arrows*). (B) Interphase fluorescence in situ hybridization (FISH) of the same specimen with a dual-color DEK-NUP214 fusion probe.

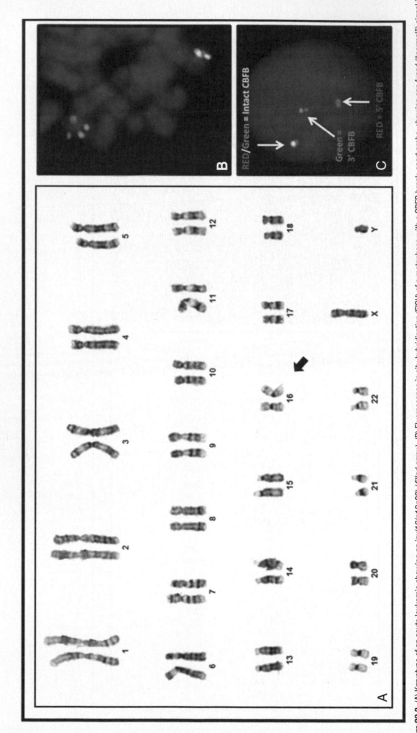

Figure 23.3 (A) Karyotype of an acute leukemia showing an inv(16)(p13q22) (*filled arrow*). (B) Fluorescence in situ hybridization (FISH) of a metaphase with a CBFB break-apart probe, showing one fused ("normal") signal in the lower right, and two split (rearranged) gray and bright white signals (*pink* and *green* fluorescent probes, respectively) on the upper left. (C) Interphase FISH with the same probe showing one fused and one split signal, indicative of a CBFB rearrangement.

4. **What are the different *BCR-ABL1* translocations and their associated conditions, and how does the specific translocation affect diagnostic testing and monitoring for these conditions?**
The genomic breakpoints involved in *BCR-ABL1* translocations all involve intron 1 of *ABL1*, with three different sets of breakpoints in BCR. The *BCR* major breakpoint cluster region (M-bcr) in introns 13 and 14 results in fusions of exon 13 or 14 with exon 2 or, less commonly, because of alternative splicing, with exon 3 of *ABL1* (e13a2, e13a3, e14a2 and e14a3), which encode the "p210" (approximately 210kd) BCR-ABL1 fusion protein, associated with chronic myeloid leukemia (CML). The minor breakpoint cluster region, in intron 1 of *BCR* produces the e1a2 and e1a3 fusion transcripts, which encode the p190 BCR-ABL1 fusion protein, characteristic of Philadelphia chromosome positive ALL (Ph+ ALL). The least common micro breakpoint cluster in intron 19 (μ-bcr) results in e19a2 and e19a3 fusions, which encode the p230 BCR-ABL1 protein seen in patients with a CML variant with increased neutrophils ("chronic neutrophilic leukemia" or "neutrophilic CML") and, rarely, typical CML.
Molecular tests, especially RT-PCR based tests, should detect the specific fusions and because of occasional overlap (e.g., CML in lymphoid blast phase presenting as Ph+ ALL, or rare p190 positive p210-negative CML), negative results for one fusion may need to be followed up with additional testing for the other fusions.

5. **What genes are commonly involved in Langerhans cell histiocytosis and related conditions, and what are their implications for therapy?**
Activation of the *RAS/RAF/MEK/ERK* (MAP kinase) pathway is a common finding in Langerhans cell histiocytosis (LCH) and in the non-Langerhans cell histiocytoses, Erdheim Chester disease (ECD), juvenile xanthogranuloma (JXG), and, to a lesser extent, in Rosai Dorfaman disease (RDD). *BRAF* V600E mutations are predominant in LCH and JXG, followed by *MAP2K1* and non-V600E *BRAF* mutations. *NRAS/KRAS* mutations predominate in RDD, whereas activation of MAPK signaling in JXG is more heterogenous with *CSF1R, KIT, ALK, MET, CSF3R, MAPK2K1, KRAS,* and *NRAS* mutations and fusions involving *NTRK1, BRAF, RET,* and *ALK*. Targeting with BRAF and MEK inhibitors is associated with transient responses in tumors with activating mutations in the MAP kinase pathway. Kinase fusions may respond to specific inhibitors.

6. **How do molecular alterations impact neuroblastoma risk classification?**
According to the 2021 International Neuroblastoma Risk Group Staging System (INRGSS), *MYCN* amplification, a diploid genome (46 chromosomes), and segmental chromosomal alterations worsen risk groups as follows. Excluding fully resected, localized tumors with no imaging defined risk factors, all *MYCN* amplified tumors are classified as high risk. Among *MYCN* nonamplified stage M (stage IV) tumors in children younger than 18 months, segmental chromosomal alterations (e.g., 11p losses), diploidy, or unfavorable histology alter the risk category from intermediate to high risk. Activating *ALK* mutations are unrelated to outcome, but germline *ALK* mutations and loss-of-function *PHOX2B* mutations are associated with hereditary neuroblastoma syndromes.

7. **What are the fusions associated with Ewing family and related tumors?**
Ewing sarcomas (ES) are characterized by fusions of *EWSR1*, or rarely *FUS*, with members of the ETS family of transcription factors (*FLI1, ERG, ETV1, ETV4,* and, *FEV*), most frequently t(11;22) (q24;q12) (*EWSR1-FLI*) at 85% and t(21;22) (q22;q12) (*EWSR1-ERG*). Ewing-like sarcomas histologically resemble ES but lack EWSR1-ETS fusions. They include CIC-rearranged sarcomas (*CIC-DUX4* most common), BCOR-rearranged sarcomas (*BCOR-CCNB3* most common), and sarcomas with *EWSR1* or *FUS* fused to a non-ETS gene (*NFATc2* or *PATZ1*). The latter are more common in young adults than in children. Desmoplastic small round cell tumor (DSRCT), with a similar morphology but characteristic immunophenotype harbors a t(11;22) (p13;q12), *EWSR1-WT1* fusion.

8. **Which subtypes of rhabdomyosarcomas are associated with recurrent gene fusions, and what are the fusions?**
Recurrent gene fusions are commonly found in alveolar rhabdomyosarcomas, and the most common fusions are *PAX3-FOXO1*/t (2;13) and *PAX7-FOXO1*/t (1;13). Embryonal rhabdomyosarcomas do not commonly harbor fusions, and karyotype is more likely to show losses and gains of chromosomes. There is still debate as to whether this fusion is a pathognomonic feature of alveolar rhabdomyosarcomas; histologically appearing embryonal rhabdomyosarcomas have been found to harbor one of these fusions in rare cases. *FOXO1* fusion-positive rhabdomyosarcomas are associated with a poor prognosis. A subset of spindle cell-sclerosing rhabdomyosarcomas in infants show *VGLL2, TEAD1,* or *SRF* fusions.
Table 23.1 shows common sarcomas and their associated fusions.

9. **Rhabdomyosarcomas are commonly found in which hereditary tumor syndromes?**
Rhabdomyosarcomas have been identified in many familial cancer syndromes, including Li-Fraumeni syndrome (*TP53*), neurofibromatosis type 1 (*NF1*), *DICER1* syndrome, Gorlin syndrome (*PTCH1*), Beckwith-Wiedemann syndrome (11p15.5 gene locus), Noonan syndrome (*PTPN11*), and Costello syndrome (*HRAS*).

10. **What is the molecular abnormality associated with Beckwith-Wiedemann syndrome, and what neoplasms commonly occur in these patients?**
Beckwith-Wiedemann syndrome is an overgrowth disorder of genomic imprinting because of genetic or epigenetic defects at two separate imprinted regions on 11p15.5, the paternally methylated telomeric imprinting control region 1 (IC1) and the more centromeric, maternally methylated IC2. Genes at this locus that may be related to the condition

Table 23.1 Common Sarcomas and Associated Fusions

SARCOMA	FUSION
Ewing sarcoma	*FLI1-EWSR1*, t(11;22)(q24;q12) (90%) *ERG-EWSR1*, t(12;22)(q22;q12) (5–10%)
Alveolar rhabdomyosarcoma	*PAX3-FOXO1*, t(2;13)(q35;q14) (75%) *PAX7-FOXO1*, t(1;13)(p36;q14) (10%)
Spindle cell sclerosing rhabdomyosarcoma	*VGLL2-NCOA2*, t(6;8)(q22;q13) *SRF-NCOA2*, t(6;8)(p21;q13) *VGLL2-CITED2*, t(6;6)(q22;q24)
Desmoplastic small round cell tumor	*EWSR1-WT1*, t(11;22)(p13;q12) (95%)
Alveolar soft part sarcoma	*ASPSCR1-TFE3*, t(X;17)(p11;q25)
Synovial sarcoma	*SS18-SSX1*, t(X;18)(p11;q11) *SS18-SSX2*, t(X;18)(p11;q11) *SS18L1/SSX2*, t(X;20)(p11;q13)
Mesenchymal chondrosarcoma	*HEY1-NCOA2*, t(8;8)(q13;q21) *IRF2BP2-CDX1*, t(1;5)(q42;q32)
Undifferentiated sarcoma	*CIC-DUX4*, t(4;19)(q35;q13)* *CIC-DUX4*, t(10;19)(q26.3;q13) *BCOR-CCNB3*, inv(X)(p11.4;p11.22)
Clear cell sarcoma	*ATF1-EWSR1*, t(12;22)(q13;q12) *CREB1-EWSR1*, t(2;22)(q32.3;q12)
Angiomatoid fibrous histiocytoma	*ATF1-EWSR1*, t(12;22)(q13;q12) *ATF1-FUS* t(12;16)(q13;q11)
Myxoid chondrosarcoma	*EWSR1-NR4A3*, t(9;22)(q22;q12)
Myxoid liposarcoma	*FUS-DDIT3*, t(12;16)(q13;p11) *EWSR1-DDIT3*, t(12;22)(q13;p12)
Low-grade fibromyxoid sarcoma	*FUS-CREB3L2*, t(7;16)(q33;p11) *FUS-CREB3L1*, t(11;16)(p13;p11)
Sclerosing epithelioid fibrosarcoma	*EWSR1-CREB3L1*, t(11;22)(p11;q12) *EWSR1-CREB3L2*, t(7;22)(q34;q12)
Infantile fibrosarcoma (and cellular congenital mesoblastic nephroma)	*ETV6-NTRK3*, t(12;15)(p13;q25) *EML4-NTRK3*, t(2;15)(2p21;15q25)

Data from Pytel P, Cipriani NA. Soft tissue and bone neoplasms. In Furtado LV, Husain AN (eds). *Precision Molecular Pathology of Neoplastic Pediatric Diseases*. Molecular Pathology Library; Sbaraglia M, Righi A, Gambarotti M, Dei Tos AP. Ewing sarcoma and Ewing-like tumors. *Virchows Arch.* 2020;476(1):109–119; Huret, JL. EWSR1 (Ewing sarcoma breakpoint region 1). *Atlas Genet Cytogenet Oncol Haematol.* 2011;15(5):395–407; and Storlazzi, Clelia T. Soft tissue tumors: t(X;20)(p11.23;q13.33) in biphasic synovial sarcoma. *Atlas Genet Cytogenet Oncol Haematol.* 2007;11(4):340–339.

include the maternally expressed *CDKN1C* and the paternally expressed *IGF2*. DNA methylation abnormalities (gain of methylation on IC2, or loss of methylation on IC1) account for 55% to 60% of cases, and 20% are because of mosaic segmental *paternal* uniparental isodisomy (UPD). Additional mechanisms include chromosomal abnormalities and *CDKN1C* loss of function mutations on the maternal allele. A molecular cause is not found in approximately 20% of patients. Cancer risk is greatest with IC1 gain of methylation and paternal UPD and lowest with IC2 loss of methylation. The most common embryonal tumor seen in these patients is Wilms tumor (WT; nephroblastoma), followed by hepatoblastoma, neuroblastoma, rhabdomyosarcoma, and adrenal cortical tumors. The risk of developing embryonal tumors is greatest in the first 2 years of life.

11. **How do the syndromic associations of WT inform germline genetic testing in children with WT?**
Ten to fifteen percent of unselected WTs and a third of familial WTs have detectable germline genomic abnormalities. The most common of these involve *WT1* mutations (nonsyndromic WT and Denys Drash syndrome) and deletions (WAGR: Wilms tumor, aniridia, growth abnormalities, and mental retardation syndrome), *TRIM28* mutations, *REST* mutations, and 11p15 methylation abnormalities. In addition, heterozygous mutations involving *ASXL1, CDC73, CTR9, DICER1, FBXW7, KDM3B,* and *TP53*; biallelic mutations involving *BLM, BRCA2, BUB1B, DIS3L2, NYNRIN, PALB2, TRIM37,* and *TRIP13*; hemizygous mutations in *GPC3*; and mosaic *PIK3CA* mutations are also seen. Variants in *TRIM28, REST, WT1, CTR9,* 11p.15, *CDC73, BRCA2,* and *NYNRINI* are also seen in familial cases.

11p.15 abnormalities are best investigated with methylation analysis and testing for paternal uniparental disomy, and *WT1* contiguous gene deletions (which also involve *PAX6* in the WAGR syndrome) with fluorescence in situ hybridization (FISH), DNA microarray, and next-generation sequencing assays that detect copy number changes. Gene sequencing panels can be used to identify point mutations and small indels in known genes, and, if negative, deletion duplication analysis will detect mutations in most of the remaining cases.

12. **What tumors in children are commonly associated with loss of INI1/SMARCB1?**
SMARCB1 is a tumor suppressor gene, and therefore, loss of function of both alleles may result in SMARCB1-deficient tumors. The prototypical SMARCB1-deficient tumor is the malignant rhabdoid tumor (MRT). The majority of MRTs are diagnosed in infants less than 1 year of age and can arise in the kidney, other visceral organs, soft tissue, or central nervous system (CNS). When it arises in the CNS, it is referred to as an atypical teratoid rhabdoid tumor (AT/RT). Other SMARCB1-deficient pediatric tumors include epithelioid sarcomas, renal medullary carcinoma, and a subset of myoepithelial carcinomas, chordomas, malignant peripheral nerve sheath tumors, and schwannomatosis.

13. **What cytogenetic abnormality in renal cell carcinoma is more frequently present in the pediatric population than in the adult population?**
Approximately 40% of renal cell carcinomas (RCCs) in children (less than 5% in the adult population) harbor a fusion involving a member of the microphthalmia transcription factor (MiTF) family, usually the *TFE3* gene located at Xp11.2. The most common fusion partners are *ASPL* (ASPSCR1) resulting from t(X;17) (p11.2; q25) and *PRCC* resulting from t(X;1) (p11.2;q21). Regardless of the partner, these fusions result in constitutive activation of TFE3. The prognosis of MiTF translocation RCC is highly variable, ranging from indolent to rapidly progressive disease, and there is evidence that the specific translocation affects the clinical outcome, with distant metastasis more common in patients with the *ASPL-TFE3* fusions. Note that the *ASPL-TFE3* gene fusion is the same as that seen in alveolar soft part sarcoma.

14. **What are the common molecular alterations in low- and high-grade glial neoplasms frequently seen in children?**
Pediatric low-grade gliomas (PLGG) are characterized by genomic alterations that activate the MAP kinase signaling. Seventy-five percent of pilocytic astrocytomas (PAs) harbor *KIAA1549-BRAF* fusions; loss of function *NF1* mutations or *BRAF* V600E mutations are seen in most of the remaining PAs. *BRAF* V600E is common in pleomorphic xanthoastrocytomas (50%–60%), and gangliogliomas (40%), and less frequent in pilomyxoid astrocytomas and other low-grade gliomas. Rare PLGGs show *RAS* mutations or fusions involving *NTRK1, FGFR1, ALK, MYB,* or *MYBL1*. *CDKN2A* deletions or mutations often accompany progression to high-grade gliomas.

Most infratentorial pediatric diffuse high-grade gliomas carry "H3K27M" mutations in histone H3 (encoded by *H3F3A or HIST1H3B*) resulting in loss of histone H3K27 trimethylation, a chromatin change associated with gene silencing. *H3F3A* G34 mutations are seen in a subset of hemispheric high-grade gliomas prevalent in adolescents and young adults. *BRAF* V600E mutations characterize epithelioid glioblastomas, a rare extremely aggressive glial tumor.

Note that because the methionine translated from the initiation codon is removed from the mature histone, "K27" and "G34" are reported as "K28" and "G35" based on their order during translation.

15. **What are the genomic subtypes of medulloblastomas, and what are their prognostic implications?**
Medulloblastomas, the most common CNS embryonal tumors, account for approximately 25% of intracranial pediatric neoplasms. Prognosis is determined by a combination of clinical and genomic features. High-risk disease is associated with age 3 years and under, subtotal resection, and leptomeningeal spread. The four major genomic medulloblastoma subgroups are:

Group 1 WNT-activated (approximately 10%–15%): They present in older children (peak 10–12 years) and have the most favorable prognosis. Somatic activating *CTNNB1* (beta catenin) exon 3 mutations characterize 85% to 90% of cases, and predominantly germline *APC* loss of function mutations are present in most remaining cases.

Group 2 SHH-activated (approximately 30%): They show a peak incidence in infancy, and a second in children over 16 years of age. Mutually exclusive loss of function mutations of *PTCH1* (all ages) and *SUFU* (infants) or activating *SMO* mutations (older children/adults) result in activation of the SHH (sonic hedgehog) pathway. *TP53* mutations (somatic or germline) worsen prognosis in this group. Germline mutations account for 20% of cases, with *PTCH1* and *SUFU* seen predominantly in infants and *TP53* germline mutations in childhood. *TP53* mutations in this group alter the risk from intermediate (5-year survival approximately 76% without *TP53* mutations) to high risk (5-year survival approximately 41%). Smoothened (*SMO*) inhibitors (vismodegib and sonidegib) have shown efficacy in clinical trials of SHH medulloblastoma; *SUFU* mutations or *GLI2* amplification, which are downstream of SMO, cause resistance to *SMO* inhibitors.

Groups 3 and 4: non-WNT/non-SHH mutated medulloblastomas make up groups 3 and 4, accounting for 20% and 40% of cases, respectively. Amplification of *MYC* (group 3) or *MYCN* (group 4) and activation of *GFI1* or *GFI1B* is typically present. Overall, non-WNT/non-SHH medulloblastomas have the worst prognosis with metastatic disease frequently identified at presentation.

16. **What recurrent chromosomal alteration defines a subset of ependymomas and in what location does this subset arise?**
    Recent studies determined supratentorial and infratentorial ependymomas are distinct disease entities with different molecular profiles. The *C11orf95-RELA* fusion is specific for supratentorial ependymomas, present in approximately 70% of cases. The presence of a *RELA* fusion does not appear to affect prognosis. *YAP1* fusions have also been identified in a minority of supratentorial ependymomas. No recurrent genetic alterations have been identified in infratentorial ependymomas.

17. **What constitutional tumor syndrome is characterized by somatic mosaicism, and how does this affect genetic testing?**
    Ollier syndrome, a type of metaphyseal enchondromatosis (called Maffucci syndrome when accompanied by vascular malformations), is characterized by somatic mosaicism for activating *IDH1* or *IDH2* mutations (mutations at *IDH1* R132 or *IDH2* R140 or R172) that alter the activity of these enzymes resulting in aberrant production of 2-hydroxyglutarate, instead of alpha-ketoglutarate. The former is an inhibitor of multiple enzymes including TET (Ten-eleven translocation methyl cytosine dioxygenase) and histone demethylases, resulting in increased DNA and histone methylation. Identical *IDH1* or *IDH2* mutations are seen in all tumors in an individual. Gliomas that develop in this setting also show the same variants. Standard germline tests do not show these mutations, although highly sensitive tests, like droplet digital PCR, have shown low levels of mutations (less than 1% mutant) in nontumor tissues

18. **How can testing mitigate the hematopoietic toxicity of thioguanines?**
    Loss-of-function mutations in thiopurine methyl transferase (*TPMT*) or *NUDT15* (nucleoside diphosphate-linked moiety X motif 15), enzymes involved in purine metabolism, cause increased risk of hematopoietic toxicity from 6-mercaptopurine or azathioprine. *TPMT* *2 or *3 variants account for almost 95% loss of function alleles in Whites; *NUDT15* R139C is seen in Asians. One in 300 Whites have virtually no detectable TPMT activity in their blood, and one in 50 Asians are *NUDT15* poor metabolizers. Molecular testing will detect only the variants tested. Tests for TMPT activity will identify poor metabolizers irrespective of genetic mutation; however, in the post-transfusion setting, results are affected by TMPT activity in donor red blood cells. Reduced drug dosage for individuals who are homozygous for *TPMT* or *NUDT15* loss of function variants or with absent *TPMT* activity in the blood can reduce toxicity without affecting antileukemic activity.

BIBLIOGRAPHY

1. Amary MF, Damato S, Halai D, et al. Ollier disease and Maffucci syndrome are caused by somatic mosaic mutations of IDH1 and IDH2. *Nat Genet.* 2011;43(12):1262–1265.
2. Arboleda VA, Xian RR. An overview of DNA analytical methods. In Yong W (ed). *Biobanking. Methods in Molecular Biology.* 1897. Humana Press, 2019.
3. Argani P. MiT family translocation renal cell carcinoma. *Semin Diagn Pathol.* 2015;32(2):103–113.
4. Brioude F, Kalish JM, Mussa A, et al. Expert consensus document: clinical and molecular diagnosis, screening and management of Beckwith-Wiedemann syndrome: an international consensus statement. *Nat Rev Endocrinol.* 2018;14(4):229–249.
5. Cole BL. Neuropathology of pediatric brain tumors: a concise review. *Neurosurgery.* 2021:nyab182. doi: 10.1093/neuros/nyab182. Epub ahead of print.
6. Dome JS, Huff V. Wilms tumor predisposition. 2003 Dec 19 [Updated 2016 Oct 20]. In Adam MP, Ardinger HH, Pagon RA, et al. (eds). *GeneReviews®* [Internet]. University of Washington, Seattle, 1993-2021.
7. Faulkner C, Ellis HP, Shaw A, et al. BRAF fusion analysis in pilocytic astrocytomas: KIAA1549-BRAF 15-9 fusions are more frequent in the midline than within the cerebellum. *J Neuropathol Exp Neurol.* 2015;74(9):867–872.
8. Hijiya N, Suttorp M. How I treat chronic myeloid leukemia in children and adolescents. *Blood.* 2019;133(22):2374–2384. Epub 2019 Mar 7.
9. Iacobucci I, Kimura S, Mullighan CG. Biologic and therapeutic implications of genomic alterations in acute lymphoblastic leukemia. *J Clin Med.* 2021;10(17):3792.
10. Irwin Meredith, Naranjo Arlene, Zhang Fan, et al. Revised neuroblastoma risk classification system: A report from the Children's Oncology Group. *J Clin Oncol.* 2021;39(29):3229–3241.
11. Jarzembowski JA. Molecular methods in oncology: genomic analysis. In Furtado L, Husain A (eds). *Precision Molecular Pathology of Neoplastic Pediatric Diseases.* Molecular Pathology Library, 2018.
12. Jarzembowski JA. Molecular methods in oncology: targeted mutational analysis. In Furtado L, Husain A (eds). *Precision Molecular Pathology of Neoplastic Pediatric Diseases.* Springer, Cham: Molecular Pathology Library, 2018.
13. Liang WH, Federico SM, London WB, et al. Tailoring therapy for children with neuroblastoma based on risk group classification: past, present, and future. JCO Clin Cancer Inform. 2020; 4:895-905. Pawel BR. SMARCB1-deficient Tumors of Childhood: A Practical Guide. *Pediatr Dev Pathol.* 2018;21(1):6–28.
14. Pui CH, Nichols KE, Yang JJ. Somatic and germline genomics in paediatric acute lymphoblastic leukaemia. *Nat Rev Clin Oncol.* 2019;16 (4):227–240.
15. Relling MV, Schwab M, Whirl-Carrillo M, et al. Clinical Pharmacogenetics Implementation Consortium guideline for thiopurine dosing based on TPMT and NUDT15 genotypes: 2018 update. *Clin Pharmacol Ther.* 2019;105(5):1095–1105.
16. Strom SP. Fundamentals of RNA analysis on biobanked specimens. In Yong W (ed). *Biobanking. Methods in Molecular Biology.* Vol 1897. Humana Press, 2019.
17. Sbaraglia M, Righi A, Gambarotti M, Dei Tos AP. Ewing sarcoma and Ewing-like tumors. *Virchows Arch.* 2020;476(1):109–119.
18. Shern JF, Yohe ME, Khan J. Pediatric rhabdomyosarcoma. *Crit Rev Oncog.* 2015;20(3-4):227–243.

19. Suttorp M, Millot F, Sembill S, Deutsch H, Metzler M. Definition, Epidemiology, Pathophysiology, and Essential Criteria for Diagnosis of Pediatric Chronic Myeloid Leukemia. *Cancers (Basel).* 2021;13(4):798.
20. Tran G, Huynh TN, Paller AS. Langerhans cell histiocytosis: A neoplastic disorder driven by Ras-ERK pathway mutations. *J Am Acad Dermatol.* 2018;78(3):579–590.e4.
21. Zhang Y, Le Beau MM, Jon C, Aster JC. *Classification, cytogenetics, and molecular genetics of acute lymphoblastic leukemia/lymphoma. In T.W. Post, A.G. Rosmarin, R.A. Larson (eds). Up to Date*; 2020. https://www.uptodate.com/contents/classification-cytogenetics-and-molecular-genetics-of-acute-lymphoblastic-leukemia-lymphoma.

CHAPTER 24

SURVIVORSHIP AND LATE EFFECTS

Lenat Joffe, MD, MS and Jennifer Levine, MD, MSW

1. **Describe the goals of survivorship care and the role of the survivorship clinic.**

   Childhood cancer survivors are at an increased risk for significant adverse health effects and impaired quality of life after disease-related therapy. Multimodal regimens, consisting of chemotherapy, radiation, and surgery, can result in a myriad of severe chronic health conditions, secondary malignancies, physical limitations, psychological and neurocognitive dysfunction, infertility, and premature frailty and death. Many of these therapy-related late effects do not present until years after completion of therapy. With childhood cancer survival rates exceeding 80%, the need for survivorship-focused health care is becoming increasingly recognized. Survivorship clinics provide standardized, comprehensive, risk-based follow-up care to decrease exposure-related health risks and improve quality of life among pediatric cancer survivors. Timely screening and intervention, health education, anticipatory guidance, and promotion of healthy lifestyle are all critical to promoting long-term health in this population. Among adolescents and young adults, the survivorship program plays an important role in facilitating the successful transition from a pediatric to an adult healthcare system.

2. **Describe the etiology of cardiac late effects and current screening recommendations for survivors.**

   Cardiotoxicity is one of the most common late effects seen among childhood cancer survivors and results in increased morbidity and mortality in this population. Chemotherapy agents, namely anthracyclines, and radiotherapy, which includes the heart in the radiation field (chest, abdomen, thoracic/whole spine), both independently and in combination with one another, are the primary causes of cardiac late effects among survivors. Chronic progressive cardiotoxicity may appear early after completion of therapy or decades later. Depending on the type and dose of exposure, potential cardiotoxic late effects are vast and include hypertension, heart failure (notably cardiomyopathy, subclinical left ventricular dysfunction, and congestive heart failure), pericardial disease, valvular disorders, atherosclerosis, coronary artery disease, and arrhythmias. During their yearly survivorship visits, patients who received any dose of anthracyclines and/or less than 15 Gy of radiotherapy should be evaluated for shortness of breath, dyspnea or exertion, orthopnea, chest pain, palpitations, and, if younger than 25 years, abdominal symptoms such as nausea/vomiting. Physical examination should include blood pressure (BP) monitoring and a complete cardiac examination, and other risk factors such as glucose and lipid levels should be monitored. Patients should be counseled on a heart-healthy diet and exercise habits. A baseline electrocardiogram (ECG; including QTc interval) should be obtained for every patient who enters survivorship. Echocardiogram screening should be conducted as per Table 24.1.

Table 24.1 Recommended Echocardiogram Frequency

ANTHRACYCLINE (DOXORUBICIN ISOTOXIC EQUIVALENT) DOSE	RADIATION DOSE (CHEST, ABDOMEN, THORACIC/WHOLE SPINE, TOTAL BODY IRRADIATION [TBI])	ECHOCARDIOGRAM FREQUENCY
None	<15 Gy or none ≥15 Gy – <35 Gy ≥35 Gy	No screening needed Every 5 years Every 2 years
<250 mg/m²	<15 Gy or none ≥15 Gy	Every 5 years Every 2 years
≥250 mg/m²	Any or none	Every 2 years

From the Children's Oncology Group. Long-Term Follow-Up Guidelines for Survivors of Childhood, Adolescent, and Young Adult Cancers. 2018. www.survivorshipguidelines.org.

3. **Describe the occurrence and risk factors associated with secondary malignancies.**
The risk of malignancy among survivors over the age of 40 is at least twice that of adult counterparts in the general population who have not had previous exposures. Secondary malignancies are associated with significant morbidity and are the most common cause of nonrelapse late mortality among 5-year survivors, accounting for nearly half of nonrelapse deaths. The risk of developing a second neoplasm is dependent on patient-related factors such as original cancer diagnosis and age at treatment (younger age is a greater risk), genetic susceptibility, and therapeutic exposures received during primary cancer treatment. Specifically, the risk is greatest for those patients who were exposed to radiation and increased doses of chemotherapeutic agents, including alkylating agents, anthracyclines, and epipodophyllotoxins. Among the most common types of secondary cancers are those of the breast, thyroid, central nervous system, bone, and soft tissues. Other secondary malignancies that are also important to screen for are leukemia, lymphoma, melanoma, and gastrointestinal malignancy.

4. **What are the screening recommendations for the most common secondary malignancies?**
For the most common second malignant neoplasms and associated screening recommendations, see Table 24.2.

Table 24.2 Secondary Malignancy Screening Recommendations

SECONDARY MALIGNANCY	ASSOCIATED THERAPEUTIC EXPOSURE(S)	SCREENING RECOMMENDATIONS
Breast cancer	Radiation to chest, axilla, total body irradiation (TBI)	• Yearly survivorship clinical breast exam beginning at puberty until age 25, then every 6 months • Breast self-exam monthly starting at puberty • Mammogram yearly beginning 8 years after radiation OR at age 25, whichever occurs last • Breast magnetic resonance imaging (MRI) yearly as an adjunct to mammogram, to be performed at the same timing
Thyroid cancer	Radiation to head/brain, neck, spine (cervical or whole), TBI systemic MIBG (metaiodobenzylguanidine)	• Yearly survivorship clinical thyroid exam • Ultrasound of palpable thyroid nodules • Fine-needle aspiration (FNA) as clinically indicated
Central nervous system (CNS) tumors	Radiation to head/brain, TBI	• Yearly survivorship history and physical exam: Headaches, vomiting, cognitive, motor or sensory deficits, seizures, and other new onset neurological symptoms • Brain MRI if symptomatic
Sarcomas	Radiation to any field, TBI	• Yearly survivorship history and physical exam: Bone pain, persistent thickening or lump of soft tissue or bone at radiation site • X-ray or other imaging as needed for concerning lesions
Leukemia (acute myeloid leukemia [AML])	Alkylating agents, Anthracyclines, Epipodophyllotoxins, autologous hematopoietic cell transplant (HCT)	• At risk for up to 10 years after drug exposure • Yearly survivorship history and physical exam: Fatigue, bone pain, easy bruising, bleeding, petechiae, pallor, purpura • Complete blood count (CBC) and marrow examination as clinically indicated
Lung cancer	Radiation to chest, axilla, TBI	• Yearly survivorship history and physical exam: cough, wheezing, shortness of breath, dyspnea on exertion • Spiral computed tomography (CT) scan for patients at high risk (smokers)

Continued on following page

Table 24.2 Secondary Malignancy Screening Recommendations (*Continued*)

SECONDARY MALIGNANCY	ASSOCIATED THERAPEUTIC EXPOSURE(S)	SCREENING RECOMMENDATIONS
Skin cancer (melanoma, basal cell carcinoma, squamous cell carcinoma)	HCT Chronic graft versus host disease (GVHD) Radiation to any field, TBI	• Yearly survivorship history and physical exam: New skin lesions, changing moles (asymmetry, bleeding, increasing size, indistinct borders) • Monthly skin self-exam • Yearly dermatologic exam
Colorectal Cancer	Radiation to abdomen, pelvis, spine (lumbar, sacral, or whole), TBI	• Colonoscopy every 5 years OR multitargeted stool DNA test every 3 years (followed by colonoscopy if positive) beginning 5 years after radiation OR at age 30, whichever occurs last
Bladder cancer	Alkylating agents, radiation to pelvis or spine (sacral or whole)	• Yearly survivorship history and physical exam: Hematuria, urinary urgency/frequency, incontinence/retention, dysuria, nocturia, abnormal urinary stream • Urinalysis, urine culture, spot urine calcium/creatinine ratio for concerning history • Ultrasound of kidneys and bladder for microscopic hematuria on at least 2 occasions

Data from the Children's Oncology Group. Long-Term Follow-Up Guidelines for Survivors of Childhood, Adolescent, and Young Adult Cancers. 2018. www.survivorshipguidelines.org.

5. **Describe the endocrinopathies that can occur in childhood cancer survivors.**
Endocrine complications are extremely common among childhood cancer survivors, and approximately 50% of survivors will contend with a hormonal dysfunction during their lifetime. Most of these disorders can be mitigated with timely screening and intervention, thereby preventing significant physical and psychological burden in this population. Endocrinopathies can primarily be attributed to radiation therapy (RT) and surgical interventions. RT to the head/brain may result in pituitary dysfunction, including altered pubertal timing; growth hormone, thyroid-stimulating hormone (TSH), adrenocorticotropic hormone (ACTH), luteinizing hormone (LH), and follicle-stimulating hormone (FSH) deficiency; altered body composition (reduced lean muscle mass and increased fat mass resulting in being overweight or obese); hyperprolactinemia; and metabolic syndrome. Noncentral hypothyroidism or hyperthyroidism can result from radiation exposure to the neck, spine, or thorax. Finally, radiation to the abdomen/pelvis or genitourinary system may result in impaired glucose metabolism/diabetes mellitus and impaired production of male and female sex hormones. Neurosurgical procedures affecting the hypothalamic pituitary axis may also result in altered body composition and overweight/obesity, as well as development of diabetes insipidus. Among females, unilateral oophorectomy results in ovarian hormone deficiencies leading to delayed or arrested puberty, as well as premature ovarian insufficiency/menopause, whereas bilateral oophorectomy may result in the absence of puberty and loss of ovarian follicular pool and infertility. Among males, unilateral or partial orchiectomy can result in testosterone deficiency/insufficiency and delayed/arrested puberty, whereas bilateral orchiectomy results in the absence of puberty and azoospermia (infertility). Lastly, thyroidectomy, radioiodine therapy, and therapeutic doses of systemic MIBG lead to hypothyroidism, and certain chemotherapeutic exposures, such as alkylating agents, corticosteroids, and tyrosine kinase inhibitors, are linked to endocrine dysfunction.

6. **What treatments pose a risk for reproductive function for males, and what interventions are available for preservation?**
Dose-related risks of infertility for males from radiation and chemotherapy are outlined in Table 24.3. Additional risks to permanent infertility come from surgical resection of the testes. Sperm banking in postpubertal males is a longstanding and very successful method of preserving fertility in males. The most common method of obtaining sperm is through masturbation, but when this is not possible, sperm may be obtained via electroejaculation or biopsy of the testicular tissue. Intracytoplasmic sperm injection, where a single sperm is injected directly into an egg, makes banking even small numbers of sperm worthwhile. Because many males will experience temporary azoospermia from an array of chemotherapy agents, it is prudent to consider sperm banking for all postpubertal males because sperm banking may not be an option in the setting of a relapse. Timing is also important, with the goal of obtaining sperm before starting treatment as the quality of the sperm can be affected by exposure to chemotherapy. Fertility preservation in prepubertal males is limited to testicular tissue biopsy. At this time, this is an experimental procedure because no human births have occurred from this intervention. Other strategies that can be invoked in males include shielding of the testes during radiation.

Table 24.3 Male Level of Risk for Gonadal Failure/Infertility Above That for the General Population

		MINIMALLY INCREASED RISK	SIGNIFICANTLY INCREASED RISK	HIGH LEVEL OF INCREASED RISK
Alkylators cyclophosphamide equivalent dose (CED) gm/m^2		CED <4		CED ≥4
Hematopoietic stem cell transplant				Alkylator +/-Total body irradiation myeloablative and reduced intensity regimens
Heavy metal mg/m^2		Cisplatin Carboplatin	Cisplatin >500	
Radiation exposure	Testicular	0.2–0.6 Gy	0.7–3.9 Gy	≥4.0 Gy
	Hypothalamus	26–29.99 Gy	>30–39.9 Gy	>40 Gy
Surgery			Retroperitoneal lymph node dissection (RPLND)	

From Green DM, Nolan VG, Goodman PJ, et al. The cyclophosphamide equivalent dose as an approach for quantifying alkylating agent exposure: a report from the Childhood Cancer Survivor Study. Pediatr Blood Cancer. 2014;61(1):53–67.

7. **What treatments pose a risk for reproductive function for females, and what interventions are available for preservation?**
The age and dose-related exposures to radiation and chemotherapy that increase a female patient's risk for adverse reproductive effects are outlined in Table 23.4. Female fertility is also affected by surgery involving the ovaries or uterus. Nonexperimental options for fertility preservation in the postpubertal patient include cryopreservation of embryos, oocytes, and ovarian tissue. Generally, embryo cryopreservation is not common in pediatrics given the requirement for fertilization with sperm. Clinical pregnancy rates with thawed oocytes range from approximately 4% to 12% per oocyte, with a clinical pregnancy rate of 36% to 61% per embryos created from thawed oocytes, successfully transferred to the uterus. Oocyte cryopreservation requires approximately 10 to 14 days of ovarian hyperstimulation and subsequent oocyte retrieval. There are two time periods when oocyte cryopreservation can be considered for females. The first is at diagnosis before the start of treatment because chemotherapy can affect the

Table 24.4 Female Level of Risk for Gonadal Failure/Infertility Above That for the General Population

		MINIMALLY INCREASED RISK	SIGNIFICANTLY INCREASED RISK	HIGH LEVEL OF INCREASED RISK
Alkylators cyclophosphamide equivalent dose (CED) gm/m^2	Prepubertal	CED <8	8–12	>12
	Pubertal	CED <4	4–8	>8
Heavy metal		Cisplatin, carboplatin		
Hematopoietic stem cell transplant				Alkylator +/- Total body irradiation myeloablative and reduced intensity regimens
Radiation exposure	Ovary Prepubertal		<15 Gy	≥15 Gy
	Pubertal		<10 Gy	≥10 Gy
	Hypothalamus	22–29.9 Gy	>30–39.9 Gy	>40 Gy

From Green DM, Nolan VG, Goodman PJ, et al. The cyclophosphamide equivalent dose as an approach for quantifying alkylating agent exposure: a report from the Childhood Cancer Survivor Study. Pediatr Blood Cancer. 2014;61(1):53–67.

ability of ovaries to respond to stimulation and potentially can affect the integrity of the oocytes. The second is after the completion of treatment, once the acute effects of treatment have resolved, for those individuals who have retained ovarian function but demonstrate a risk for premature ovarian insufficiency. Ovarian tissue cryopreservation (OTC), now considered nonexperimental, is a laparoscopic procedure that can be combined with other procedures to help mitigate cost and can be performed after the start of chemotherapy. Of these procedures, OTC is the only intervention that is available to prepubertal patients. To date, there is one report of a live birth from oocytes removed in a prepubertal female and one in a peri-pubertal female. Although the designation of OTC as nonexperimental is not age-specific, concerns do remain about considering this a standard of care procedure in young girls. Additional strategies include fertility-sparing surgeries and transposition of the ovaries out of the field of radiation.

8. **Describe the etiology of pulmonary toxicity and how patients with respiratory compromise should be evaluated.**
   Pulmonary toxicity and late effects may result from surgical intervention involving the thorax; RT to the chest, axilla, or total body irradiation (TBI); exposure to chemotherapeutic agents, including bleomycin, busulfan, carmustine, and lomustine; and in patients who have a history of chronic graft versus host disease (GVHD) after high-dose allogeneic hematopoietic stem cell transplant (HSCT). Depending on the exposure, patients may be at risk for pulmonary fibrosis (any of the aforementioned chemotherapies or RT), interstitial pneumonitis (bleomycin, RT), restrictive or obstructive lung disease (RT), bronchiolitis obliterans/chronic bronchitis/bronchiectasis (HSCT with chronic GVHD), pulmonary dysfunction after surgical intervention (chest wall, pulmonary), and, very rarely, acute respiratory distress syndrome (bleomycin). At-risk patients should have a yearly survivorship visit to assess for cough, wheezing, shortness of breath, and dyspnea on exertion. Additionally, they should have pulmonary function testing with DLCO (diffusing capacity of carbon monoxide) and spirometry at baseline when first transitioning to the long-term follow-up clinic, with repeat testing in those where there is concern for one of the aforementioned pathologies. It is important to remember that risk increases in patients who received a combination of any of the aforementioned therapies, including higher doses of chemotherapy and/or radiation, who were younger when exposed to RT, have an atopic history, and who smoke or use inhaled illicit drugs. In addition to counseling this patient population on healthy lifestyle habits, you should ensure that these patients have repeat pulmonary function tests (PFTs) before general anesthesia and receive the influenza and pneumococcal vaccines.

9. **Describe the neurocognitive and educational late effects associated with cancer care.**
   Therapy exposures that are associated with neurocognitive sequelae are high-dose cytarabine (1000 mg/m^2 or more), high-dose methotrexate (1000 mg/m^2 or more), intrathecal methotrexate, cranial RT (particularly with increased doses, larger radiation field, greater cortical volumes, and having the temporal lobe within the field), and neurosurgical intervention. These, either individually or in combination with one another, may result in:
   - Functional deficits in executive function (planning and organization), sustained attention, memory (particularly visual, sequencing, and temporal memory), processing speed, visual-motor integration, and fine motor dexterity
   - Learning deficits in math and reading (especially reading comprehension)
   - Diminished intelligence quotient (IQ)
   - Behavioral changes

   Younger age at treatment (<3 years), female sex, and family history of learning or attention problems puts patients at increased risk for developing treatment-related neurocognitive late effects. Risk is also increased in those who receive any of the aforementioned therapies in combination with one another, with TBI, or with corticosteroids. Patients with this exposure history should undergo yearly evaluation of educational and vocational progress in the survivorship clinic and a formal baseline neuropsychological evaluation at entry to survivorship. In cases where an educational impairment is detected, a school liaison, school counselor, psychologist, or social worker should be involved to facilitate acquisition of educational resources and/or social skills training.

10. **Describe the adverse psychosocial effects associated with the childhood cancer experience.**
    Adverse psychosocial outcomes are a common occurrence among pediatric cancer survivors and are not associated with any one disease or treatment type. These may manifest in a number of ways, including social withdrawal and relationship problems, which extends to intimate partnerships; educational challenges and potential employment limitations; psychosocial disability because of pain and other physical limitations related to cancer and its treatment; mental health disorders such as anxiety, depression, post-traumatic stress, and even suicidal ideation; and financial strain and poor access to insurance and other healthcare resources. Patients experiencing psychosocial distress frequently present with fatigue and sleep disturbance, in which case other physiologic etiologies like anemia, cardiopulmonary disease, endocrinopathies, and nutritional deficiencies must be ruled out first. Moreover, psychosocial late effects often confer an impaired quality, and patients are prone to participating in risk-taking behaviors, such as smoking, alcohol, and illicit drug use. Thus yearly psychosocial assessment in the survivorship clinic is needed in this population. Social work and psychology resources either within the clinic or in the community must be identified to address these issues in a timely manner.

11. **Discuss late effects related to treatment with corticosteroids.**
    Corticosteroids, namely prednisone and dexamethasone, are frequently used in the treatment of childhood leukemia and lymphoma. Late effects associated with the use of corticosteroids include reduced bone mineral density, osteonecrosis, and cataracts. As such, to ensure long-term bone health, patients treated with corticosteroids should all have a baseline dual-energy x-ray absorptiometry (DXA) scan to evaluate bone density at entry into

survivorship. Additionally, all patients should be encouraged to participate in weight-bearing exercise and, particularly among pediatric patients, you must ensure that they are receiving the recommended dietary intake of calcium and vitamin D (400 IU/day or higher if they are deficient). Patients should be instructed to avoid smoking and limit intake of alcohol and carbonated beverages. However, even with appropriate lifestyle interventions, a subset of patients who develop osteoporosis or frequent fractures may need evaluation and follow-up with an endocrinologist. Although osteonecrosis is well-recognized as an adverse effect of corticosteroid use in the acute phase of therapy, it may progress over time and manifest during survivorship as well. Bone morbidities are more likely to occur in the older population (adolescents and young adults) than younger kids. Patients should be evaluated for joint pain, swelling, immobility, and limited range of motion yearly. To assess for cataracts, patients should have a visual acuity and fundoscopic exam yearly.

12. **Describe late effects associated with radiation therapy to the chest.**
Chest RT includes the mediastinum, hila, whole lung, and chest wall in the radiation field. As with any radiation exposure, RT to the chest is a risk factor for dermatologic late effects and secondary benign or malignant neoplasm near the radiation field. Of these second malignancies, breast cancer is most notable among females, whereas lung cancer is more likely to occur in those who smoke or have exposure to secondhand smoke, asbestos, arsenic, or further radiation. In addition to breast cancer, chest RT in females, particularly those who are prepubertal at the time of treatment, may result in permanent breast tissue hypoplasia, necessitating breast reconstruction for those who desire it. Musculoskeletal growth problems, fractures, and deformity/asymmetric growth may also be attributed to thoracic radiation. Scoliosis and kyphosis are one such example, although they are less likely to occur with contemporary treatment. Thus assessing growth pattern and examining the spine for curvature yearly is especially important in patients who had this exposure before puberty. Cardiotoxicity and pulmonary toxicity are also well-known late effects of chest RT.

13. **Describe late effects associated with cranial radiotherapy.**
Cranial RT is employed in the treatment of a number of pediatric malignancies, including brain tumors, leukemia and lymphoma involving the central nervous system, and a subset of extracranial solid tumors located in that region. There are many late effects associated with cranial RT including the following:
- Malignant and nonmalignant second neoplasms
- Endocrinopathies, including growth hormone deficiency, precocious puberty, hyperprolactinemia, central or noncentral hypothyroidism, hyperthyroidism, thyroid nodules, gonadotropin deficiency, and central adrenal insufficiency
- Neurocognitive deficits
- Dermatologic toxicity, including permanent alopecia, altered skin pigmentation, telangiectasias, or fibrosis
- Clinical leukoencephalopathy presenting as spasticity, ataxia, dysarthria, dysphagia, hemiparesis, or new-onset seizures
- Cerebrovascular complications presenting as stroke, moyamoya, occlusive cerebral vasculopathy, and cavernomas
- Carotid artery disease
- Craniofacial abnormalities resulting in psychosocial distress
- Chronic sinusitis
- Overweight or obese body habitus
- Ocular toxicity presenting with orbital hypoplasia, lacrimal duct atrophy, xerophthalmia, keratitis, telangiectasias, retinopathy, optic chiasm neuropathy, enophthalmos, chronic painful eye, maculopathy, papillopathy, glaucoma, or cataracts
- Ototoxicity (if dose received is 30 Gy or more) presenting with tympanosclerosis, otosclerosis, eustachian tube dysfunction, conductive hearing loss, sensorineural hearing loss, tinnitus, or vertigo
- Xerostomia and salivary gland dysfunction
- Dental abnormalities presenting with tooth/root agenesis, root thinning/shortening, enamel dysplasia, microdontia, ectopic molar eruption, dental caries, periodontal disease, or malocclusion
- Temporomandibular joint dysfunction (TMJD)
- Osteoradionecrosis of the jaw (if dose received is 40 Gy or more)

14. **Describe late effects associated with total body irradiation.**
Total body irradiation (TBI) is employed before HSCT in the treatment of relapsed/refractory malignancies and is associated with numerous late effects affecting nearly all body systems, including the following:
- Secondary benign or malignant neoplasms at or near the radiation field, including those of the brain, breast, thyroid, lung, and colorectal region
- Dermatologic toxicity
- Neurocognitive deficits
- Clinical leukoencephalopathy
- Endocrinopathies, including growth hormone deficiency, gonadotropin deficiency, hypothyroidism, thyroid nodules, and impaired glucose metabolism
- Cataracts
- Dry mouth and salivary gland dysfunction

- Dental abnormalities and TMJD
- Breast tissue hypoplasia in females
- Pulmonary toxicity
- Dyslipidemia
- Renal toxicity
- Reproductive dysfunction including impaired spermatogenesis in males and ovarian hormone deficiencies, reduced ovarian follicular pool, and uterine vascular insufficiency in females
- Musculoskeletal growth problems

15. **Describe late effects associated with chronic graft versus host disease.**

GVHD is a complication that can occur after allogeneic stem cell transplantation, wherein the donor T cells view the host cells as "foreign" and attack them. Chronic GVHD may arise up to several years after transplant and can affect one or multiple body systems (Table 24.5).

Table 24.5 Chronic Graft Versus Host Disease (GVHD) Late Effects and Follow-Up

LATE EFFECT	PRESENTATION AND EVALUATION
Dermatologic toxicity • Permanent alopecia • Nail dystrophy • Vitiligo • Sclerodermatous changes • Squamous cell carcinoma • Melanoma	• Monthly skin self-exam • Yearly exam of hair, nails, and skin in survivorship clinic
Xerophthalmia	• Yearly evaluation for symptoms of dry eyes (burning, itching, foreign body sensation, inflammation) and eye exam in survivorship clinic • Yearly evaluation by optometrist or ophthalmologist
Oral toxicity • Xerostomia • Salivary gland dysfunction • Dental caries • Periodontal disease • Oral cancer	• Yearly evaluation for xerostomia and oral exam in survivorship clinic • Dental exam and cleaning every 6 months
Pulmonary toxicity • Bronchiolitis obliterans • Chronic bronchitis • Bronchiectasis	• Yearly evaluation for cough, wheezing, shortness of breath, and dyspnea on exertion in survivorship clinic • Pulmonary function tests (PFTs) with diffusing capacity of the lungs for carbon monoxide (DLCO) and spirometry at transition to survivorship clinic
Immunologic complications • Secretory immunoglobulin A (IgA) deficiency • Hypogammaglobulinemia • Decreased B cells • T-cell dysfunction • Chronic infections	• Yearly evaluation for chronic conjunctivitis, sinusitis, or bronchitis, recurrent or unusual infections, and sepsis
Functional asplenia (if currently active chronic GVHD)	• Physical exam, blood culture, and potential administration of broad spectrum antibiotics at the time of febrile illness (temperature $\geq 101°F$ or $38.3°C$)
Esophageal stricture	• Yearly evaluation for dysphagia and heartburn in survivorship clinic
Vulvar scaring, vaginal fibrosis/stenosis	• Yearly evaluation for dyspareunia, postcoital bleeding, difficulty with tampon insertion, vaginal dryness, vulvar pain, vulvovaginal burning or pruritus, and dysuria in the survivorship clinic • Yearly physical exam of genitalia for lichen planus-like features, erosions, fissures, and ulcers
Joint contractures	• Yearly musculoskeletal exam in the survivorship clinic

Data from the Children's Oncology Group. Long-Term Follow-Up Guidelines for Survivors of Childhood, Adolescent, and Young Adult Cancers. 2018. www.survivorshipguidelines.org.

16. **Why are lifestyle habits, including diet and exercise, critical for maintaining overall health in the survivor population?**
The vast majority of childhood cancer survivors will develop a treatment-related chronic health condition in the years after therapy, with about one-third of survivors having a severe, disabling, or life-threatening condition. A critical role of late effect care is to promote healthy lifestyle habits among survivors to mitigate against poor health outcomes, such as through:
   - Tobacco cessation or avoidance: Particularly in those at risk for female health and reproductive complications (alkylator, RT, oophorectomy exposure), pulmonary toxicity (alkylator, bleomycin, RT, chronic GVHD, thoracic surgery exposure), lung cancer (RT exposure), urinary tract toxicity (alkylator exposure), bladder malignancy (alkylator, RT exposure), reduced bone mineral density (antimetabolite, corticosteroid, HCT exposure), cardiotoxicity (anthracycline, RT exposure), and vasospastic attacks (plant alkaloid exposure).
   - Maintenance of a proper diet and weight management and participation in regular physical activity: Particularly in those at risk for cardiotoxicity (anthracycline, RT exposure), becoming overweight/obese (RT, neurosurgery exposure), carotid or subclavian artery disease (RT exposure), impaired glucose metabolism/dyslipidemia (RT exposure), reduced bone mineral density (antimetabolite, corticosteroid, HCT exposure), and complications of limb-sparing procedures.
   - Moderation of alcohol consumption: Particularly in those at risk for urinary tract toxicity (alkylator exposure), bladder malignancy (alkylator, RT exposure), reduced bone mineral density (antimetabolite, corticosteroid, HCT exposure), and hepatic toxicity (RT, HCT exposure).
   - Avoidance of inhaled or other illicit drug use: Particularly in those at risk for pulmonary toxicity (alkylator, bleomycin, RT, chronic GVHD, thoracic surgery exposure) and vasospastic attacks (plant alkaloid exposure).
   - Protect skin from sun exposure using sunscreen and protective clothing: Particularly in those at risk for skin toxicity and cancer (RT, GVHD exposure).

17. **How has the increased focus on survivorship issues impacted long-term outcomes?**
Survivorship care and research has been instrumental in shaping the way that we treat pediatric cancer patients, aiming not only to increase cure rates but also to reduce the burden of late effects that contribute to long-term morbidity and early mortality among childhood cancer survivors. Broadening our understanding has enhanced delivery of risk-stratified care by reducing treatment exposures, including cumulative doses of chemotherapy and RT, while preserving treatment efficacy. These critical, ongoing treatment modifications, along with increased early screening and intervention for late effects, have resulted in an appreciable decline in late mortality among 5-year survivors of childhood cancer over the past several decades.

BIBLIOGRAPHY

1. Armstrong GT, Chen Y, Yasui Y, et al. Reduction in late mortality among 5-year survivors of childhood cancer. *N Engl J Med.* 2016;374 (9):833–842.
2. Burns KC, Hoefgen H, Strine A, Dasgupta R. Fertility preservation options in pediatric and adolescent patients with cancer. *Cancer.* 2018;124(9):1867–1876.
3. Children's Oncology Group. Long-Term Follow-Up Guidelines for Survivors of Childhood, Adolescent, and Young Adult Cancers. 2018. www.survivorshipguidelines.org.
4. Green DM, Nolan VG, Goodman PJ, et al. The cyclophosphamide equivalent dose as an approach for quantifying alkylating agent exposure: a report from the Childhood Cancer Survivor Study. *Pediatr Blood Cancer.* 2014;61(1):53–67.
5. Hudson MM, Hester A, Sweeney T, et al. A model of care for childhood cancer survivors that facilitates research. *J Ped Oncol Nurs.* 2004;21(3):170–174.
6. Robison LL, Hudson MM. Survivors of childhood and adolescent cancer: life-long risks and responsibilities. *Nat Rev Cancer.* 2014;14 (1):61–70.
7. Phillips SM, Padgett LS, Leisenring WM, et al. Survivors of childhood cancer in the United States: prevalence and burden of morbidity. *Cancer Epidemiol Biomarkers Prev.* 2015;24(4):653–663.
8. Scholz-Kreisel P, Spix C, Blettner M, et al. Prevalence of cardiovascular late sequelae in long-term survivors of childhood cancer: A systematic review and meta-analysis. *Pediatr Blood Cancer.* 2017;64(7).
9. Lipshultz SE, Adams MJ, Colan SD, et al. Long-term cardiovascular toxicity in children, adolescents, and young adults who receive cancer therapy: pathophysiology, course, monitoring, management, prevention, and research directions: a scientific statement from the American Heart Association. *Circulation.* 2013;128(17):1927–1995.
10. Meacham LR, Burns K, Orwig KE, Levine J. Standardizing risk assessment for treatment-related gonadal insufficiency and infertility in childhood adolescent and young adult cancer: The Pediatric Initiative Network Risk Stratification System. *J Adolesc Young Adult Oncol.* 2020;9(6):662–666.
11. Nahata L, Woodruff TK, Quinn GP, et al. Ovarian tissue cryopreservation as standard of care: what does this mean for pediatric populations? *J Assist Reprod Genet.* 2020;37(6):1323–1326.
12. Practice Committee of the American Society for Reproductive Medicine. Fertility preservation in patients undergoing gonadotoxic therapy or gonadectomy: a committee opinion. *Fertil Steril.* 2019;112(6):1022–1033.
13. Turcotte LM, Liu Q, Yasui Y, et al. Temporal trends in treatment and subsequent neoplasm risk among 5-year survivors of childhood cancer, 1970-2015. *JAMA.* 2017;317(8):814–824.
14. Turcotte LM, Neglia JP, Reulen RC, et al. Risk, Risk factors, and surveillance of subsequent malignant neoplasms in survivors of childhood cancer: a review. *J Clin Oncol.* 2018;36(21):2145–2152.
15. van Santen HM, Chemaitilly W, Meacham LR, Tonorezos ES, Mostoufi-Moab S. Endocrine health in childhood cancer survivors. *Pediatr Clin North Am.* 2020;67(6):1171–1186.

CHAPTER 25

INTEGRATIVE THERAPIES

Elena J. Ladas, PhD, RD and Michelle Bombacie, MS, LAc, LMT

1. **Describe complementary and integrative health therapies.**
   Complementary and integrative health therapies (CIHTs) are nonmainstream practices used in combination or together with conventional medicine. CIHTs are divided into three categories: natural products, mind and body practices, and whole-systems. Natural products include dietary supplements such as botanicals, vitamins and minerals, and probiotics. Mind and body practices include acupuncture, acupressure, aromatherapy, healing touch, hypnotherapy, massage therapy, movement therapies, tai chi, and qigong. Whole-system approaches include traditional Chinese medicine (TCM), Ayurvedic medicine, homeopathy, and naturopathy.

2. **Why do patients often seek treatment with CIHT?**
   Surveys have found up to 84% of children with cancer use CIHT, but this varies by geographical location. Parents of children and adolescents with cancer often seek the use of CIHT to help manage the side effects associated with cancer therapy, to augment the efficacy of conventional therapy, or to provide support for coping with the diagnosis of cancer. A smaller number of families may choose to seek the use of CIHT to treat the cancer itself. Most commonly, this is observed among children diagnosed with a malignancy that is associated with a poor prognosis or tumors that have not been responsive to frontline therapy. Of most concern are families that choose CIHT in lieu of conventional medicine; however, this is a small subset of families. Parents report pursuing the use of CIHT to ensure that they have left "no stone unturned" and feel as if they are doing all they can to help their child fight cancer or support them during cancer therapy.

3. **Are there special considerations for using CIHT in children with cancer?**
   There are several unique factors to consider when counseling patients on the use of CIHT during and after treatment for a pediatric malignancy. In contrast to adult oncology, common childhood tumors are more sensitive to chemotherapy with survival exceeding 90% for acute lymphoblastic leukemia (ALL), Hodgkin lymphoma, and other localized and low-risk malignancies. Children also undergo treatment for a longer period of time, tend to tolerate chemotherapy better, and are less likely to have comorbid conditions. Therefore it is imperative that the use of CIHT therapies not interfere with or encourage the refusal or delay of conventional therapy. The type of CIHT and its appropriateness for the developmental age and planned conventional treatment of the child must be considered *a priori.* Therapies that may exacerbate common treatment-related toxicities (TRTs) should undergo detailed evaluation so as to not further increase the risk or severity of TRTs. Sociodemographic factors are important considerations in selecting the type of CIHT. The economic impact of CIHT can have detrimental effects on a family, which is especially concerning for CIHTs that have limited scientific evidence supporting efficacy. Other influential factors may be a family's lifestyle and cultural and religious practices.

4. **Where can I find reliable information on the use of CIHT?**
   The most reliable resources for information and scientific research on CIHTs are the National Center for Complementary and Integrative Health (NCCIH) (https://www.nccih.nih.gov) and the National Cancer Institute's Physician Data Query (https://www.cancer.gov/publications/pdq/information-summaries/cam) on CIHT. Medline is the U.S. National Library of Medicine (NLM) database and can also provide peer-reviewed information.

5. **Are there strategies to employ when counseling patients on CIHT?**
   Parents often seek advice to determine whether a CIHT is safe and reasonable. As health care practitioners, it is important to help parents weigh the risks with the potential benefits, evaluate interactions with treatment and medications, determine recommended doses and frequency, and find qualified licensed or certified practitioners who have experience working with children. It is especially important to keep communication open by assuming a nonjudgmental approach. Patients and their families who choose to use CIHT often want individualized counseling considering a myriad of factors including patient/family preferences, sociodemographic factors, and intended benefit of a CIHT.

6. **Is there guidance on evaluating the safety and efficacy of CIHT?**
   The NCCIH and the National Cancer Institute (NCI) provide an introductory overview of factors to consider when evaluating CIHT approaches. Emphasis is placed on relying on gold-standard scientific approaches to assess conventional therapies. However, this can be challenging because of the paucity of evidence in pediatric oncology and unorthodox study designs (e.g., N = 1 trials, sham acupuncture) inherent to many trials evaluating CIHT. A commonly used 2 by 2 grid may be used to rank safety and efficacy along separate axes. When safety and efficacy is strong, the therapy can be encouraged. When safety and efficacy is weak, it makes sense to discourage it. When evidence supports safety but efficacy is inconclusive, or when there is evidence of efficacy, but not safety, then the therapy

should be considered with caution and monitored closely for effectiveness or safety. The dilemma arises when there is no evidence on either safety or efficacy. Each therapy needs to be considered individually alongside the goals of the patient and their family.

7. What is the evidence for the use of acupuncture in pediatric oncology, hematology, and HSCT?
Acupuncture is a CIHT based on the principles and philosophies of Traditional Chinese Medicine. The primary objective of acupuncture is to regulate qi, the vital life force, and promote balance and overall wellbeing. This is done by accessing "acupoints" located along energetic pathways in the body known as meridians with single-use, small, fine needles. Upon stimulation, a therapeutic effect is conferred. Several TRTs may be effectively managed with acupuncture or acupressure (applying pressure on acupoints without needle penetration) in circumstances where a licensed acupuncturist is not available. The National Institutes of Health recommend the use of acupuncture for the management of pain, nausea/vomiting, fatigue, and anxiety. In the setting of pain, acupuncture may be a safer alternative to opioid prescriptions. This may be especially relevant for pain associated with sickle cell disease. Unfortunately, much of the research has been extrapolated from the pediatric to the oncology setting.

Acceptance of acupuncture has been demonstrated in several studies performed in children and adolescents with cancer. Acupuncture has been found to be widely accepted among children as young as 2 years of age with cancer and others undergoing hematopoietic stem cell transplant (HSCT) and is sought to treat a wide array of symptoms associated with cancer therapy. Acupuncture provides a nonpharmacologic approach to symptom management but must be provided by a well-trained, licensed acupuncturist, thereby limiting its access in many medical settings. In patients with sickle cell disease, acupuncture can offer a substitute for opioid medications. Clinical studies have found a reduction in self-reported measures of pain when acupuncture is delivered either in lieu of or as an adjunct treatment to adolescents in sickle cell crisis. Existing studies also suggest that acupuncture may reduce the frequency of visits to the pediatric emergency department and inpatient admissions.

CASE ILLUSTRATION 18-Year-Old Male With Relapsed Hodgkin Lymphoma Who Was Undergoing a Second Hematopoietic Stem Cell Transplant (HSCT).

In preparation for his HSCT, he was complaining of persistent anxiety/stress that often led to feelings of nausea and vomiting (N/V). This greatly impacted his quality of life and his motivation to maintain a healthy and positive approach to his transplant. Upon referral, acupuncture treatments were administered before and continued throughout the conditioning phase and after infusion of his HSCT. Additional complementary and integrative health therapies modalities were provided to mask the unpleasant odor of preservatives in the stem cell product while acupressure was taught to the patient to help him manage anxiety/stress and N/V when an acupuncturist was not available. The patient reported a significant improvement in symptoms and shorter durations of anxiety/stress and N/V.

CASE ILLUSTRATION 15-Year-Old Female With Sickle Cell Anemia Hemoglobin (Hb SS) and Acute Anemia Admitted for Lower Back Pain, Bilateral Thigh Pain, and Bilateral Knee Pain Because of Sickle Cell Pain Crisis

A 15-year-old female was referred to an acupuncturist with a history of prolonged pain crisis, multiple visits to the emergency room, prolonged hospital stays, and pain that was not entirely controlled by oxycodone. She also was being considered as a candidate for hematopoietic stem cell transplant. Upon consultation, she was groggy and complained of constipation that was attributed to opioids. She wanted to explore alternative treatments. She was administered acupuncture based on the location of her pain and other diagnostic features inherent to Traditional Chinese Medicine. Heat was also applied locally to her lower back, thighs, and knees. During her treatment, her pain decreased from an eight to five out of ten. She continued to receive acupuncture during subsequent visits, which was associated with reduced visits to the emergency room, improved quality of life, and an overall reduction of pain.

8. Is acupuncture safe in children with thrombocytopenia or neutropenia?
There are several studies that have documented the safety of acupuncture in childhood cancer. One of the largest studies found that the delivery of acupuncture was safe in children with cancer who were also experiencing either severe, moderate, or mild thrombocytopenia. There were no reports of increased bleeding, infections, or bruising when clean needle technique protocols are employed to deliver acupuncture.

9. What are common indications for the use of massage therapy in children with cancer?
Massage therapy is a therapeutic intervention that involves manipulation of the soft tissues of the body. Massage therapists who specialize in pediatric oncology often draw from a variety of techniques including Swedish massage, reflexology, and pediatric Tuina. Massage may reduce pain, alter metabolism, alleviate stress, improve circulation and lymph flow, and promote muscle tone and flexibility. Biopsy, lumbar puncture, bone marrow aspiration, and central venous-catheter placement can illicit pain and anxiety that can be lessened with massage therapy. Studies performed among children with cancer have found that massage therapy can improve mood, reduce heart rate, reduce diastolic blood pressure, and reduce constipation.

CASE ILLUSTRATION 10-Year-Old Boy With T-Cell Lymphoblastic Leukemia Experiencing Jaw Pain and Bilateral Leg Pain From Chemo-Induced Neuropathy, Which Led to Uncontrollable Crying

Upon consultation, he was found to be in distress from pain and anxiety but refused treatment with acupuncture. The massage therapist began treatment with aromatherapy (blended oils consisting of lavender, lemon, and rosemary essential oils) and proceeded with an aromatic massage therapy. The treatment focused on the muscles of the face and scalp, which created a sense of calmness and reduced pain associated with neuropathy. The treatments also benefited his parents after seeing his response to massage therapy and learning self-massage techniques when a therapist was not available. Massage continued to be an essential complementary and integrative health therapies throughout the course of his cancer treatment, and he referred to his treatment as "his potion of healing blend!"

10. Are there contraindications for the use of massage in children with cancer?
    When administered by a licensed massage therapist, massage therapy is a safe CIHT approach with a high safety profile. It is often necessary for massage therapists to adjust and modify practice according to the age and diagnosis of the patient. For example, applying minimal pressure to weakened bone structures, areas of minimal sensation, and severe neutropenic patients is a recommended practice. In all circumstances, massage therapist should avoid massaging sites of active tumor growth, open wounds, radiation burns, cutaneous infection, and areas where deep vein thrombosis is a concern.

11. Should a child with cancer follow a special diet?
    It is well-established that nutrition is a critical component of cancer care. Children and adolescents with undernutrition or overnutrition have increased risk of TRTs and are at risk for reduced survival. For example, children with ALL or acute myeloid leukemia (AML) who are overweight or obese have a 31% and 35% increased risk of mortality compared with their healthy weight counterparts, respectively. In children with undernutrition, an increased risk of infection and prolonged hospital stays has been reported. To date, there is no single diet that has been found to improve outcomes or reduce TRTs in children with cancer. Dietary quality has become an increasingly important aspect of nutrition counseling both during and after treatment for cancer. A diet high in nutritious foods has been found to be associated with reduced TRTs and late-effects. For survivors, diets high in nutritious foods may reduce the risk for several adult-onset malignancies such as breast and colon cancer. Guidance on the component of high-quality diets may be found at the American Institute for Cancer Research/World Health Cancer Research Foundation (www.aicr.org).

12. Can dietary supplements interact with chemotherapy or radiation?
    The potential for an interaction between a dietary supplement and either chemotherapy or radiation is largely based on anecdotal evidence. To date, most studies have found that dietary supplementation, within the Dietary Reference Intakes (DRI), is likely safe during treatment for cancer. This includes patients that may supplement with folate-containing multivitamins and are receiving antifolate chemotherapy (e.g., methotrexate). Studies have also found that supplementation with micronutrients may not confer an increased beneficial effect over and above dietary intakes that are rich in phytonutrients, including foods high in antioxidants. The risk of an interaction with chemotherapy/radiation is less certain when administering herbal (e.g., milk thistle, echinacea) or nutrition supplements without a DRI (e.g., pycnogenol, l-carnitine). In these circumstances, weighing the available evidence with the potential for interaction is the most thorough approach to determining safety.
    It is worth highlighting the potential role of probiotic therapy in children with cancer or undergoing HSCT. Probiotics are nutritional supplements that contain a defined number of viable microorganisms and upon administration confer a benefit to the host. There are hundreds of species/strains of probiotics, making the safety determination of a single or multitude of species difficult. There has been a lot of patient interest in supplementation with probiotics as they are widely touted in the media as being healthy for the gut, thereby improving weight management, reducing depression, and reducing gastrointestinal upset. This is especially true in children undergoing treatment with antibiotics, which are known disrupters of a healthy microbiome.
    Probiotics have been found to be safe in children undergoing HSCT and receiving chemotherapy. In adults, probiotics have been found to reduce radiation-induced diarrhea. Moreover, a healthy microbiome has been associated with improved outcomes among adults undergoing HSCT. Based on the existing evidence, it is likely that some probiotics may be safe in the setting of oncology and HSCT, but additional research on the underlying mechanisms and safety of various species/strains is needed.

BIBLIOGRAPHY

1. Adams D, Spelliscy C, Sivakumar L, et al. CAM and pediatric oncology: where are all the best cases? *Evid Based Complement Alternat Med.* 2013;2013:1–6.
2. Bhula R, Nieder M, Jubelirer T, Ladas EJ. Gut microbiome and pediatric cancer: current research and gaps in knowledge. *J Natl Cancer Inst Monogr.* 2019;2019(54):169–173.
3. Chokshi SK, Ladas EJ, Taromina K, et al. Predictors of acupuncture use among children and adolescents with cancer. *Pediatr Blood Cancer.* 2017;64(7). https://doi.org/10.1002/pbc.26424.

4. Hughes D, Ladas E, Rooney D, et al. Massage therapy as a supportive care intervention for children with cancer. *Oncol Nurs Forum.* 2008;35(3):431–442.
5. Jacobs S, Mowbray C, Cates LM, et al. Pilot study of massage to improve sleep and fatigue in hospitalized adolescents with cancer. *Pediatric Blood Cancer.* 2016;63(5):880–886.
6. Jong MC, Boers I, Van Wietmarschen H, et al. Development of an evidence-based decision aid on complementary and alternative medicine (CAM) and pain for parents of children with cancer. *Support Care Cancer.* 2020;28(5):2415–2429.
7. Ladas EJ, Chen L, Bhatia M, et al. The safety and feasibility of probiotics in children and adolescents undergoing hematopoietic cell transplantation. *Bone Marrow Transplant.* 2016;51(2):262–266.
8. Ladas E, Rooney D, Taromina K, et al. The safety of acupuncture in children and adolescents with cancer therapy-related thrombocytopenia. *Support Care Cancer.* 2010;18(11):1487–1490.
9. National Center for Complementary and Integrative Health. Acupuncture: In Depth. 2016. https://www.nccih.nih.gov/health/acupuncture-in-depth.
10. National Center for Complementary and Integrative Health. Complementary, Alternative, or Integrative Health: What's In a Name? 2018. https://www.nccih.nih.gov/health/complementary-alternative-or-integrative-health-whats-in-a-name.
11. Zia F, Olaku O, Bao T, et al. The National Cancer Institute's conference on acupuncture for symptom management in oncology: state of the science, evidence and research gaps. *JNCI Monographs.* 2017;2017(52):68–73.

CHAPTER 26

PALLIATIVE CARE

Linda Granowetter, MD and Joyce Varkey, MD

1. **What are the differences between palliative care, end-of-life care, and hospice care?**
   Palliative care for children and adolescents is an evolving field but can be defined as an interdisciplinary collaborative approach to improve the quality of life of children with life-threatening or profoundly challenging conditions, as well as that of their families, inclusive of physical, emotional, social, and spiritual elements.

   Hospice, or end-of-life care, is focused on the comfort of a dying child and bereavement support for the child's loved ones. Hospice care may take place in the home or in an institutional setting. In most locales, there is a dearth of inpatient pediatric hospice care facilities. For adults, acceptance into a hospice program requires an estimated life expectancy of 6 months or less, and the patient must forego curative treatment. In pediatrics, the time course is more flexible and ongoing disease-directed therapy is permitted.

2. **What are some key differences when providing palliative care to a pediatric patient compared with care for an adult patient?**
   Although the fundamental principles are the same, execution is markedly different. Developmental factors that affect physiology, pharmacokinetics, cognition, and emotional maturity must be evaluated and addressed. Pediatric palliative care must consider not only the needs of the patient but also of the entire family as well. The impact of chronic illness and/or the death of a child on siblings and parents cannot be overestimated. The death of a child, in particular, challenges societal expectations and often transforms family relationships and functioning on a long-term basis. Lastly, the etiologies of life-threatening illnesses are different between the two populations, which inform the therapies selected.

3. **What are the key components of effective palliative care?**
   - An interdisciplinary team, which typically includes:
     - Social worker
     - Child life specialists
     - Chaplains
     - Physician
     - Clinical nurse specialists
   - A strong relationship between the medical team and the patient and family
   - Effective communication, including:
     - Respect for the family's beliefs and expectations
     - Awareness of what the patient and family understands
     - The imparting of knowledge at an appropriate level and pace
     - Remaining open to questions
   - Shared decision-making based on a holistic approach to the child and goals of care
   - Addressing psychosocial and spiritual elements
   - Anticipation, prevention, and management of symptoms
   - Preparation for end-of-life care

4. **For which patients would palliative care be appropriate?**
   In the simplest terms, palliative care is appropriate for any child and family facing any severe life-threatening or life-altering chronic disease. Examples include:
   - When cure is possible but treatment is complex and possibly prolonged over time and may fail (i.e., complex congenital heart disease)
   - A chronic, progressive condition requiring life-intensive treatments (i.e., cystic fibrosis)
   - Static conditions with susceptibility to significant morbidity (i.e., hypoxic brain injury)
   - Conditions without chance of cure (i.e., severe neurodegenerative syndromes, cancer unresponsive to therapy)
     The following categories of conditions are most often seen by pediatric palliative care teams: genetic or congenital disease (41%), neuromuscular disorders (39%), cancer (20%), respiratory diseases (13%), and gastrointestinal (GI) diseases (11%).

5. **What are the symptoms most commonly experienced by children with cancer? How can they be managed?**
See Table 26.1 for management suggestions.

6. **What are methods used to treat anorexia and weight loss? What are some considerations to take into account when deciding about artificial hydration and nutrition?**
Periactin, olanzapine, and dronabinol are medications that have shown effect in improving appetite in many patients. Where legal, medicinal marijuana may be useful in improving appetite and is best considered for adolescents already comfortable with its effects. Nevertheless, appetite stimulants should be used with caution in end-of-life care because patients may not want to eat.

Table 26.1 Pharmacological and Pharmacological Interventions for Common Pediatric Symptoms

SYMPTOM	PHARMACOLOGICAL INTERVENTIONS	NONPHARMACOLOGICAL INTERVENTIONS
Pain	Please see questions 7–16	• Cognitive behavioral measures[a] • Physical measures[b]
Dyspnea	• Opioids: Morphine can be given sublingually, or nebulized (has not been shown to be superior to orally [PO]) • Oxygen: By mask or blow-by • Lorazepam • Bronchodilators • For cough: Dextromethorphan and/or opioids • For sialorrhea: Humidifier, nebulized saline, antihistamines, or anticholinergics • Terminal dyspnea ("death rattle") is a gurgling noise caused by pooled secretions in those who are too weak to swallow or cough: Subcutaneous or transdermal scopolamine	• Cool air from a fan or open window directed at the face • Repositioning • Hypnosis
Sleep Disturbance	• Melatonin clonidine • Used rarely: Haloperidol (in small doses), tricyclic antidepressants, trazodone • Benzodiazepines: Especially if anxiety contribute to sleep disturbance; except at end-of-life, it should only be used in a time-limited manner.	• Cognitive behavioral measures[a] • Proper sleep hygiene
Constipation	**All patients receiving opioids should receive a laxative pre-emptively.** Choices include: • Peg-Glycol (MiraLAX): Patient must be able to take a minimum of 4 oz liquid orally to use this • For reduced motility: Stimulant (i.e., Senna) • For hard stool: Softener • If opioid-induced and unresponsive to other laxative: SC methylnaltrexone • If paraplegia: Always combination softeners and glycerin suppository • Oral lactulose • Glycerin suppository • Enema if absolutely required Enemas should not be given to patients with neutropenia.	N/A
Diarrhea	• Fluid management • Antimicrobial therapy as indicated • Pancreatic enzyme replacement • Loperamide if infectious etiologies are excluded • For severe high-output diarrhea at end-of-life, can use octreotide	N/A

Continued on following page

Table 26.1 Pharmacological and Pharmacological Interventions for Common Pediatric Symptoms *(Continued)*

SYMPTOM	PHARMACOLOGICAL INTERVENTIONS	NONPHARMACOLOGICAL INTERVENTIONS
Oral discomfort	• Soothing mouthwashes • Oral candidiasis: Nystatin, miconazole gel, PO fluconazole artificial saliva (i.e., Glandosane) • Aphthous ulcers: Triamcinolone or hydrocortisone lozenges • Sodium bicarbonate rinses	• Sponges or gauze dipped in mouthwash or water applied to gums and teeth • Clean tongue with soft toothbrush or effervescent mouthwash tablet • Humidifier with oxygen • Petroleum jelly • Stimulate salivation with ice chips, chewing gum
Nausea and vomiting	Treat the underlying cause, including opioid-induced nausea: First-line agent: 5HT antagonists (ondansetron, granisetron, and palonosetron are all in the same class, but patients may respond differently to each, so you may need to try each) Second-line agents: • Antihistamine blockers (Benadryl intravenous [IV] or PO; PO Atarax) • Prochlorperazine: Sedating, high doses may cause extrapyramidal symptoms • Olanzapine • Metoclopramide • Dronabinol (cannabinoids): Dysphoria may occur Special situations: • Anticipatory nausea: Lorazepam (benzodiazepine) • Raised intracranial pressure: Steroids • Liver damage: Metoclopramide, steroids • Vestibular symptoms: Scopolamine patch	• Make food more palatable (use smaller portions, use smaller plates) • Smaller, more frequent meals • Be flexible about meal timing • Make food easier to eat (i.e., soft foods) • Emphasize comfort and enjoyment of food rather than focusing on nutrition • Try to reduce anxiety and tension around mealtimes
Anorexia and cachexia	Please see question 6	
Fatigue	• Methylphenidate, timed to coincide with important events during the day	• Treatment of depression, anxiety, and/or sleep disturbances as relevant • Exercise programs within the child's tolerance level • Rest and frequent naps • Modifying activities
Depression and anxiety	• Selective serotonin reuptake inhibitor • Methylphenidate: May be helpful for depression combined with fatigue • Benzodiazepines: Short-term benefit for anxiety	• Cognitive behavioral measures
Delirium and agitation	• Treat the underlying cause when possible, including pain • Antipsychotic medications • Switch from short-acting to long-acting opioids	• Environmental manipulations (i.e., provide clocks, calendars, windows with outside view) • Verbal reorientation • Cognitive stimulation during the day • Sleep hygiene • Frequent touch • Do not endorse or challenge delusions

Table 26.1 Pharmacological and Pharmacological Interventions for Common Pediatric Symptoms *(Continued)*

SYMPTOM	PHARMACOLOGICAL INTERVENTIONS	NONPHARMACOLOGICAL INTERVENTIONS
		• Constant observation • Physical restraints as a last resort • Pay attention to commonly implicated medications (i.e., benzodiazepines)
Anemia and bleeding	• Red blood cell transfusion if symptomatic • PO or IV aminocaproic acid • Topic fibrin sealants • May require platelet transfusion	N/A
Seizures	• Transmucosal administration of antiepileptic drugs	N/A

[a]Cognitive behavioral/psychosocial measures may include meditation, hypnosis, distraction, music, art, storytelling, relaxation training, stimulus control, guided imagery, and pet therapy.
[b]Physical measures may include massage, cuddling, heat, cold, and physical/occupational therapy.
Adapted from Hain R, Jassal S. Oxford Specialist Handbook of Paediatric Palliative Medicine. *2nd ed. Oxford University Press, 2016.*

Feeding a child is a basic parental instinct, and thus many parents wish to institute parenteral or enteral nutrition for their child if the child cannot eat normally. The decision to begin artificial nutrition must be approached individually for each child and requires the consideration of multiple factors, including risks (such as nausea, vomiting, aspiration, edema, and the infection risk inherent with foreign bodies). Increased caloric intake may not reverse cachexia because it is often related to the disease process in addition to reduced caloric intake. Families should know that children can live comfortably for extended periods of time with minimal nutrition and hydration. Most importantly, you should incorporate the child's goals of care in the conversation.

7. How should you assess pain in children?
   Use the QUEST approach to elicit more details.

Question the child	Use PQRST to assess: Palliative or precipitating factors Quality of pain Radiation or region of pain Subjective descriptions of pain and severity of pain Timing of pain

Use pain-rating tools	Use an age-appropriate tool
	    There are two main methods of assessing pain in children: self-reporting and behavioral observational.
	Age 3–8 years: visual analog pain scale
	Age 8–11 years: visual analog pain scale; numerical scale
	Age 11+ years: numerical scale; can give descriptions; pain location tool
	    In patients who are unable to self-report: Use observational tools (scores assigned in different domains, such as how they respond consolation, facial expressions, motor responses). An example is the R-FLACC tool. For children with neurological impairments, it's important to combine the score with input from a consistent caregiver, who can provide normative information.

Evaluate behavior	I.e., grimacing, stiffening
Sensitize parents & staff	Ask a parent and bedside nurse to report the child's pain
Take action	Administer medications and nonpharmacological therapies

• Do a thorough examination (Is there tachycardia? Tachypnea? Hypertension? Erythema at the site of an intravenous (IV) catheter? Mucositis? Pressure sores?)
• Review the medication administration record, including the patient-controlled analgesia (PCA) pump.
• Classify the pain
  • Pain should be classified by:
    • The pathophysiology (i.e., nociceptive, neuropathic)

- The etiology (i.e., soft tissue, bone, nerve, central, muscle, or total)
- The temporal pattern (i.e. acute, recurrent)
- The patient's responsiveness to opiates (i.e., responsive or resistant)

Total pain refers to the role of emotional/spiritual/interpersonal turmoil on a patient's perception of pain. Categorizing the pain helps guide the selection of appropriate medications.

8. **What are the basic principles and phases of pain management?**
The approach to pain management is built on the following pillars:
- The ladder: Use a stepwise approach to treatment (Figure 26.1).
- The clock: The duration of action of the specific drug should guide the regular scheduling of the medication. For example, the duration of action of IV morphine is 2 to 4 hours; thus to prescribe it every 6 hours is not appropriate. Providing steady pain relief and avoiding high peaks of pain lessens the total amount of analgesic medications needed.
- The route: Use the least invasive route of administration.
- The child: Tailor treatment to the individual's experience of pain and, when possible, the child's choice

9. **How should you optimize opioid medications?**
- Select a starting dose: This can be either an empiric weight-based dose or an equianalgesic dose of an alternative opioid if the patient is already on another medication. The total daily dose should be divided and given on schedule based on the medications' duration of action ("by the clock"), with an as needed (PRN) dose equivalent to one-sixth to one-third of the total daily dose, available every 2 to 4 hours. Although you do not need to remember the dose of every medication, morphine is the gold standard; the starting IV dose of morphine for a narcotic-naïve patient is 0.1 mg/kg/dose. If a patient is in pain and has been using an opioid, the starting dose should be 10% to 20% higher than the patient's usual dose.
- Titrate the dose: Adjust the dose to provide effective relief. If the patient is taking more than 1 to 2 PRN doses, then the total daily dose (and concurrently the PRN dose) should be increased.
- If there are significant adverse effects with adequate pain control, change to a new opioid *with* reduction of the new dose of opioid by 25% to 50%.
- If there are significant adverse effects without adequate pain control, change opioid agents *without* reduction of the equianalgesic dose.
- Maintenance: Once the patient has adequate pain relief, change the medications to a more convenient form (i.e., converting IR [immediate release] to SR [sustained release] formulation).

10. **What are the different methods of analgesic administration?**
The most common routes of delivering pain medication are oral and IV. In the absence of vomiting, mouth pain, nausea, and vomiting, oral medication can deliver pain control just as well as IV delivery. However, nausea, vomiting, and mouth pain may render oral delivery unfeasible. Other effective routes of delivery are as follows:
- Sublingual: Small doses of liquid opioids such as concentrated morphine or hydromorphone may be rapidly absorbed sublingually
- Transdermal: Fentanyl is currently available as a transdermal patch. Morphine can be compounded to a gel.
- Subcutaneous (SC): If the dose can be concentrated, SC injection or infusion may be effective. Infusions of up to 5 cc/hour and injections of less than 1 mL are generally tolerated. A topical anesthetic such as lidocaine/prilocaine cream can minimize injection site pain. For infusions, an insuflon may be used.
- Epidural, intraspinal, or intraventricular: May be considered for patients who require high doses of opioids not tolerated systemically. Indwelling catheters may be placed for ongoing delivery.

		Add standing opioid titrate to effect
	0.1 mg/kg OME q1-4hr PRN breakthrough pain	1/6 total standing dose q4hr PRN breakthrough pain
Non-opioids +/- adjuvants	Non-opioids +/- adjuvants	Non-opioids +/- adjuvants
MILD PAIN	MODERATE PAIN	SEVERE PAIN

Figure 26.1 Stepwise approach to pain management. Modified WHO ladder of pain management. *OME*, Oral morphine equivalents; *PRN*, as needed; *WHO*, World Health Organization. (Adapted from Pergolizzi J, Raffa R. The WHO pain ladder: Do we need another step? *Practical Pain Management.* 2015;14(1), and from Hain R, Jassal S. *Oxford Specialist Handbook of Paediatric Palliative Medicine.* 2nd ed. Oxford University Press, 2016.)

- Rectal: Medications given per rectum are generally avoided in neutropenic and/or thrombocytopenic patients to avoid infection or bleeding. However, some patients receiving palliative care may not be myelosuppressed, so rectal delivery is a viable option. Several opioids are available in a PR form.

    Note that intramuscular administration of analgesia should be avoided because of unpredictable absorption and the pain of the injection.

11. **How are changes between opioids made?**
    There are several equianalgesic dose charts and validated online dose calculators. We have provided one for general reference (Table 26.2) and a table of opioid duration of action (Table 26.3). Opioid doses must always be checked with a validated reference. The use of an online verified opioid calculator is recommended.
    1. Determine the total daily doses of current opioid medications.
    2. Convert each dose into morphine milligram equivalents (MMEs) by multiplying the dose by the conversion factor.
    3. Determine equivalent daily dose of new opioid by dividing the calculated MMEs of current opioid by new opioid's conversion factor.
    4. Opioid-tolerant patients should start at a dose of 25% to 50% less than the calculated equianalgesic dose (because cross-tolerance between opioids is incomplete) and then divide into appropriate intervals.

Table 26.2 Calculating Morphine Equivalents	
OPIOID (DOSES IN MG/DAY EXCEPT WHERE NOTED)	**CONVERSION FACTOR**
Codeine	0.15
Fentanyl transdermal (in mcg/hr)	2.4
Hydrocodone	1
Hydromorphone	4
Methadone 1–20 mg/day 21–40 mg/day 41–60 mg/day 61–80 mg/day	4 8 10 12
Morphine	1
Oxycodone	1.5
Oxymorphone	3

These dose conversions are estimated and cannot account for all individual differences in genetics and pharmacokinetics.
From CDC. *Calculating Total Daily Dose of Opioids for Safe Dosage.* https://www.cdc.gov/drugoverdose/.

Table 26.3 Opioid Duration of Action	
OPIOID	**DURATION OF ACTION (HOURS)**
Intravenous morphine	2–4
Oral morphine intermediate release (IR)	3–4
Morphine slow release	8–12
Oxycodone	4–6
Oxycodone slow release	8–12
Hydrocodone (available in a fixed combination with acetaminophen)	3–5
Methadone	variable half-life (ranging from 6–190 hours depending on the dosage

Adapted from AAFP Opioid Conversion Table. https://www.aafp.org/dam/AAFP/documents/patient_care/pain_management/conversion-table.pdf.

Example
Sarah is a 30-kg patient receiving intravenous (IV) morphine at 4 mg every 4 hours. How would you convert her to oral (PO) hydromorphone?

Calculate the total daily morphine requirement: $4 \times 6 = 24$ mg/day of IV morphine
Convert IV morphine to oral morphine: $24 \times 3 = 72$ mg PO morphine
Convert PO morphine to PO hydromorphone: $72/7.5 = 18$ mg PO hydromorphone
Dose-reduce this amount by 25% to 50% $= 9$ mg/day PO hydromorphone
Divide this amount by 6 (for every 4 hour interval): 1.5 mg every 4 hours PO hydromorphone

---

12. **What is PCA?**
    PCA is an acronym for patient-controlled analgesia, which refers to IV administration of analgesia using a programmable pump. The pump can deliver medications in different schedules (i.e., standing medication with the option to press a button for a PRN bolus or only for boluses). It also has a maximum allowable dose, so as to prevent oversedation. Most pumps register both the doses given and the number of attempts, which allows providers to more objectively assess pain management effectiveness. If the pump is used by a child who cannot reliably use a PCA to administer boluses, either a nurse or a parent can use it.

13. **What are advantages and disadvantages of methadone?**
    Methadone is a medication that not only binds to the μ-receptor (like morphine) but the N-methyl-D-aspartate (NDMA) receptor as well. This allows us to use it for simple analgesia and neuropathic pain as well; it is also well known for its use in detoxification programs for chronic opioid use. Nevertheless, titration is complicated because of rapid distribution and slow variable elimination. Therefore conversion to methadone should only be undertaken by those with experience.

14. **What are adjuvants?**
    Adjuvants are not necessarily analgesics, nor are they more potent, but some are more specific. Therefore they should be chosen based on the etiology of the pain and added to opioid therapy.
    • Neuropathic pain: Gabapentinoids, antidepressants
    • Bone pain: Nonsteroidal anti-inflammatory drugs (NSAIDs), bisphosphonates, dexamethasone
    • Muscle spasm: Muscle relaxants, antispasmodics
    • Cerebral irritation: Benzodiazepines
        General nonmedicinal adjuvants such as play therapy, physical therapy, and music, art, and pet therapy may also be very useful.

15. **What are the side effects of opioids, and how are they managed?**
    See Table 26.4.

16. **What is neuropathic pain, and what is the most commonly used medication to relieve it?**
    The International Association for the Study of Pain defines neuropathic pain as "pain arising as a direct consequence of a lesion or disease affecting the somatosensory system." It can be described as a burning, shooting, electric, or tingling sensation. The etiology is varied; it may be caused by compression, transection, infiltration, ischemia, or metabolic injury. Specifically in oncology, neuropathic pain can be caused by chemotherapy (most commonly vincristine), compression by the tumor itself, and/or as a complication of surgery. Gabapentin and tricyclic antidepressants (particularly nortriptyline) are effective in treating neuropathic pain. Gabapentin should be titrated up to optimal dosing slowly, with each change happening every 3 days. Similarly, nortriptyline should be titrated to effect as well. Gabapentin has fewer side effects compared with tricyclics and are thus employed more often.

17. **What are the differences between dependence, addiction, pseudoaddiction, and tolerance?**
    • Dependence is a phenomenon in which physical changes occur during long-term use of a drug, precipitating withdrawal if the medication is abruptly stopped.
    • Addiction is a complex phenomenon characterized by physical and psychosocial dependence of a drug; it is considered a mental illness. True psychological addiction rarely occurs among patients receiving therapy for pain.
    • Tolerance is a shift in the dose-response curve, which creates a need for increasing doses of the medication for equal effect.
    • Pseudoaddiction is the onset of apparent addiction and drug-seeking behavior (i.e., changing the way they request pain medications) in patients who have been inadequately treated for pain

18. **What are the different forms of withdrawing or withholding life-prolonging therapy, and are they legal? What is euthanasia?**
    The word "euthanasia" evokes a wide range of responses regarding its ethical and legal underpinnings. In Greek, the word means "a good death"; it can be defined as the painless termination of life for an individual whose disease is fatal or unbearable to the patient. There are different types of euthanasia, and legality varies by type and region. There is no place for active euthanasia for children and adolescents in the United States; active euthanasia requires the consent

Table 26.4 Management of Side Effects of Opioids

SIDE EFFECT	MANAGEMENT
Constipation	• Any patient receiving scheduled opioids should receive constipation prophylaxis, titrated to effect (a soft bowel movement at least every 48 hours) • Please see Table 26.1 for more details
Nausea, vomiting	• Often related to untreated constipation • If there is no evidence of constipation, antiemetics may be effective; please see Table 26.1 • Many patients become tolerant over time or respond to a different opioid
Pruritus	• May respond to a change of opioids • Ondansetron and nalbuphine at standard doses • Antihistamines are not effective
Urinary retention	• Occurs infrequently • Usually responds to running water or bladder massage • Intermittent straight catheterization may be required; patient often resumes normal urination after 1 to 2 catheterizations • A decrease in dose or change of opioid may be required • If retention persists, consider other etiologies
Respiratory depression	• Although respiratory depression is fairly uncommon, fear of oversedation often results in undermanaged pain • If there is true respiratory depression, stimulate the patient and decrease by the dose of opioid to 30% of original dose • If required, naloxone may be given (can induce a severe withdrawal reaction, use with caution)
Confusion, hallucinations, and dizziness	• Usually transient, may not be necessary to titrate the opioids to a lower dose • Rule out electrolyte abnormalities, especially hypercalcemia
Fatigue	• A common complaint, but the illness itself may be an equal culprit

and intent of the dying individual. In contrast, life-sustaining interventions may be withdrawn or withheld for children; however, although by definition this is "passive euthanasia," this is not commonly referred to as such among families or providers because the term evokes considerable controversy.

ACTIVE
• Deliberately administering a lethal dose of medication with the intent of causing death
• Legality: As of December 2020, active human euthanasia for requesting adults is legal in Belgium, Canada, Colombia, Luxembourg, the Netherlands, Spain, and Western Australia. In Belgium and the Netherlands, euthanasia is permitted for children under some conditions.
• Subtype: Medical aid in dying (MAID; in the past referred to as physician assisted aid in dying or physician assisted suicide)
  • Legal in Germany, Switzerland, and Victoria (Australian state). In the United States, it is legal in California, Colorado, District of Columbia, Hawaii, Maine, New Jersey, Oregon, and Vermont
  • Medical aid in dying in the United States is restricted to requesting adults.

PASSIVE
Withdrawing or withholding life-sustaining interventions; this may be restricted to certain forms of care such as do not intubate (DNI) or do not resuscitate (DNR). Patients and their guardians may request specific interventions and eschew others. For example, a family may want transfusions and antibiotics if indicated but not more heroic interventions such as intubation, chest compressions, and medical resuscitation with vasopressors.

19. **What is a DNR/DNI order, and what are some key components of a discussion revolving around a DNR?**
   DNR/DNI means "do not resuscitate/do not intubate." Before a life-threatening event, the primary health care provider should take the responsibility to discuss resuscitative and life-sustaining efforts and how they align with the patient's and family's wishes and goals. It is important to remind the family that although resuscitative efforts may not be done, therapies will continue that provide comfort and quality of life.
   The MOLST (Medical Orders for Life Sustaining Treatment) is a document that should be prepared in advance to clarify the patient's (or parent's if the child does not have capacity) wishes. This document details the interventions desired or to be declined and may be updated/changed over time if the patient's wishes and/or condition changes.

The MOLST is part of the medical record and should also be available for any patient who is at home and may require emergency treatment so that a family can document their wishes.

20. **What is "double effect" in relation to analgesia at the end of life, and how does this contrast to the "ceiling effect"?**
The ceiling effect is the concept that a medication has a maximum dose above which no additional benefit is seen; for example, acetaminophen (paracetamol) has a ceiling effect after 15 mg/kg. In contrast, there no ceiling effect for opioids. One must simply monitor for intolerable side effects. Double effect refers to the concept of medication given to prevent suffering having the possible, unintended (but not avoided) effect of shortening life. This is not considered to be medical aid in dying because the primary goal is to reduce suffering, and it is therefore ethically justifiable.

21. **What should one do if there is an ethical conflict between provider and patient or between providers?**
Usually, resolution of the conflict will transpire with continued discussion among the involved parties. Social workers, psychologists, psychiatrists, and pastoral counselors may all be called on to provide guidance and mediation. All hospitals have ethics boards that are available as well for consultation.

22. **What can health care providers do to help families with bereavement?**
Parents, siblings, and extended family all experience grief, albeit in different ways. Key elements of care during the bereavement process include continued contact with the care team (for both medical information such as autopsy results and for general psychosocial support), providing educational materials about the process, and helping to connect them to support groups and/or grief counseling.

23. **How is pathological grief defined?**
A child's death will profoundly and permanently change all members of the family. The timeframe in which a parent may process the loss is very individual. Historically, pathological grief was defined as grief occurring more than 1 year after the loss. However, the current model suggests that it may take years for a parent to evolve through grief. At most, abnormal grief is an equivocal concept, and grief may be considered abnormal if the individual does not progress through the stages and instead is unable to participate in normal activities. The DSM-5 has a new definition for a disabling or a prolonged response to loss. This diagnosis is not without some controversy, particularly in relation to the time course that is stated as 6 months for children and adolescents and one year for adults. Multiple other factors are also considered including, but not limited to, a sense of disbelief about the death, feeling numb, difficulty with reintegration in normal activities, and feeling that life is meaningless. This diagnosis should be considered only in the context of providing additional help and support for the bereaved, rather than stigmatizing anyone whose grief seems prolonged and disabling.

BIBLIOGRAPHY

1. Anghelescu D, Tesney JM. Neuropathic pain in pediatric oncology – a clinical decision algorithm. *Paediatr Drugs*. 2019;21(2):59–70.
2. Hain R, Jassal S. *Oxford Specialist Handbook of Paediatric Palliative Medicine*. 2nd ed. Oxford University Press, 2016.
3. NYU. Integrating Palliative Care and Symptom Relief Into Pediatrics: A WHO Guide for Health Care Planners, Implementers, and Managers. 2018. https://www-who-int.ezproxy.med.nyu.edu/health-topics/palliative-care.
4. Larcher V, Craig F, Bhogal K, et al. Making decisions to limit treatment in life-limiting and life-threatening conditions in children: a framework for practice. *Arch Dis Child*. 2015;100(Suppl 2), s3.
5. Lichtenthal W, Sweeney C, Roberts K, et al. Bereavement follow-up after the death of a child as a standard of care in pediatric oncology. *Pediatr Blood Cancer*. 2015;50(4):375–382.
6. Pergolizzi J, Raffa R. The WHO pain ladder: do we need another step? Practical Pain. *Management*. 2015;14(1).
7. Rapoport A, Shaeed J, Newman C, et al. Parental perceptions of foregoing artificial nutrition and hydration during end-of-life care. *Pediatrics*. 2013;131(5):861–869.
8. Stanford Palliative Care Training Portal. Opioid Conversion. 2021. https://palliative.stanford.edu/opioid-conversion/.
9. Upshaw NC, Roche A, Gleditsch K, et al. Palliative care considerations and practices for adolescents and young adults with cancer. *Pediatr Blood Cancer*. 2021;68(1):e28781.

AN OVERVIEW OF THE EMOTIONAL AND EDUCATIONAL NEEDS OF CHILDREN WITH HEMATOLOGICAL AND ONCOLOGICAL CONDITIONS

Dara M. Steinberg, PhD, Gabriella E. George, PsyM, Caitlin Constantino, MAEd, Evelyn M. Ramirez, PhD, and Meghan F. Tomb, PhD

CHAPTER 27

1. **What are the emotional and educational needs of children with hematological/oncological conditions?**
   Although every child is different, there are certain considerations when it comes to the emotional well-being of children with chronic and acute medical conditions. A group of psychosocial experts came together to establish standards of care for children with oncological conditions, many which are applicable across pediatric medical conditions. They highlight, among other areas, the importance of psychosocial screening, psychological intervention, neuropsychological assessment, academic support, support for parents and siblings, addressing adherence, and procedural support.

2. **How do children with hematological/oncological conditions typically adjust to their diagnoses?**
   There are various factors that influence how children will adjust to medical conditions, including preexisting vulnerabilities, genetic predisposition, and environmental factors. The Pediatric Psychosocial Preventative Health Model by Anne Kazak proposes that children with acute or chronic medical illness may be categorized into three groups:
   - Universal group: The majority of children adjust with limited psychological intervention, may experience some distress but adapt, and benefit from limited screening and information.
   - Target group: Children in this group may experience some distress and have characteristics that put them at higher risk; thus they benefit from intervention focused on the symptoms experienced.
   - Clinical/Treatment group: Children in this group experience significant levels of distress and benefit from mental health treatment.

3. **How can caregivers help their children adjust to new medical diagnoses and treatments?**
   Families should be encouraged to help children integrate their diagnosis into their daily lives and form a new routine and sense of normalcy. This includes being open with others so as to not be burdened by keeping their diagnosis a "secret," having set expectations around medications and treatment, and engaging in the typical daily activities of childhood (e.g., school work, chores, remaining connected to peers) to the extent medically possible. Caregivers may have questions as to how much misbehavior to allow. It is important to encourage them to expect their children to behave in a developmentally appropriate way (to the extent medically feasible) to encourage their overall positive adjustment.

4. **Identify the reasons for common referrals to a pediatric clinical psychologist or mental health professional**
   It is expected that when faced with a new diagnosis/treatment/prognosis, a child will exhibit a range of emotional and behavioral reactions. When their reactions do not lessen or begin to interfere with their ability to engage in care and other aspects of daily life, referral to a pediatric clinical psychologist or other mental health professional may be warranted. Adjustment disorders, in which an individual has significant and enduring distress related to an expected stressor, may occur. Some children may develop persistent sadness that leads to diagnoses of depression, or persistent worries that are diagnosed as anxiety. At times, children with medical conditions may experience behavioral difficulties. Changes in setting (e.g., being hospitalized) and routines may lead them to act out. At times, it may be difficult to disentangle side effects of the medical condition/treatment from a psychological symptom such as irritability, pain, disruption in sleep, and loss of appetite. Thus close collaboration between mental health and medical professionals is optimal.

5. **What types of treatment might a licensed clinical psychologist or other mental health professional provide?**
Children with medical conditions may benefit from routine screenings of mood and overall wellbeing. Those with more significant concerns can benefit from a psycho-diagnostic evaluation. It may be recommended that they engage in psychotherapy. Cognitive behavioral therapy (CBT) is an empirically based intervention that focuses on the intersection between thoughts, feelings, and behaviors. Treatment that has shown to be effective for addressing behavioral difficulties include parent management training (PMT) and parent child interaction therapy (PCIT). An important factor that promotes therapeutic success is the involvement of the child's caregivers in treatment to provide reinforcement of therapy skills in the child's home environment. At times, there may need to be an evaluation with a psychiatrist to determine whether psychopharmaceutical intervention would be beneficial.

6. **What should be assessed if adherence is problematic?**
When addressing adherence, important areas to explore include the family's access to the medical treatment, the family's understanding of the medical treatment, and the family/child's motivation to comply with the medical treatment. Assessing these areas will allow for treatment targeting the specific needs of the family/child.

7. **Why might feeding difficulties emerge in children with hematological/oncological conditions?**
Children who take certain medications, including chemotherapy, may experience difficulties with feeding. This may be because of delay in developing age-appropriate eating skills depending on age of diagnosis and treatment, as well as associations they may develop between food and nausea or food and certain tastes. Behavioral strategies to increase oral intake can be addressed by a psychologist in collaboration with a dietician. For more significant difficulties, feeding therapy can be pursued.

8. **Should children be told about their diagnosis/treatment/prognosis?**
Sharing clear and developmentally appropriate information with children is important. Often, children will have a greater awareness of what is occurring, thus open communication will give them a sense of security and allow them to maintain trust in their families and medical teams. Sharing information can enable children to ask questions and misconceptions can be clarified. Additionally, informing children about what to expect (e.g., before procedure, treatment) enables them to prepare themselves and engage in coping mechanisms to better tolerate the procedure. At times, children benefit from coaching in how to tolerate certain procedures. Parents, child life specialists, psychologists, and other members of the treatment team can help them in such cases.

9. **What are risk factors for long-term neurocognitive effects?**
Hematological/oncological conditions and the treatments for them can lead to neurocognitive sequela. Long-term neurocognitive effects are most common when the disease or its required treatment directly involves the central nervous system (CNS). Children with hematological conditions that cause restriction of blood flow and may lead to transient ischemic attacks (TIAs) or stroke are at risk. Additionally, children diagnosed with brain tumors, acute lymphoblastic leukemia (ALL), non-Hodgkin lymphoma, or any tumor of the eye, ear, or face are often at higher risk for late effects. The Children's Oncology Group (COG) indicates that specific types of treatment are known to impact learning and memory, which include, but are not limited to, cranial, craniospinal, or total body irradiation (TBI), any surgery involving the brain, intrathecal methotrexate, and high-dose intravenous (IV) cytarabine.

10. **What factors increase the risk for academic challenges?**
There are many factors in addition to the medical diagnosis and treatment that may affect a child's academic progress. Children who are diagnosed at a very young age are at a higher risk for academic challenges later in life because of the effect of treatment on the developing brain. Students with premorbid learning challenge may see a further decline in educational progress. It is also important to consider that these students will miss a significant amount of school because of hospitalizations or the inability to attend because of a weakened immune system and high risk for illness exposure.

11. **Why might a neuropsychological evaluation be beneficial?**
Due to the late effects and academic challenges that can emerge, children may benefit from a neuropsychological evaluation. Neuropsychological evaluations are assessments of skills and abilities linked to brain function. Neuropsychological evaluations target strengths and weaknesses in various areas of cognitive functioning, including attention, working memory, executive functioning, verbal and nonverbal learning, short-term memory, working memory, visual and auditory processing, problem solving, processing speed, and motor functioning.
    Depending on the need and timing, the scope of the evaluation may be a brief screening assessment, targeted assessment, or more comprehensive evaluation. Evaluations are recommended approximately 1 year after completion of oncological treatment and again at 3 to 5 years post-treatment or at any point where clinical decline is noted. Findings from these serial evaluations can help inform educational planning (e.g., school placement, classroom accommodations, and access to special education services) and emotional and psychological well-being, social needs, and medical intervention if needed (e.g., recommendations for psychopharmacological treatment).

12. What are interventions that could be put in place in a school setting to address academic, cognitive, and emotional needs?

In the United States, there are laws that protect children with medical conditions and that federally funded schools must comply with. These include the Individuals with Disabilities Education Act (IDEA), Section 504 of The Rehabilitation Act of 1973, and the Americans with Disabilities Act (ADA). Thus there are various mechanisms through which children with medical conditions can receive accommodations and services in the academic setting.

Early Intervention (birth to age 3) is a publicly funded program that provides services at a free or reduced cost. Any child can be referred based on concerns for developmental delay or disability and will receive an evaluation after which appropriate services will be provided. A 504 plan for school-age children is a document developed by the school with support from the medical team and details accommodations a child will need throughout the school day. An Individualized Education Program (IEP) for preschool and school-age children is a legal document developed for every child eligible for special education services. Many children with hematological/oncological conditions are eligible for special education services under the classification "Other Health Impaired" (OHI). The Office of Disability or Accessibility Services (college/postsecondary school) provides support for children in college or postsecondary school.

BIBLIOGRAPHY

1. Castellino SM, Ullrich NJ, Whelen MJ, Lange BJ. Developing interventions for cancer-related cognitive dysfunction in childhood cancer survivors. *J Natl Cancer Inst.* 2014;106(8):dju186.
2. Cheung YT, Krull KR. Neurocognitive outcomes in long-term survivors of childhood acute lymphoblastic leukemia treated on contemporary treatment protocols: a systematic review. *Neurosci Biobehav Rev.* 2015;53:108–120.
3. Hay GH, Nabors M, Sullivan A, Zygmund A. Students with pediatric cancer: a prescription for school success. *Physical Disabilities.* 2015;34(2):1–13.
4. Kazak AE. Pediatric Psychosocial Preventative Health model (PPPHM): Research, practice, and collaboration in pediatric family systems medicine. *Families Systems & Health.* 2006;24(4):381–395.
5. Kazak AE, Rourke MT, Alderfer MA, Pai A, Reilly AF, Meadows AT. Evidence-based assessment, intervention and psychosocial care in pediatric oncology: a blueprint for comprehensive services across treatment. *J Pediatr Psychol.* 2007;32(9):1099–1110.
6. Roberts MC, Steele RG (eds). *Handbook of Pediatric Psychology.* 5th ed. The Guilford Press, 2017.
7. Wiener L, Kazak AE, Noll RB, Patenaude AF, Kupst MJ. Standards for the psychosocial care of children with cancer and their families: an introduction to the special Issue. *Pediatr Blood Cancer.* 2015;62(Suppl 5(Suppl 5)):S419–S424.
8. Weiner LS, Pao M, Kazak AE, Kupst MJ, Patenaude AF, Arceci RJ (eds). *Pediatric Psycho-Oncology: A Quick Reference on the Psychosocial Dimensions of Cancer Symptom Management (APOS Clinical Reference Handbooks).* 2nd ed. Oxford University Press, 2015.

CHAPTER 28

GLOBAL HEALTH ISSUES IN PEDIATRIC ONCOLOGY

Elena J. Ladas, PhD, RD and Nader Kim El-Mallawany, MD

1. How does the epidemiology of childhood cancer vary in different geographic regions of the world?

Variation in the epidemiology of childhood cancer worldwide is largely influenced by the impact of infection-associated malignancies (Figure 28.1). Although acute lymphoblastic leukemia (ALL) is the most common pediatric malignancy observed in most geographic regions of the world, equatorial sub-Saharan Africa has long been characterized by the uniquely high incidence of Burkitt lymphoma in children. Although Epstein-Barr virus (EBV) was originally discovered from a tumor sample taken from a Ugandan child with Burkitt lymphoma in the 1960s, the geographic distribution of endemic Burkitt lymphoma is geographically linked with holoendemic prevalence of plasmodium falciparum infection rather than EBV-specific factors. Additional epidemiological drivers of unique distinctions in childhood cancer patterns in sub-Saharan Africa include the disproportionate burden of human immunodeficiency virus (HIV) infection and the high prevalence of human herpesvirus-8 (HHV-8), which is the causative agent of Kaposi sarcoma (KS). Both of these factors contribute to the remarkably high incidence of KS in children in eastern, central, and southern Africa—regions of the continent with the highest rates of HHV-8 infection—where KS is ranked among the five most common childhood cancers overall.

Although EBV is equally ubiquitous in worldwide prevalence, there are geographic distinctions in the distribution of several EBV-related malignancies. EBV-related Burkitt lymphoma and Hodgkin lymphoma are more prominent in low- and middle-income countries (LMIC); however, the explanation for this phenomenon remains uncertain. Although rare in comparison, the distinct spectrum of EBV-related T- and natural killer (NK)-cell lymphomas and lymphoproliferative disorders (LPD) occur at disproportionately higher rates in East Asia, Mexico, and Central and South America. This heterogeneous group of lymphoid neoplasms includes the extranodal NK/T-cell lymphoma nasal type, the systemic EBV+ T-cell lymphoma of childhood, aggressive NK-cell leukemia, hydroa vacciniforme-like LPD, severe mosquito bite allergy, systemic T/NK-cell chronic active EBV, and EBV-associated hemophagocytic lymphohistiocytosis (HLH). Ultimately, the impact of infection-associated malignancies is more profound in adult oncology, highlighted by extreme numbers of patients with *Helicobacter pylori*-associated gastric cancer, human papillomavirus-associated cervical carcinoma, hepatitis B/C virus-associated hepatocellular carcinoma, and EBV-associated nasopharyngeal carcinoma. Nevertheless, notable variations in the epidemiology of childhood cancer are also attributable to the relationship between infection and malignancy (Table 28.1).

2. What are some of the factors contributing to the glaring disparities in curative outcomes for children with cancer in LMIC?

Globally, greater than 400,000 children and adolescents are estimated to develop cancer each year.[11] More than 85% of these patients live in LMIC, where the estimated survival is less than 30%, contrasting starkly with the 80% survival achieved for the approximately 45,000 children diagnosed with cancer in high-income countries (HIC). Although innumerable factors contribute to this unacceptable disparity in survival, the relationship between poverty and poor survival is inseparable. One of the biggest limitations is the failure to recognize and diagnose cancer in children at all, with an estimated 50% of children who develop cancer in LMIC never even being diagnosed, compared with an estimated 6% in HIC (Figure 28.2). Challenges along the cancer diagnosis and treatment spectrum include the following:

- General lack of access to both primary care and specialized health care; societal perception of cancer as incurable (including among health care workers)
- Late clinical presentation by the time a diagnosis is achieved
- Lack of diagnostic and therapeutic technologies
- Lack of access to essential anticancer and other supportive care medications
- Lack of financial cushion for families to support themselves through the time-intense commitment to complete therapy
- Relative emphasis on priorities of public health leadership within given countries
- Presence of severe comorbidities such as malnutrition or infection
- Inherent challenges in delivering anticancer treatment and supportive care amid severe limitations in medical resources

Whether basic daily needs or sophisticated technological advances, severe societal limitations for masses of people marginalized by extreme poverty contribute to the dismal survival rates for children with cancer living in LMIC.

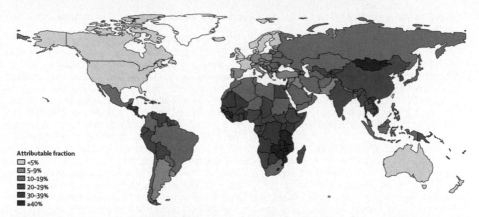

Figure 28.1 Attributable fraction of cancer related to infection, 2012. (From Plummer M, de Martel C, Vignat J, Ferlay J, Bray F, Franceschi S. Global burden of cancers attributable to infections in 2012: a synthetic analysis. *Lancet Glob Health.* 2016;4(9):e609–e616.)

Table 28.1 Geographical Distinctions in the Epidemiology of Childhood Cancer

GEOGRAPHICAL REGION	MALIGNANCIES WITH DISPROPORTIONATELY HIGHER INCIDENCE	INFECTIOUS LINKS
Equatorial Africa	Endemic Burkitt lymphoma	Malaria, EBV
Eastern, Central, and Southern Africa	Kaposi sarcoma	Human Herpesvirus-8, HIV
Central & South America plus East Asia	1. Extranodal NK/T-cell Lymphoma, Nasal Type 2. Systemic EBV+ T-cell Lymphoma of Childhood 3. Aggressive NK-cell Leukemia 4. Systemic T/NK-cell Chronic Active EBV 5. Hydroa Vacciniforme-like LPD 6. Severe Mosquito Bite Allergy 7. EBV-associated HLH	EBV

EBV, Epstein-Barr virus; *HIV,* human immunodeficiency virus; *HLH,* hemophagocytic lymphohistiocytosis; *LPD,* lymphoproliferative disorder; *NK,* natural killer cell.

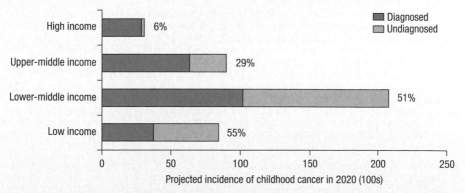

Figure 28.2 Projected incidence of childhood cancer for 2020, by country income group. Incidence categorized by World Bank income group. Percentages indicate the proportion of children with cancer who will not be diagnosed. (From Atun R, Bhakta N, Denburg A, et al. Sustainable care for children with cancer: A Lancet Oncology Commission. *Lancet Oncol.* 2020;21(4):e185–e224.)

3. **What are some of the limitations in multidisciplinary medical services that hamper curative outcomes in LMIC?**
Successful treatment of childhood cancer depends on a wide spectrum of multidisciplinary teams working in collaboration. Ranging from the essential service of pathologists to render definitive diagnoses to reliance on surgical expertise and anesthesiology to obtain tumor samples for histological evaluation to radiology support for comprehensive staging evaluation, the basis for cancer diagnosis is rooted in multidisciplinary teamwork. Oncology-specific therapy is also multidisciplinary in its approach. For hematological malignancies with exceptionally high cure rates in HIC such as ALL and pediatric lymphomas, ability to deliver the intensity of therapy required to optimize curative outcomes is compromised by lack of adequate supportive care, arising from deficiencies in specialized oncology nursing, pharmacy support, and laboratory services. For solid tumors, curative therapy depends on access to highly specialized surgical expertise and surgical technology to completely resect anatomically complex masses such as brain tumors, retinoblastoma, neuroblastoma, Wilms tumor, germ cell tumors, osteosarcoma, and hepatoblastoma. Curative intent for often unresectable solid tumors such as Ewing sarcoma, rhabdomyosarcoma, and nasopharyngeal carcinoma requires radiation therapy. Additional teams that provide essential support for childhood cancer patients include specialists in critical care, infectious disease, nutrition, social work, and palliative care; however, these are not routinely accessible in many LMIC. This is especially true for low-income countries where often one trained pediatric oncologist may be accessible for the entire country. Delivering optimal care for childhood cancer can be especially challenging in these circumstances.

To address disparities in resources between pediatric cancer centers located in HIC and LMIC, modified treatment strategies have been developed to enable centers to optimize cure within the resources available. For example, adjustments of methotrexate dosing, infusion duration, leucovorin rescue, and/or monitoring parameters for the treatment of Burkitt lymphoma or ALL may be necessary depending on available supportive care resources. Several international working groups have focused on disease-specific adapted regimens leveraging regional networks of pediatric oncology programs and global twinning relationships. Selection of the optimal therapy depends heavily on the local personnel capacity and their training as well as institutions' timely access to laboratory values, pathology reports, and blood cultures. At a given institution, capacity-building is an essential component of sustainable development. Adapted treatment regimens have been developed for several common childhood malignancies including ALL and acute myeloid leukemia (AML), lymphomas, neuroblastoma, Wilms tumor, sarcomas, and medulloblastoma; additionally, supportive care, radiation therapy, and medical nutritional therapy guidelines have been recently published among numerous other collaborative efforts across the globe.

4. **How does the management of treatment-related toxicities in the LMIC setting differ from that of the HIC setting?**
Treatment-related toxicities (TRT) are an expected result of successful treatment of childhood cancer with the number and duration of TRT primarily driven by the intensity of treatment. In the LMIC setting, adapted regimens that provide lower intensity treatments are often delivered because of limited or inconsistent access to routine supportive care treatments including antiemetics, agents for the prevention/management of mucositis, access to routine nutrition support, blood products for transfusion, and antimicrobial therapies. In the setting of mucositis, pain management can be especially challenging because of no or extremely limited access to opioid medications. Management may be further impeded by limited access to parenteral nutrition, especially pediatric formulations, or lack of staff knowledge of its administration in the pediatric setting. Infectious complications are an additional challenge facing physicians in LMIC and are often more common because of high endemic rates of infectious disease. Many patients and families are often exposed to poor sanitation, contaminated water, and food safety practices that further elevate the risk of developing an infectious toxicity among immunocompromised children. The combination of lower intensity regimens, twinning programs, and rigorous patient education interventions have been effective at reducing the risk of infectious toxicities; however, advocacy remains critical to further improving consistent access to supportive care interventions so that optimal doses of treatment are administered. One aspect of supportive care that has been especially effective in improving access to consistent care is nutrition. A tiered approach to advance education in the provision of nutritional care, increase clinical capacity in pediatric cancer centers located in LMIC, and advance high-quality research in LMIC has been effective at improving the quality of nutritional care to children with cancer across the globe. Educational sessions target improving knowledge among medical, nursing, and nutrition staff, and adapted clinical guidelines have been established based on institutional access to nutritional resources. Taken together, these efforts have reduced the incidence of new-onset severe acute malnutrition and minimized the risk of recidivism among children at high-risk for its onset. Other successful efforts are underway within the nursing and palliative care disciplines.

5. **Describe the impact of the human immunodeficiency virus (HIV) epidemic on childhood cancer.**
The story of HIV and childhood cancer can be broken down into two distinct chapters demarcated by time and space. Much of the data originating from the pre-antiretroviral therapy (ART) era is derived from HIV Cancer Registries from the United States and Europe. In those early Western experiences dating back to the 1970s to 1990s, greater than 70% of HIV-related cancers reported in children were non-Hodgkin lymphomas (NHLs), with Burkitt lymphoma and diffuse large B-cell lymphoma (DLBCL) representing the most common pathological entities. EBV-associated leiomyosarcoma represented approximately 10% of HIV-related cancers in children, and KS and Hodgkin lymphoma

were rare. Since that time, the emergence of ART and the prevention of maternal-to-child transmission through prenatal screening and treatment programs has dramatically decreased the incidence of HIV infection in children in HIC; however, the burden of pediatric HIV has disproportionately affected sub-Saharan Africa, which is home to over 90% of the world's two million children living with HIV. The epidemiology of HIV-related pediatric cancers in Africa has been completely different than the experience in the United States and Europe, with KS accounting for the vast majority of diagnoses. The dramatic difference in disease epidemiology is directly linked to the geographic variation in HHV-8 prevalence, the causative agent for KS. Although the United States and Europe are characterized by less than 5% seroprevalence, infection rates in eastern, central, and southern Africa range from 10% in South Africa up to 60% in Tanzania (East Africa). Accordingly, KS has accounted for up to 90% of HIV-related pediatric malignancies in countries like Uganda and Malawi and ranks as one of the most common overall childhood cancers overall across the region. The incidence of Burkitt lymphoma has not increased dramatically despite the impact of HIV on Africa, whereas its impact on other HIV-associated lymphomas such as DLBCL, Hodgkin lymphoma, primary central nervous system lymphoma, primary effusion lymphoma, plasmablastic lymphoma, and HHV-8-associated multicentric Castleman disease remains undefined.

6. **Is the clinical presentation of KS in children similar to that seen in adults?**
   Similar to many other malignancies that occur in both the pediatric and adult populations, there are distinct differences in the clinical phenotype observed in children. Pediatric KS was originally described over 50 years ago in HHV-8 endemic regions of Africa, long before the HIV epidemic began. This epidemiologic variant of KS is referred to as endemic KS, and early reports in children described the predominance of primary lymph node involvement, sparse and anomalous presence of prototypical hyperpigmented skin lesions, and fulminant clinical courses in children that remained untreated with chemotherapy. The contemporary experience with HIV-related epidemic KS in children in HHV-8 endemic regions of Africa has been similar in all accounts, with lymphadenopathic KS representing the most common clinical subtype. Other distinct features include the relative frequency of presentation with normal CD4 counts, frequent presentation with severe thrombocytopenia and/or anemia, and the rare observation of treatment response with ART alone. The vast majority of children with KS in Africa require chemotherapy in addition to ART, and those with lymphadenopathic KS typically exhibit a favorable response to even moderate chemotherapy regimens such as bleomycin and vincristine. Other clinical phenotypes include presentation with woody edema (typically in adolescents and often with a chronic, persistent disease course) and visceral disease involving the lung or gastrointestinal tract (typically associated with unfavorable response to chemotherapy and high mortality rates).

7. **Are there differences in characteristics between endemic Burkitt lymphoma in sub-Saharan Africa and sporadic Burkitt lymphoma seen elsewhere in the world?**
   Endemic Burkitt lymphoma is the most common overall childhood cancer in equatorial sub-Saharan Africa, whereas sporadic Burkitt lymphoma is the most common pediatric NHL everywhere else in the world (Table 28.2). The endemic variant shares geographic overlap with the incidence of malaria, and chronic antigenic stimulation from plasmodium falciparum is thought to play a role in the malignant transformation of this germinal center mature B-cell lymphoma. Although clinical presentation with a jaw mass is clinically striking and unmistakable, a large percentage of children in Africa present with abdominal involvement. Sporadic Burkitt lymphoma refers to disease outside of equatorial Africa and occurs worldwide. Patients typically present with intrabdominal disease and jaw masses are rarely appreciated. Another distinction includes the relative frequency of EBV association, nearly all endemic cases are EBV+ compared with approximately 30% for sporadic. Both epidemiologic variants share the same histological

Table 28.2 Comparison of Endemic Versus Sporadic Burkitt Lymphoma

FEATURES	ENDEMIC BURKITT	SPORADIC BURKITT
Disease Epidemiology	Most common childhood cancer in equatorial sub-Saharan Africa	Most common pediatric NHL everywhere else in the world
Common Clinical Presentations	Intra-abdominal involvement, jaw mass	Intra-abdominal involvement
Pathology Characteristics	Intermediate-sized CD20+ mature B cells, scant cytoplasm with lipid vacuoles, apoptotic bodies engulfed by macrophages impart 'starry sky" appearance	
Cytogenetics	*C-MYC*/Ig Gene translocation is the defining characteristic	
EBV Association	Nearly always EBV+	approximately 30% EBV+
Risk-Stratification Platform	Central nervous system and/or bone marrow involvement (stage IV) is highest risk, abdominal involvement (stage III) with elevated LDH intermediate-high risk	

EBV, Epstein-Barr virus; LDH, lactate dehydrogenase; NHL, non-Hodgkin lymphoma.

features and translocation of the *C-MYC* oncogene partnered with an immunoglobulin gene is the defining biologic characteristic of this malignancy. Although greater than 90% of children with Burkitt lymphoma in the United States and Europe are cured with contemporary treatment regimens combining the monoclonal anti-CD20 antibody rituximab plus intensive multiagent chemotherapy, survival in sub-Saharan Africa remains poor and is limited by failure to effectively intensify therapy according to disease stage. Survival disparities for Burkitt lymphoma are emblematic of the injustice in child health outcomes that persist in LMIC versus HIC and represent a critical opportunity to bridge the survival gap that persist more than 50 years after the original descriptions by Denis Burkitt.

8. What are the reasons for the high rates of abandonment in LMIC?

Abandonment of treatment (e.g., failure to either start or complete curative treatment for childhood cancer) is accountable for approximately one-third of the survival gap between rates observed in HIC compared with LMIC. Causes for abandonment are multifactorial, but the presence of poverty significantly increases the likelihood of discontinuing treatment across multiple continents. Other factors predisposing families to abandon treatment are poor nutritional status, low parental education, and the use of traditional medicine. A challenging issue in many LMIC is the limited number of medical centers providing treatment for childhood cancer, which often necessitates that families travel for several hours or days to visit a pediatric cancer center. Several published approaches have been established to minimize abandonment, including establishing short-term housing for patients and families who live far from the pediatric cancer center; however, loss of income and minimal ability to care for other children remain as challenges for families from underserved backgrounds. Other interventions aimed at minimizing abandonment include providing proactive nutritional care for patients with severe acute malnutrition and educating traditional healers on the signs and symptoms of pediatric malignancies so that prompt referral and bidirectional care may be provided. This has proven to be especially beneficial in sub-Saharan Africa where hospital staff have implemented field work to educate local healers throughout Cameroon to avoid delays to the hospital. Finally, the direct (e.g., cost of medications, supportive care) and indirect (e.g., income loss, childcare needs) costs of treatment remain a barrier for families with restricted resources. Advocacy at the government-level to improve coverage of services for treatment and partnering with local community hospitals to avoid lengthy travel for monitoring of laboratory values or to enable the administration of agents that do not necessitate admission have been instrumental in reducing abandonment and improving the odds of survival of childhood cancer in LMIC.

BIBLIOGRAPHY

1. Chagaluka G, Paintsil V, Renner L, et al. Improvement of overall survival in the Collaborative Wilms Tumour Africa Project. *Pediatr Blood Cancer*. Sep 2020;67(9):e28383.
2. de Martel C, Georges D, Bray F, Ferlay J, Clifford GM. Global burden of cancer attributable to infections in 2018: a worldwide incidence analysis. *Lancet Glob Health*. 2020;8(2):e180–e190.
3. El-Mallawany NK, Wasswa P, Mtete I, et al. Identifying opportunities to bridge disparity gaps in curing childhood cancer in Malawi: malignancies with excellent curative potential account for the majority of diagnoses. *Pediatr Hematol Oncol*. 2017;34(5):261–274.
4. Friedrich P, Lam CG, Itriago E, Perez R, Ribeiro RC, Arora RS. Magnitude of treatment abandonment in childhood cancer. *PloS one*. 2015;10(9):e0135230.
5. Howard SC, Davidson A, Luna-Fineman S, et al. A framework to develop adapted treatment regimens to manage pediatric cancer in low- and middle-income countries: The Pediatric Oncology in Developing Countries (PODC) Committee of the International Pediatric Oncology Society (SIOP). *Pediatr Blood Cancer*. 2017;64(Suppl):5.
6. Israels T, Renner L, Hendricks M, et al. SIOP PODC: recommendations for supportive care of children with cancer in a low-income setting. *Pediatr Blood Cancer*. 2013;60(6):899–904.
7. Ladas EJ, Gunter M, Huybrechts I, Barr R. A global strategy for building clinical capacity and advancing research in the context of malnutrition and cancer in children within low- and middle-income countries. *J Nat Cancer Inst Monogr*. 2019;2019(54):149–151.
8. Ladas EJ. A global approach addressing the double burden of malnutrition in pediatric oncology: a bench to bedside paradigm. A report from the State of the Science Meeting, Children's Oncology Group. *J Nat Cancer Inst Monogr*. 2019;2019(54):125–126.
9. Lam CG, Howard SC, Bouffet E, Pritchard-Jones K. Science and health for all children with cancer. *Science*. 2019;363(6432):1182–1186.
10. Magrath IT. African Burkitt's lymphoma. History, biology, clinical features, and treatment. *Am J Pediatr Hematol Oncol*. 1991;13(2):222–246.
11. Navarrete M, Rossi E, Brivio E, et al. Treatment of childhood acute lymphoblastic leukemia in central America: a lower-middle income countries experience. *Pediatr Blood Cancer*. 2014;61(5):803–809.
12. Ozuah NW, Lubega J, Allen CE, El-Mallawany NK. Five decades of low intensity and low survival: adapting intensified regimens to cure pediatric Burkitt lymphoma in Africa. *Blood Adv*. 2020;4(16):4007–4019.
13. Plummer M, de Martel C, Vignat J, Ferlay J, Bray F, Franceschi S. Global burden of cancers attributable to infections in 2012: a synthetic analysis. *Lancet Glob Health*. 2016;4(9):e609–e616.
14. Shannon-Lowe C, Rickinson A. The global landscape of EBV-associated tumors. *Front Oncol*. 2019;9:713.
15. Stefan DC. Patterns of distribution of childhood cancer in Africa. *J Trop Pediatr*. 2015;61(3):165–173.
16. Sullivan R, Kowalczyk JR, Agarwal B, et al. New policies to address the global burden of childhood cancers. *Lancet Oncol*. Mar 2013;14(3):e125-35.
17. Mansell R, Purssell E. Treatment abandonment in children with cancer in Sub-Saharan Africa: systematic literature review and meta-analysis. *J Adv Nurs*. Apr 2018;74(4):800-808.
18. Parkes J, Hess C, Burger H, et al. Recommendations for the treatment of children with radiotherapy in low- and middle-income countries (LMIC): a position paper from the Pediatric Radiation Oncology Society (PROS-LMIC) and Pediatric Oncology in Developing Countries (PODC) working groups of the International Society of Pediatric Oncology (SIOP). *Pediatr Blood Cancer*. 2017;64(Suppl 5).

19. Parkes J, Hendricks M, Ssenyonga P, et al. SIOP PODC adapted treatment recommendations for standard-risk medulloblastoma in low and middle income settings. *Pediatr Blood Cancer.* Apr 2015;62(4):553-64.
20. Parikh NS, Howard SC, Chantada G, et al. SIOP-PODC adapted risk stratification and treatment guidelines: recommendations for neuroblastoma in low- and middle-income settings. *Pediatr Blood Cancer.* 2015;62(8):1305–1316.
21. Tukei V, Kekitiinwa A, Beasley R. Prevalence and outcome of HIV-associated malignancies among children. *Aids.* 2011;25:1789–1793.
22. Ward ZJ, Yeh JM, Bhakta N, Frazier AL, Girardi F, Atun R. Global childhood cancer survival estimates and priority-setting: a simulation-based analysis. *Lancet Oncol.* 2019;20(7):972–983.
23. World Health Organization. Global Update on HIV Treatment 2013: Results, Impact, and Opportunities. 2013. http://apps.who.int/iris/handle/10665/85326.

CHAPTER 29

PRINCIPLES OF PEDIATRIC SURGICAL ONCOLOGY

Erica M. Fallon, MD and Angela V. Kadenhe-Chiweshe, MD

1. **What are the surgical guidelines for the treatment of neuroblastoma? How does stage affect operative management decisions?**
   Surgical goals include establishing a definitive diagnosis, accurate staging, and gross total resection, if possible. For stage I to II disease, upfront resection is encouraged with complete dissection of the primary tumor site, regional lymph nodes, and adjacent vasculature. En-bloc resection and/or injury to surrounding vital structures is discouraged. Surgical approach depends on tumor characteristics, location, and relation to surrounding structures. For extensive stage III to IV, initial surgery should be limited to biopsy of tumor tissue, staging, and placement of a vascular access device. After four to five cycles of chemotherapy, surgical resection is re-evaluated after repeat imaging is obtained.

2. **What staging systems are used for neuroblastoma?**
   The International Neuroblastoma Staging System (INSS) evaluates tumor size and location relative to midline, the presence and extent of metastatic disease, and the extent of surgical resection of the primary tumor. The International Neuroblastoma Risk Group (INRG) is a classification system that determines pretreatment risk stratification based on age, image defined risk factors (IDRF), and histological and biological factors of the tumor.

3. **Define the principles used for staging Wilms tumor.**
   Wilms tumor is assigned a local and disease stage. Local stage is determined clinicopathologically by the surgeon at the time of operation and confirmed by the pathologist. Intraoperative assessment for the presence and quality of peritoneal fluid and/or studding, assessment of the tumor capsule, and palpation of renal vein and vena cava provide essential information for staging.

4. **Describe the surgical guidelines for the treatment of Wilms tumor.**
   Upfront resection of the tumor is the mainstay of surgical therapy, without preoperative biopsy. Complete unilateral radical nephroureterectomy with lymph node sampling and without tumor spillage or rupture is the main goal. Visualization and palpation of the contralateral kidney is not necessary, if imaging is normal. The extent of contamination by "spilled" tumor (e.g., limited spill after biopsy versus widespread after tumor rupture) is crucial to accurate staging because it determines adjuvant chemotherapy and the extent of radiation therapy directed at the abdomen (e.g., flank versus whole abdominal radiation).

5. **What are the contraindications to primary nephrectomy in Wilms tumor?**
   Contraindications to upfront resection in Wilms tumor include extension of caval tumor thrombus into the retrohepatic vena cava and/or above the hepatic veins; involvement of contiguous structures (e.g., pancreas); bilateral tumors; tumor in a solidary kidney; syndromic Wilms; and/or pulmonary compromise because of extensive pulmonary metastases. Treatment involves neoadjuvant chemotherapy and resection is anticipated after week six reimaging. Biopsy before treatment initiation is considered when the diagnosis of Wilms is uncertain.

6. **Describe the staging and surgical management of hepatoblastoma.**
   The goal of surgery in hepatoblastoma is complete removal of the tumor by standard resection, if feasible. The PRETEXT (PRETreatment EXTent of Disease) staging system was developed to help define surgical resectability and classifies tumors into four groups based on the number of liver "sections" free of tumor. If the tumor is not amenable to resection upfront by standard hepatectomy, then pretreatment biopsy is obtained for diagnostic purposes. An image-guided core needle biopsy is the preferred method of tumor sampling and should not result in contamination of liver uninvolved with tumor. Neoadjuvant chemotherapy is then administered, and tumor burden is reassessed after two cycles. If an advanced hepatic resection or total hepatectomy with transplant is anticipated, the patient should be referred to a tertiary center before completing an additional two cycles of chemotherapy.

7. **Describe staging and surgical principles for the management of rhabdomyosarcoma.**
   Rhabdomyosarcoma is staged preoperatively and grouped postoperatively. Stage, group, and histology will then determine risk stratification. Complete resection with confirmed margin (at least 0.5 cm) is recommended, provided that surgery does not lead to disfigurement nor substantial functional compromise or organ dysfunction. Delayed primary excision (DPE) can be performed after chemotherapy, if substantial tumor shrinkage occurs, to reduce the radiation dose postoperatively. Lymph node biopsy is indicated to confirm clinically or radiographically positive nodes and is required,

Table 29.1 Staging of Rhabdomyosarcoma

STAGE	SITE OF PRIMARY TUMOR	TUMOR SIZE	LYMPH NODES	METASTASES
I	Orbit; Head/neck (non-PM); GU non-bladder/prostate; biliary tract	Any size	N0, N1	M0
II	Bladder/prostate; extremity; cranial PM, other (trunk, retroperitoneum)	<5 cm	N0	M0
III	Same as stage II	<5 cm	N1	M0
		>5 cm	N0 or N1	M0
IV	Any site	Any size	N0 or N1	M1

GU, Genitourinary; *PM*, parameningeal.

preferable as SLNB, in all extremity tumors and in paratesticular tumors in patients older than 10 years. The extent of surgical resection is important and affects prognosis. See Table 29.1 for clinical staging information.

8. **Describe the surgical guidelines for ovarian germ cell tumors (GCTs).**
The goal of surgery is to evaluate the extent of disease, stage appropriately, and completely resect the tumor. Ovary-sparing tumor resection can be considered based on the status of tumor markers, predictors of malignancy (e.g., size, tumor extent), and/or imaging characteristics. Staging intraoperatively consists of thorough inspection and palpation (including the contralateral ovary); collection of peritoneal fluid washings; biopsy of suspicious peritoneal, omental, liver lesions, and/or lymph nodes; and removal of the primary tumor. If the fallopian tube is involved, it should be removed with the ovary.

9. **List the guidelines for surgical management of testicular GCTs.**
Preoperative status of tumor markers must be investigated. Preoperative imaging of chest, abdomen, and pelvis will determine extent of disease. For malignant GCTs, indicated resection of the primary tumor is radical high *inguinal* orchiectomy with ligation of the spermatic cord. Transscrotal approach for biopsy and/or resection is contraindicated. Resection is followed by chemotherapy then reimaging to assess for residual tumor burden. Surgical management of persistent lung metastases and/or retroperitoneal lymph node dissection is indicated in the presence of residual nodal disease or if tumor markers do not normalize.

10. **What are the surgical guidelines for treatment of malignant lung tumors?**
Bronchoscopic examination with biopsy (EBUS) should be considered, depending on tumor location. Thoracoscopic biopsy and/or resection can additionally be considered to achieve histologic diagnosis. Treatment of primary malignant lesions depends on histology and location. Pulmonary metastases are considered for resection once the primary tumor is eradicated with no evidence of recurrence or additional metastases, and the extent of metastatic lung disease is amenable to resection. The surgical approach varies depending on the disease process, patient age, and whether the metastatic disease is responsive to chemotherapy or radiation.

11. **Describe the goals of surgical intervention for brain tumors.**
Obtaining a histologic diagnosis, debulking, and/or removing as much tumor as possible with avoidance of neurologic compromise and reestablishing or redirecting normal cerebrospinal fluid pathways are the goals of surgical management. Biopsy can be performed by stereotactic technique or craniotomy. Intraoperative imaging, electrophysiologic recording and stimulation, and microsurgical techniques can be used intraoperatively to aid the neurosurgeon during the procedure.

12. **What vascular access devices are available for pediatric patients with cancer, and how should the correct device be chosen?**
The correct device is the one that will most reliably permit infusion of therapeutic agents and blood sampling, with minimal discomfort, restriction of normal activity, and risk of infection. Considerations in choosing a device include diagnosis, age and size of the patient, and the type and duration of therapy being contemplated. Devices include completely implanted, accessible units with subcutaneous reservoirs (e.g., port), externally accessed catheters with implanted "cuffs" (e.g., Broviac, pheresis catheter), and peripherally inserted central catheters (PICCs).

13. **Discuss special considerations involved in wound healing in patients with cancer.**
Cytotoxic and antiproliferative treatment, including radiation therapy, can impair tumor cell growth and prohibit the physiologic proliferation of the cells that support normal healing, including fibroblasts, endothelial cells, and enterocytes. Patients must be monitored for alterations in healing, including increased incidence of wound or device infection and/or failure of healing, such as abdominal wall closure after laparotomy or intestinal anastomoses.

14. **How should tumor tissue be handled in the operating room?**
    Samples should be placed in sterile saline (not formalin) and immediately collected by the pathologist for transport to the laboratory. Fixatives, contamination, and tissue decay compromise the retrieval of tissue for biological evaluation.

SUGGESTED READING

1. Aldrink JH, Heaton TE, Dasgupta R, et al. Update on Wilms tumor. *J Pediatr Surg.* 2019;54(3):390–397.
2. Cohn SL, Pearson AD, London WB, et al. The International Neuroblastoma Risk Group (INRG) classification system: an INRG Task Force report. *J Clin Oncol.* 2009;27(2):289–297.
3. Kieran K, Ehrlich PF. Current surgical standards of care in Wilms tumor. *Urol Oncol.* 2016;34(1):13–23.
4. Lautz TB, Chi YY, Li M, et al. Benefit of delayed primary excision in rhabdomyosarcoma: a report from the Children's Oncology Group. *Cancer.* 2021;127(2):275–283.
5. Matei D, Brown J, Frazier L. Updates in the management of ovarian germ cell tumors. *Am Soc Clin Oncol Educ Book.* 2013.
6. Murphy JM, La Quaglia MP. Advances in the surgical treatment of neuroblastoma: a review. *Eur J Pediatr Surg.* 2014;24(6):450–456.
7. Newman EA, Abdessalam S, Aldrink JH, et al. Update on neuroblastoma. *J Pediatr Surg.* 2019;54(3):383–389.
8. Rhee DS, Rodeberg DA, Baertschiger RM, et al. Update on pediatric rhabdomyosarcoma: a report from the APSA Cancer Committee. *J Pediatr Surg.* 2020;55(10):1987–1995.
9. Wilms Tumor and Other Childhood Kidney Tumors Treatment (PDQ(R)): Health Professional Version. In: *PDQ Cancer Information Summaries.* National Cancer Institute, 2002.
10. Yang T, Whitlock RS, Vasudevan SA. Surgical management of hepatoblastoma and recent advances. *Cancers (Basel).* 2019;11(12).

III

ONCOLOGIC DISEASES

CHAPTER 30

ACUTE LYMPHOBLASTIC LEUKEMIA

Chana L. Glasser, MD and Justine M. Kahn, MD, MS

1. **Describe the frequency of acute lymphoblastic leukemia of childhood.**

   Acute lymphoblastic leukemia (ALL) is the most common malignancy in children, accounting for one-fourth of all childhood cancers and 72% of all childhood leukemia. The annual incidence rate is 3 out of 100,000 children. About 4900 children are diagnosed with ALL each year in the United States. Peak incidence is 3 to 5 years old.

2. **What is the cause of ALL?**

   The etiology for most ALL cases is unknown. There is an increased risk for development of ALL in individuals with Down syndrome, Schwachman syndrome, Bloom syndrome, and ataxia-telangiectasia. Factors associated with an increased risk for ALL include male sex, age 2 to 5 years, Hispanic race, and radiation exposure. The interaction of multiple environmental and host factors is likely involved in the etiology of ALL.

3. **List the common presenting signs and symptoms of a child with ALL.**

   The signs and symptoms of ALL reflect the degree of bone marrow infiltration by leukemic cells and the extent of disease outside the bone marrow. These include:
   - Marrow infiltration by leukemic blasts restricting normal hematopoiesis leading to anemia, thrombocytopenia, and neutropenia
   - Systemic symptoms resulting from low blood counts including fatigue, pallor, petechiae, purpura, bleeding, and fever
   - Lymphadenopathy and hepatosplenomegaly, which are signs of extramedullary involvement
   - Leukemic infiltration of the periosteum and bone resulting in bone pain with associated limp or refusal to walk in up to 25% of children
   - Central nervous system (CNS) disease presenting as focal neurologic signs or cranial nerve deficits, and boys potentially presenting with testicular involvement, although this is rare

4. **What diagnostic studies are necessary in a child suspected of having ALL?**
   - A complete blood count with differential may provide the first clues that a child has ALL.
     - An elevated leukocyte count is seen in close to 50% of cases and is greater than $50,000/mm^3$ in 17% of cases.
     - Anemia is observed 90% of the time.
     - Platelet counts of less than $100,000/mm^3$ are observed in 75%.
   - Morphologic assessment of the peripheral smear may reveal lymphoblasts.
   - Flow cytometry: Immunophenotyping of the peripheral blood leukocytes using a panel of monoclonal antibodies directed against early B- or T-cell antigens expressed on the blast surface may confirm the diagnosis.
   - Bone marrow aspirate and biopsy: To definitively establish a diagnosis of ALL, a bone marrow aspirate is required. The finding of at least 25% blast cells in the marrow is necessary to differentiate ALL from acute lymphoblastic lymphomas.
     - Cytogenetic analysis and fluorescent in situ hybridization (FISH) of the leukemic blasts provides important prognostic information.
   - A lumbar puncture with prophylactic chemotherapy is performed during diagnostic workup to screen for CNS leukemia.
     - Cerebrospinal fluid is examined after cytocentrifugation to concentrate the leukemic cells and increase the diagnostic sensitivity. Evidence of CNS leukemia is present in less than 5% of children at the time of diagnosis.
   - A chest radiograph to ascertain the presence of mediastinal involvement, which is most prevalent in patients with T-cell ALL (T-ALL), should be obtained.

5. **List the characteristics of T-cell ALL.**

   T-ALL is more common in male patients and is more often found in older children. It is frequently associated with the following clinical characteristics:
   - Splenomegaly
   - Lymphadenopathy
   - Large anterior mediastinal mass
   - Increased risk for initial CNS involvement or relapse
   - Initial leukocyte count of at least $50,000/mm^3$
   - Hemoglobin of at least 10 g/dL

Table 30.1 National Cancer Institute (NCI) Risk Classification for B-Cell Acute Lymphoblastic Leukemia (ALL)		
RISK	**DEFINITION**	**PERCENTAGE OF B-CELL ALL PATIENTS**
Standard	Age 1–9.99 years and white blood cell (WBC) count <50,000/mm³	68%
High	Age ≥10 years or WBC ≥50,000/mm³	32%

6. **Describe the National Cancer Institute (NCI)/Rome Criteria Risk Groups for B-ALL.**
   Age and leukocyte count at diagnosis are important predictors associated with ALL outcome (Table 30.1).

7. **What clinical or pathologic features are prognostic in ALL?**
   See Table 30.2.

8. **Describe features and prognosis of infant ALL.**
   Infants tend to have a type of leukemia that is biologically different from the ALL seen in older children.
   - The leukemic blasts are more likely to have an unfavorable translocation, such as t(4;11) involving chromosome 11q23, the location of the *KMT2A* (MLL) fusion gene.
   - Immunophenotyping is usually consistent with an early B-cell precursor origin, with CD10 (common ALL antigen) negativity.
   - Infants often present with elevated leukocyte counts and CNS disease and frequently have massive hepatosplenomegaly.
   - The prognosis is particularly poor in infants younger than 6 months.

9. **Define event-free survival and overall survival.**
   - Event-free survival (EFS) is generally defined as the time from remission to disease recurrence or relapse, second malignant neoplasm, or death from any cause.
   - Overall survival (OS) is the time from treatment to death from any cause.

10. **What is the prognosis for children with ALL?**
    The outcomes for children with ALL have improved dramatically over the last several decades because of refinements in risk stratification, improved diagnostics and high-level minimal residual disease (MRD) detection, and novel targeted therapies. Despite these advances, prognostic factors such as NCI risk group, molecular and genetic signature, patient characteristics, and early response to therapy continue to play important roles in prognosis.
    - Children with NCI standard risk B-cell ALL (B-ALL) have 5-year EFS rates of approximately 85% to 90% and a 5-year OS rate of approximately 97%.

Table 30.2 Prognostic Features in B-Cell and T-Cell ALL		
	FAVORABLE	**UNFAVORABLE**
Immunophenotype	B-cell	T-cell
Central nervous system disease	Negative (CNS1 status)	Positive (CNS3 status)
Cytogenetics/FISH	• *ETV6-RUNX1 (TEL/AML1)*; t(12;21) • Double trisomy 4 and 10 • Hyperdiploid karyotype (51–65 chromosomes per leukemia cell)	• iAMP21: Intrachromosomal amplification of chromosome 21 • MLL (*KMT2A*) gene rearrangements • *E2A-HLF* t(17;19) • *BCR-ABL* t(9;21) • Ph-like ALL • *CRLF2* rearrangement • *IKZF1* deletions • Hypodiploid karyotype (<45 chromosomes per leukemia cell)
Residual disease after Induction chemotherapy	MRD level <0.01%	Detectable residual disease >0.01%

These are increasingly incorporated into treatment approaches for children and adolescents with ALL.
ALL, Acute lymphoblastic leukemia; *FISH*, fluorescent in situ hybridization; *MRD*, minimal residual disease.

- Outcomes for patients with T-ALL have improved dramatically and now approach those of standard risk (SR) and favorable subgroup of high-risk (HR) B-ALL patients with 5-year EFS of approximately 85% and 5-year OS of approximately 94%.

11. **What are the phases of therapy for the treatment of ALL?**
    See Table 30.3.
    Because ALL is a heterogenous disease, the stratification of children into risk groups has a significant impact on outcome. With this risk-based approach, the treatment is divided into four main phases, with higher-risk patients receiving a more intensive backbone of chemotherapy. All therapy for ALL in the upfront setting is approximately 2 years long.

12. **What is the difference between complete morphologic remission and MRD negative remission?**
    Complete morphologic remission is defined as a bone marrow with normal cellularity and with fewer than 5% blasts by morphologic assessment (slides under microscope). An MRD negative remission is defined as a bone marrow with normal cellularity and undetectable blasts by flow cytometry evaluation to a level of less than 0.01%. An MRD negative remission at the end of induction chemotherapy is a favorable prognostic indicator.

13. **Describe the role of CNS preventative therapy**
    CNS preventative therapy is based on the concept that the CNS is a sanctuary site for previously undetected leukemic cells to be protected by the blood-brain barrier from therapeutic concentrations of systemically administered chemotherapy. Because these cells are only partially treated during some cycles of chemotherapy, resistant leukemic cells are selected out and can lead to relapse.
    For high-risk patients, intrathecal chemotherapy in conjunction with high-dose intravenous (IV) methotrexate affords a good prognosis. The addition of cranial radiation for high-risk patients improved cure rates in the 1960s and 1970s, but it was associated with an increased risk of secondary CNS tumors, delayed growth, endocrinopathies, and neurocognitive effects. CNS irradiation as a preventative therapy has since been eliminated from most treatment protocols and is reserved only for those with overt CNS disease.

14. **Why is trimethoprim-sulfamethoxazole prescribed for children with ALL?**
    Children with ALL receiving chemotherapy are at high risk for developing a potentially life-threatening pneumonia with *Pneumocystis jiroveci*. The prophylactic use of trimethoprim-sulfamethoxazole administered as infrequently as 2 to 3 days each week is effective in reducing the incidence of this complication. Alternative antibiotic agents include dapsone, atovaquone, and IV pentamidine.

Table 30.3 Phases of ALL Therapy

TREATMENT PHASE	PURPOSE	CHEMOTHERAPEUTIC AGENTS (VARY DEPENDING ON TREATMENT PROTOCOL)
Induction (∼ 4 weeks)	• Reduce burden of lymphocytes in marrow • Induce remission • Restore normal hematopoietic function	Glucocorticoid Vincristine Asparaginase +/- Anthracycline Intrathecal chemotherapy
Consolidation with CNS-directed therapy (∼2 months)	• Eradicate subclinical CNS leukemia • Treatment of sanctuary sites shielded from chemotherapy by blood-brain barrier	Intrathecal chemotherapy Systemic chemotherapy
Consolidation (intensification) therapy (∼6 months)	• Clear any drug-resistant cells • Eliminate any residual disease	Methotrexate Vincristine Asparaginase Glucocorticoid Cyclophosphamide Cytarabine Thioguanine 6-Mercaptopurine
Maintenance (∼1 – 1.5 years)	• Low-dose antineoplastics • Prevent relapse	6-Mercaptopurine Methotrexate Vincristine Glucocorticoid

ALL, Acute lymphoblastic leukemia; *CNS*, central nervous system.

15. **What is the role of molecular targeted therapy and precision medicine in upfront treatment of ALL? Give an example of molecular targeted therapy in ALL**
Recent advancements in our understanding of the genetic basis of ALL and the development of agents that target driver mutations have led to the incorporation of novel agents into ALL therapy.
    - **Patients with Ph-positive ALL** are treated with targeted therapy in addition to chemotherapy. The *BCR-ABL1* fusion caused by t(9;21) occurs in 25% of adults and 3% to 5% of children with ALL. This is termed Ph-positive ALL. Imatinib mesylate is an oral tyrosine kinase inhibitor that blocks downstream activity of the *BCR-ABL1* fusion. The addition of imatinib mesylate to cytotoxic chemotherapy is highly effective in children with Ph-positive ALL. As more data emerges about other targetable mutations in Ph+ ALL, second- and third-line kinase inhibitors are being developed and trialed in combination with chemotherapy.

16. **What is the role of immunotherapy in treating ALL?**
The use of targeted immunotherapies has led to significant advances in the treatment of relapsed/refractory B-ALL. Blinatumomab and inotuzumab ozogamicin, as described in Table 30.4, have shown the most promise.

17. **Describe the management of relapsed ALL.**
Relapse occurs in up to 20% of children with ALL. Increasing use of targeted agents has improved post-relapse outcomes significantly.
    - **Describe poor prognostic factors at the time of relapse.** Factors associated with poor outcome include early relapse (<24 months from the end of therapy), bone marrow relapse, and T-cell immunophenotype. Treatment includes intensive chemotherapy, cranial radiation if the CNS is involved, and often also includes stem cell transplantation.
    - **Describe favorable prognostic factors at the time of relapse.** For patients with an SR relapse defined as B-cell, late relapse, and end reinduction MRD less than 0.1%, treatment includes intensive chemotherapy with the addition of cranial radiation if the CNS is involved. Studies have shown that incorporation of blinatumomab and inotuzumab ozogamicin into relapse therapy is effective, well-tolerated, and associated with a high chance of complete remission, which is critical before stem cell transplant

18. **What is chimeric antigen receptor T-Cell therapy?**
Chimeric antigen receptor T-cell therapy (CAR-T) is adoptive immunotherapy using genetically modified autologous T cells from the ALL patient. These T cells are engineered to elicit a sustained antileukemic immune response.
    - **Describe the production of CAR-T cells.** After T cells are harvested from a patient by leukapheresis, they are reengineered ex vivo to contain a monoclonal antibody recognition fragment, specific for a target on the leukemic cell (most commonly CD19), linked to a T-cell signaling domain and additional costimulatory domains.
    - **Describe the mechanism of action of CAR-T.** The CAR-T cells are reinfused into the patient after lymphodepleting conditioning chemotherapy. Once infused, CAR-T cells bind to tumor antigens, activating cytotoxic effects and also promoting proliferation and persistence, leading to tumor cell death and long-term disease control. Tisagenlecleucel (Kymriah, Novartis) an anti-CD19 CAR-T cell product was the first to be approved for treatment of relapsed/refractory B-ALL in adults and children in 2017. Additional CAR-T products, including a CD22-directed CAR, are undergoing evaluation in clinical trials. Currently patients with a second relapse or primary refractory disease are eligible to receive CAR-T therapy. The necessity for post-CAR-T consolidation with hematopoietic stem cell therapy remains controversial.

19. **What are the late sequelae associated with treatment for ALL?**
Late effects of ALL therapy vary depending on the type of therapy received.
    - Glucocorticoids results in avascular necrosis of bone in about 5% to 10% of patients, particularly in adolescents.
    - Anthracycline chemotherapy (daunorubicin, doxorubicin) is associated with cardiomyopathy, especially when given in high cumulative doses. At cumulative doses of 300 to 360 mg/m^2, approximately 30% of patients will develop abnormal echo. Dexrazoxane, a cardioprotectant, prevents acute doxorubicin-induced cardiac injury and is increasingly incorporated into many protocols.
    - Cranial radiotherapy administered to children with CNS relapse is rarely associated with brain tumors, neuropsychological deficits, and endocrine abnormalities (obesity, short stature, precocious puberty).

Table 30.4 Immunotherapy for Treatment of ALL

IMMUNOTHERAPY AGENT	TARGET ANTIGEN	MECHANISM OF ACTION
Blinatumomab	CD19	Bispecific T-cell engaging (BiTE) antibody targeting CD19 on lymphoblasts
Inotuzumab ozogamicin	CD22	Humanized antibody-drug conjugate (conjugated to calicheamicin, a potent antitumor cytotoxic antibiotic) targeting CD22 on lymphoblasts

BIBLIOGRAPHY

1. Brown P, Inaba H, Annesley C, et al. Pediatric Acute Lymphoblastic Leukemia, Version 2.2020, NCCN Clinical Practice Guidelines in Oncology. *J Natl Compr Canc Netw.* 2020;18(1):81–112.
2. Hunger SP, Raetz EA. How I treat relapsed acute lymphoblastic leukemia in the pediatric population. *Blood.* 2020;136(16):1803–1812.
3. Pui CH, Pei D, Raimondi SC, et al. Clinical impact of minimal residual disease in children with different subtypes of acute lymphoblastic leukemia treated with response-adapted therapy. *Leukemia.* 2017;31(2):333–339.
4. Tran TH, Hunger SP. The genomic landscape of pediatric acute lymphoblastic leukemia and precision medicine opportunities. *Semin Cancer Biol.* 2020.
5. Tasian SK, Loh ML, Hunger SP. Childhood acute lymphoblastic leukemia: integrating genomics into therapy. *Cancer.* 2015;121 (20):3577–3590.
6. Silverman LB. Balancing cure and long-term risks in acute lymphoblastic leukemia. *Hematology Am Soc Hematol Educ Program.* 2014;2014(1):190–197.
7. Vrooman LM, Blonquist TM, Harris MH, et al. Refining risk classification in childhood B acute lymphoblastic leukemia: results of DFCI ALL Consortium Protocol 05-001. *Blood Adv.* 2018;2(12):1449–1458.
8. Vrooman LM, Silverman LB. Treatment of childhood acute lymphoblastic leukemia: prognostic factors and clinical advances. *Curr Hematol Malig Rep.* 2016;11(5):385–394.

CHAPTER 31

ACUTE MYELOID LEUKEMIA

Jaclyn D. Rosenzweig, MD and Maria Luisa Sulis, MD, MS

1. **Discuss the incidence of acute myeloid leukemia in children in the United States.**
   There are 500 to 600 new cases of pediatric acute myeloid leukemia (AML) diagnosed annually in the United States and approximately 10,000 cases diagnosed each year worldwide. The incidence is 5 to 7 cases per million people per year. AML accounts for about 25% of pediatric leukemias. There is a bimodal distribution, with a higher incidence in both children younger than 2 years of age and adolescents 15 to 20 years old. Although the incidence of childhood AML is not affected by sex and race, an ethnicity-based difference has been observed, with children of Hispanic ethnicity more commonly diagnosed compared with other ethnic groups.

2. **Which disorders are associated with an increased risk for development of AML?**
   See Table 31.1.

3. **Which environmental exposures are associated with an increased risk for development of AML?**
   - Ionizing radiation
   - Exposures during pregnancy (flavonoids in soy products, catechins in tea, and alcohol)
   - Pesticides
   - Benzenes
   - Heavy metals
   - Alkylating agents
   - Topoisomerase II inhibitors

4. **Define the World Health Organization (WHO) classification of AML.**
   See Box 31.1.

5. **List the signs and symptoms of pediatric AML.**
   - Fatigue
   - Bone pain
   - Limp
   - Lymphadenopathy
   - Hepatosplenomegaly
   - Leukemia cutis (bluish cutaneous nodules or plaques)
   - Gingival hypertrophy
   - Chloromas (tumorous aggregates of leukemic blasts)
   - Purpura, petechiae, mucosal bleeding, and hematomas
   - Headache, focal neurologic deficits, and seizures (with central nervous system [CNS] involvement)
   - Laboratory findings of anemia, thrombocytopenia, neutropenia, and coagulopathy (especially in acute promyelocytic leukemia)

6. **Which diagnostic tests and procedures are recommended as part of the initial work-up for pediatric AML?**
   - History, vital signs, and complete physical examination
   - Laboratory studies at baseline: Complete blood count (CBC) and differential count, electrolyte panel, renal and hepatic function test, coagulation profile, lactate dehydrogenase (LDH), uric acid, serum pregnancy test, type and screen, viral studies (cytomegalovirus [CMV], Epstein-Barr virus [EBV], and varicella zoster virus [VZV] titers)
   - Review of peripheral blood smear stained with Wright-Giemsa or similar stain
   - Bone marrow aspirate (BMA) smear stained with Wright-Giemsa or similar stain and bone marrow biopsy for assessment of cellularity and morphologic evaluation
   - BMA for assessment of blast lineage by multiparameter flow cytometry and/or immunohistochemistry on the bone marrow biopsy
   - BMA for karyotype, fluorescent in situ hybridization (FISH), and molecular analysis
   - Lumbar puncture for cell count and cytospin analysis
   - Echocardiogram and electrocardiogram
   - Chest x-ray
   - Human leukocyte antigen (HLA) typing

Table 31.1 Disorders Associated With Development of Pediatric Acute Myeloid Leukemia (AML)

INHERITED	ACQUIRED
Down Syndrome (Trisomy 21)	Severe aplastic anemia
Trisomy 8	Acquired amegakaryocytic thrombocytopenia
Fanconi anemia	Paroxysmal nocturnal hemoglobinuria
Bloom syndrome	
Li-Fraumeni syndrome	
Dyskeratosis congenita	
Severe congenital neutropenia	
Neurofibromatosis 1	
CEBPA-mediated AML	
Shwachman-Diamond syndrome	
Diamond-Blackfan anemia	
Familial platelet disorder	
Congenital amegakaryocytic thrombocytopenia	
Thrombocytopenia with absent radius syndrome	

Box 31.1 WHO Classification of Acute Myeloid Leukemia (AML)

1. AML with recurrent genetic abnormalities
   - AML with t(8;21)(q22;q22) (*RUNX1-RUNX1T1*)
   - AML with inv(16)(p13.1q22) or t(16;16)(p13.1;q22); *CBFB-MYH11*
   - APL with t(15;17)(q22;q12); *PML-RARA*
   - AML with t(9;11)(p21.3;q23.3); *MLLT3-KMT2A*
   - AML with t(6;9)(p23;q34); *DEK-NUP214*
   - AML with inv(3)(q21.3q26.2) or t(3;3)(q21.3;q26.2); *GATA2, MECOM*
   - AML (megakaryoblastic) with t(1;22)(p13.3;q13.3); *RBM15-MKL1*
   - AML with *BCR-ABL1*
   - AML with mutated *NPM1*
   - AML with biallelic mutations of *CEBPA*
   - AML with mutated *RUNX1*
2. AML with myelodysplastic syndrome (MDS)–related features
3. Therapy-related AML
4. AML not otherwise specified
   - AML with minimal differentiation
   - AML without maturation
   - AML with maturation
   - Acute myelomonocytic leukemia
   - Acute monoblastic/monocytic leukemia
   - Pure erythroid leukemia
   - Acute megakaryoblastic leukemia
   - Acute basophilic leukemia
   - Acute panmyelosis with myelofibrosis
5. Myeloid sarcoma
6. Myeloid proliferations related to Down syndrome
   - Transient abnormal myelopoiesis (TAM)
   - Myeloid leukemia associated with Down syndrome

7. **How is the diagnosis of AML confirmed?**
   Multiple methods are used to diagnose and classify AML on BMA and biopsy samples or from peripheral blood (if leukemic blasts are present) if bone marrow samples cannot be obtained.
   - **Morphology:** The morphologic characteristics of the myeloblasts, including size, appearance of the nucleus, granularity of the cytoplasm, and presence of intracellular structures, such as Auer rods (thin, needle-shaped, cytoplasmic protein deposits), vary according to the stage of maturation and differentiation of the cell of origin. AML is diagnosed when myeloblasts represent at least 20% of all nucleated cells in the bone marrow.
   - **Immunophenotype:** Antigens commonly expressed on AML blasts include CD11b, CD13, CD14, CD15, CD33, CD34, CD41, CD42, CD56, CD61, CD64, glycophorin A, HLA-DR, MPO, and CD117 (c-Kit).

- **Cytogenetics:** Karyotype and FISH analysis should be performed at initial assessment to evaluate for prognostically significant genetic aberrations. AML can be diagnosed regardless of the blast percentage if t(8;21)(q22;q22), t(16;16)(p13.1;q22), inv(16)(p13.1;q22), or t(15;17)(q22;q12) is identified.
- **Molecular genetics:** Mutational analysis of *NPM1, CEBPA,* and *FLT3* should be performed on the BMA sample at diagnosis for risk classification.

8. List significant prognostic factors in pediatric AML.
   See Table 31.2.

9. Discuss the diagnosis and management of CNS disease in pediatric AML.
   See Table 31.3.

10. Describe the current standard treatment for children with newly diagnosed AML.
    Children with newly diagnosed AML undergo multiple courses of intensive myelosuppressive chemotherapy, typically including cytarabine and anthracyclines, the most active agents to treat AML. Treatment begins with one to two cycles of induction chemotherapy, consisting of an anthracycline drug (daunorubicin or idarubicin) or mitoxantrone in combination with low-dose or high-dose cytarabine, with the goal to induce complete remission (CR; Table 31.4); the addition of a third drug (fludarabine or etoposide) has been studied, but its efficacy remains unclear. Induction phase chemotherapy is followed by two to three cycles of consolidation chemotherapy, typically including high-dose cytarabine with or without a second agent such as mitoxantrone, amsacrine, or etoposide. Intrathecal chemotherapy as prophylaxis or for treatment of CNS disease is delivered throughout the time of systemic therapy (see Table 31.3). The role of allogeneic hematopoietic cell transplant (HCT) as consolidation therapy in newly diagnosed pediatric AML remains controversial. Although it is generally recommended that patients with favorable-risk AML are not transplanted in first CR, patients with high-risk features should be considered as candidates for HCT, usually after two to three cycles of chemotherapy and once CR is achieved.

Table 31.2 Risk Stratification in Pediatric Acute Myeloid Leukemia (AML)

	HOST FACTORS	CLINICAL FACTORS	CYTOGENETIC/MOLECULAR ABNORMALITIES
Favorable	Trisomy 21 and age <4 years	Complete remission No MRD at EOI	Inv(16)(p13.1q22)/t(16;16)(p13.1;q22); *CBFB-MYH11* t(8;21)(q22;q22.1); *RUNX1-RUNX1T1* *NPM1* mutation Biallelic *CEBPα* mutation
			KMT2A (MLL) (11q23.3) rearrangements: • t(X;11)(q24;q23) • t(1;11)(q23;q23)
Unfavorable		WBC >100 k/µL Persistent disease Presence of MRD at EOI	Monosomy 5 Monosomy 7 Deletion 5q *FLT3*-ITD with high allelic ratio
			Complex karyotype *MECOM* (3q26.2) rearrangements: t(6;9)(p23;q34.1) *(DEK-NUP214)* *NUP98* (11p15.5) rearrangements 12p abnormalities (ETV6 rearrangement or deletion) *ETS* fusions *CBFA2T3-GLIS2* fusion *KAT6A* (8p11.21) fusion *KMT2A* (MLL) (11q23.3) rearrangements: • t(4;11)(q21;q23) • t(6;11)(q27;q23) • t(10;11)(p11.2;q23) • t(10;11)(p12;q23) • t(11;19)(q23;p13.3)

Risk stratification in AML is constantly updated as the characterization of genetic defects underlying its pathogenesis evolves. Less established criteria in childhood AML, currently under clinical investigation, are highlighted in gray.

EOI, End of induction; *MRD,* minimal residual disease; *WBC,* white blood cell.

Table 31.3 Central Nervous System Disease in Pediatric Acute Myeloid Leukemia

Diagnosis	CNS1: CSF without blasts on cytospin regardless of the WBC in an atraumatic lumbar puncture (LP) AND No neurologic deficits at diagnosis CNS2: <5 WBC/μL in CSF with blasts on cytospin in an atraumatic LP CNS3: >5 WBC/μL in CSF with blasts on cytospin in an atraumatic LP OR Presence of neurologic deficits at diagnosis OR Presence of radiographic evidence of CNS involvement OR Traumatic LP (>100 RBCs) + WBC/RBC ratio in CSF ≥2x WBC/RBC ratio in peripheral blood
Associated features at diagnosis	Age <1 year Inv(16)(p13.1q22)/t(16;16)(p13.1;q22); t(8;21)(q22;q22.1) Elevated WBC Elevated blasts in the peripheral blood
Therapy	CNS prophylaxis: One dose of intrathecal chemotherapy per cycle dosed by age (typically cytarabine alone or in combination with hydrocortisone and/or methotrexate) CNS treatment: Frequent intrathecal chemotherapy (typically cytarabine alone or in combination with hydrocortisone and/or methotrexate) with systemic chemotherapy that crosses the blood-brain barrier (i.e., high-dose cytarabine) *Cranial irradiation is not recommended for patients with newly diagnosed AML

AML, Acute myeloid leukemia; *CNS*, central nervous system; *CSF*, cerebrospinal fluid; *RBC*, red blood cell; *WBC*, white blood cell.

Table 31.4 Classification of Disease Response

CATEGORY	DEFINITION
Complete remission (CR)	Bone marrow blasts <5% in an aspirate with spicules AND Absence of extramedullary disease AND Absolute neutrophil count (ANC) >1000/mm³ AND Platelet count ≥100,000/mm³ independent of transfusions
CR with incomplete recovery (CRi)	All CR criteria except for Residual neutropenia (ANC <1000/mm³) OR Residual thrombocytopenia (platelets <100,000/mm³)
Resistant disease (RD)	Failure to achieve CR or CRi
Relapse	Reappearance of leukemic blasts in the peripheral blood OR ≥5% blasts in the bone marrow, not attributable to another cause OR Development of extramedullary disease

11. **What is the prognostic significance of minimal residual disease in AML?**
   Recent studies show that end of induction (EOI) response, as defined by presence of minimal residual disease (MRD), is a strong predictor of relapse. In children with newly diagnosed AML enrolled on COG AAML03P1 and AAML0531 trials, the presence of residual disease after the first cycle of induction chemotherapy was associated with a significantly lower disease-free survival and higher relapse rate. Multiple techniques are used to detect MRD in AML, such as multidimensional flow cytometry (MDF) and polymerase chain reaction (PCR), allowing for improved disease detection compared with morphologic assessments. Although PCR assessment of response to therapy is limited to few subtypes of AML with specific genetic defects, response assessment by MDF is feasible in all subtypes; however, the most accurate technique to detect residual disease remains controversial as does the numerical threshold predictive of survival.

12. **Which targeted agents have been studied for use in pediatric AML?**
   • **Immunotherapy:** Gemtuzumab-ozogamicin (GO) is a monoclonal antibody directed to the CD33 antigen, which is expressed on the cell membrane of most leukemic myeloblasts, conjugated with the cytotoxic agent calicheamicin. Binding of GO to CD33 leads to internalization of calicheamicin and subsequent cell death. Addition of GO to standard chemotherapy for children with newly diagnosed AML led to improved event free survival (EFS) of 53.1% from 46.9% in those patients who received standard chemotherapy alone. Additionally, Arceci et al. evaluated GO as a single agent in children with refractory and relapsed AML and found response rates of 30% and 26%, respectively. The most common adverse events were myelosuppression and hepatotoxicity, and sinusoidal obstructive syndrome was observed in patients receiving HCT after GO administration.

- **Tyrosine kinase inhibitor (TKI):** FMS-like tyrosine kinase 3 (*FLT3*) is a transmembrane receptor tyrosine kinase normally expressed on hematopoietic stem cells, critical for lymphoid and myeloid development. Internal tandem duplication mutations (*FLT3*-ITD) and mutations in the tyrosine kinase domain (*FLT3*-TKD) occur in approximately 20% of children with AML. *FLT3*-ITD mutations are the most common and confer a poor prognosis, particularly when present in high allelic ratios. Several TKIs have been designed to target *FLT3*-activating mutations and are currently being studied both alone and in combination with chemotherapy (i.e., "first-generation" *FLT3* inhibitors [sorafenib, sunitinib, lestaurtinib, and midostaurin] and "second-generation" *FLT3* inhibitors [quizartinib, crenolanib, and gilteritinib], which are more specific against *FLT3* and therefore more potent inhibitors with fewer off-target side effects). Specifically, sorafenib was evaluated in combination with standard chemotherapy and as single-agent maintenance therapy in children with *FLT3*-ITD AML; a 3-year EFS of 57.5% was seen compared with 34.3% for the historical controls, supporting its use in these patients.

13. **What are the prognostic factors predicting survival in relapsed AML?**
   Approximately 5% of children with AML will have refractory disease, and 30% to 50% will experience relapse. Length of first remission is the most important prognostic factor for patients with relapse; approximately 80% of patients who relapse more than 12 months from diagnosis achieve CR2 compared with 50% of patients who relapse less than 12 months from diagnosis. Additionally, cytogenetic features identified at diagnosis represent a strong prognostic factor affecting rate of CR2, disease-free survival, and EFS.

14. **What are the indications for HCT for pediatric patients with AML?**
   Patients with high-risk molecular and cytogenetic features and those with a poor response to induction chemotherapy (presence of MRD at EOI or failure to achieve CR) experience high rates of relapse after completion of chemotherapy. HCT has been shown to decrease the rate of relapse for patients with newly diagnosed high-risk AML; however, the overall survival benefit is not yet established. For patients who experience relapse after upfront chemotherapy, HCT is considered the optimal treatment option, with higher cure rates compared with chemotherapy alone. Post-HCT outcomes are more favorable for patients who receive a HCT in CR compared with patients who proceed to HCT with persistent disease. Children with relapsed AML who receive HCT in CR2 have a 5-year OS of approximately 60% compared with approximately 20% for children who do not achieve CR2 prior to HCT.

15. **Name distinct subtypes of AML and describe characteristics that make each unique.**
   See Table 31.5.

16. **Which antiemetic prophylaxis is recommended for use during therapy for AML?**
   Chemotherapy for treatment of pediatric AML is moderately to highly emetogenic. Scheduled antiemetic prophylaxis should be administered before and during chemotherapy administration with additional agents available as needed. First-line agents include serotonin (5-HT3) receptor antagonists (ondansetron, granisetron, and palonosetron). Additionally, dexamethasone and lorazepam can be used, but dexamethasone should be used with caution because of the increased risk of fungal infection when used for prolonged periods of time. Aprepitant, a neurokinin-1 (NK-1) receptor antagonist, can also be considered if needed for prophylaxis of nausea.

Table 31.5 Characteristics and Treatment of Unique Acute Myeloid Leukemia (AML) Subtypes

AML SUBTYPE	DISTINGUISHING CHARACTERISTICS	CYTOGENETICS/ MOLECULAR ASSOCIATIONS	TREATMENT
Acute promyelocytic leukemia (APML)	Presence of Auer rods in the cytoplasm of the blast. Frequent coagulopathy at diagnosis	t(15;17)(q22;q21.1) with *PML-RARA* fusion	Anthracyclines, all-*trans* retinoic acid (ATRA), and arsenic trioxide
Therapy-related AML	Develops after radiotherapy and/or chemotherapy, specifically alkylating agents and topoisomerase II inhibitors	11q23 (*KMT2A*) rearrangement, 5q-/-5, and 7q-/-7	AML-type induction courses followed by allogeneic hematopoietic cell transplant (HCT)
AML in Down syndrome (DS-AML)	Majority of cases are acute megakaryoblastic leukemia (AMKL)	Mutations in *GATA1*, accompanied by additional mutations in components of the cohesion complex, epigenetic regulators, and members of the RAS pathway; Trisomies 8 and 1; Monosomy 7	Cytarabine and anthracyclines

BIBLIOGRAPHY

1. Aplenc R, Elgarten C, Choi JK, Meshinchi S. Acute myeloid leukemia and myelodysplastic syndromes. In Pizzo PA, Poplack D (eds). *Principles and Practice of Pediatric Oncology.* Wolters Kluwer, 2021:454–486.
2. Cheson BD, Bennett JM, Kopecky KJ, et al. Revised recommendations of the international working group for diagnosis, standardization of response criteria, treatment outcomes, and reporting standards for therapeutic trials in acute myeloid leukemia. *J Clin Oncol.* 2003;21 (24):4642–4649.
3. Creutzig U, van den Heuvel-Eibrink M, Gibson B, et al. Diagnosis and management of acute myeloid leukemia in children and adolescents: recommendations from an international expert panel. *Blood.* 2012;120(16):3187–3205.
4. Lamble AJ, Tasian SK. Opportunities for immunotherapy in childhood acute myeloid leukemia. *Blood Adv.* 2019;3(22):3750–3758.
5. Loken M, Alonzo T, Pardo L, et al. Residual disease detected by multidimensional flow cytometry signifies high relapse risk in patients with de novo acute myeloid leukemia: a report from Children's Oncology Group. *Blood.* 2012;120(8):1581–1588.
6. Rubnitz J. How I treat pediatric acute myeloid leukemia. *Blood.* 2012;119(25):5980–5988.
7. Rubnitz J, Razzouk B, Lensing S, et al. Prognostic factors and outcome of recurrence in childhood acute myeloid leukemia. *Cancer.* 2007;109(1):157–163.
8. Sexauer A, Tasian S. Targeting FLT3 signaling in childhood acute myeloid leukemia. *Front Pediatric.* 2017;5:248.

CHAPTER 32

CHRONIC MYELOID LEUKEMIA/ OTHER LEUKEMIA

Jing Chen, MD and Nobuko Hijiya, MD

1. **What is the chromosomal abnormality associated with chronic myeloid leukemia?**
   The Philadelphia chromosome—or t(9;22)(q34.1;q11.2) resulting in a *BCR-ABL1* fusion gene—is the hallmark of 90% to 95% of chronic myeloid leukemia (CML) cases. The remaining cases consist of variant and cryptic translocations that also result in the characteristic *BCR-ABL1* fusion gene.

2. **What should be included in the initial evaluation of a patient with suspected CML?**
   - Spleen size (below costal margin) on examination
   - Complete blood count (CBC) with differential
   - Qualitative reverse transcription polymerase chain reaction (RT-PCR) for BCR-ABL
   - Bone marrow aspirate (BMA) and biopsy for morphology, karyotyping, and fluorescent in situ hybridization (FISH)

3. **Describe the three phases of CML.**
   The three phases are chronic phase (CP), accelerated phase (AP), and blast phase (BP). There is no universally agreed on definition for AP- or BP-CML. The recommendation by the Children's Oncology Group (COG) is to follow the classification by the World Health Organization (WHO; Table 32.1).

4. **Is there is a curative therapy for CML, and what is its role?**
   Stem cell transplant (SCT) was the only curative therapy for CML before tyrosine kinase inhibitors (TKIs) were introduced. Nevertheless, with the expansion of Food and Drug Administration (FDA)–approved TKIs for childhood CML, and their relatively safe profile compared with the potential risks and long-term toxicities of SCT, TKIs have replaced SCT as the primary treatment. There is no clear criteria for SCT, but it can be considered for the following conditions: BP or AP (either at diagnosis or as a progression from CP), failure of multiple TKIs, or significant toxicity from TKIs.

5. **What are the three TKIs approved by the FDA to treat pediatric CML?**
   Imatinib, dasatinib, and nilotinib.

6. **How do TKIs compare with each other with regard to efficacy?**
   Second-generation TKIs, such as dasatinib, nilotinib, and bosutinib, have shown deeper and faster molecular response compared with imatinib in adults with CML. There have been no randomized controlled trials in children directly comparing TKIs, but reported studies have shown similar tendencies.

7. **How do TKIs compare with each other in regard to side effects?**
   In general, TKIs are well tolerated. All three FDA-approved TKIs for children can cause myelosuppression, which is usually mild and self-limited. Muscle cramp, bone pain, edema, rash, diarrhea, nausea/vomiting, and impaired longitudinal growth (especially in prepubertal children) may occur with any TKI. Pleural effusion is mainly associated with dasatinib, although this has mostly been reported in adults. Vascular occlusive events such as peripheral arterial occlusive disease, cerebral ischemia, and myocardial infarction are seen with nilotinib, although they have not been reported in children. Nilotinib has also been associated with QTc prolongation, hyperglycemia, increased transaminases, and elevated lipase level associated with clinical pancreatitis.

8. **Define the three types of responses to therapy in CML.**
   According to the National Comprehensive Cancer Network (NCCN), the definition of response is based on hematological, cytogenetic, and molecular criteria.
   A. Complete hematological response:
      - No palpable splenomegaly or signs and symptoms of disease
      - Normalization of CBC with normal white blood cell (WBC) count less than 10×10^9/L; absence of immature cells such as myelocytes, promyelocytes, and blasts in the peripheral blood; and platelet count less than 450×10^9/L
   B. Cytogenetic response: Based on bone marrow metaphase cells with positive BCR-ABL
      - Complete cytogenetic response: No Ph+ metaphases
      - Partial cytogenetic response: 1% to 35% Ph+ metaphases
      - Major cytogenetic response: 0% to 35% Ph+ metaphases
      - Minor cytogenetic response: 36% to 65% Ph+ metaphases

Table 32.1 Classification of Three Phases of CML by the World Health Organization

CHRONIC PHASE: PRESENCE OF ALL OF THE FOLLOWING CRITERIA	ACCELERATED PHASE: PRESENCE OF ANY OF THE FOLLOWING CRITERIA	BLAST PHASE: PRESENCE OF ANY OF THE FOLLOWING CRITERIA
Less than 10% blasts in peripheral blood or bone marrow	10%–19% blasts in peripheral blood or bone marrow	$\geq$20% blasts in peripheral blood or bone marrow
Does not meet definition for accelerated or blast phase	Persistent or increasing WBC ($>$10 $\times$ 10^9) unresponsive to therapy	Extramedullary blast proliferation
	Persistent thrombocytosis ($>$1000 $\times$ 10^9) unresponsive to therapy or persistent thrombocytopenia ($<$100 $\times$ 10^9) unrelated to therapy	
	Blood basophils $\geq$20% in peripheral blood	
	Persistent or increasing splenomegaly, unresponsive to therapy	
	Additional clonal chromosomal abnormalities in Ph+ cells at diagnosis, including major route abnormalities (second Ph chromosome, trisomy 8, isochromosome 17q, trisomy 19), complex karyotype, and abnormalities of 3q26.2	
	Any new clonal chromosomal abnormality in Ph+ cells that occurs during therapy	
	Provisional response criteria to TKI: Failure to achieve complete hematological response to first TKI; any hematological, cytogenetic, or molecular indications of resistance to two sequential TKI treatments; or occurrence of two or more mutations in *BCR-ABL* fusion gene during TKI therapy	

CML, Chronic myeloid leukemia; *TKI*, tyrosine kinase inhibitor; *WBC*, white blood cell.

   C. Molecular response: Based on RT-PCR of BCR-ABL transcript level using the international scale (IS), a method of standardizing quantitative PCR across different laboratories with an assay sensitivity of at least 4-log reduction from the standardized baseline.
- Early molecular response: IS up to 10% at 3 and 6 months
- Major molecular response (MMR): IS up to 0.1% or at least a 3-log reduction in *BCR-ABL1* mRNA from the standardized baseline
- Complete molecular response (CMR): Variably described and is best defined by the assay's level of sensitivity

9. **How do we monitor treatment response?**
Two generally accepted practices include recommendations from the National Comprehensive Cancer Network (NCCN) and European LeukemiaNet (ELN), both of which can be applied to pediatric CML. Both the NCCN and ELN guidelines use specific time-dependent molecular monitoring thresholds based on BCR-ABL1 transcript levels. Responses by NCCN guidelines are color-coded into green (indicates adequate response without a need for treatment change), yellow (indicates closer monitoring and possible need for treatment change), and red (indicates suboptimal response that does need a treatment change). Responses by ELN guidelines are defined as optimal (continue current treatment), warning (suboptimal response with consideration for a change in treatment based on more frequent monitoring), or failure (requires a change in treatment).

10. **What are common reasons for suboptimal response to therapy?**
Noncompliance or resistance to TKI through BCR-ABL dependent (such as mutations of kinase domain) or BCR-ABL independent pathways.

11. **Is it feasible to stop TKIs in children who are in remission?**
Studies have shown that 40% to 60% of adults with CP-CML who demonstrated deep and sustained molecular remission are able to remain in at least MMR after discontinuation of TKI. According to the NCCN, TKI discontinuation outside of a clinical trial should be considered only if all of the following criteria are met:

- Age of at least 18 years old
- CP-CML (no history of AP or BP)
- On approved TKI therapy for at least 3 years
- Prior evidence of quantifiable BCR-ABL1 transcript
- Stable molecular response of MR4 (IS $\leq 0.01\%$) for at least 2 years
- Access to reliable quantitative RT-PCR testing with sensitivity of detection of at least MR4.5
- Close molecular monitoring is required after stopping TKI

Although there are limited data on stopping TKIs in children, there is a current clinical trial studying the feasibility of cessation. It is recommended that TKIs should only be stopped in children with CML in the context of prospective clinical trials.

12. **What are the BCR-ABL negative myeloproliferative neoplasms in children?**
Myeloproliferative neoplasms are very rare in children and are characterized as clonal stem cell disorders with hyperproliferation of at least one myeloid lineage. The classic BCR-ABL negative myeloproliferative neoplasms in children include essential thrombocythemia (ET), polycythemia vera (PV), and primary myelofibrosis (MF), which are characterized respectively by abnormal clonal proliferation of megakaryocytes, erythroid, and development of marrow fibrosis after PV or ET.

BIBLIOGRAPHY

1. Athale U, Hijiya N, Patterson BC, et al. Management of chronic myeloid leukemia in children and adolescents: recommendations from the Children's Oncology Group CML Working Group. *Pediatric Blood Cancer.* 2019;66:E27827.
2. Cortes JE, Gambarcorti-Passerini C, Deininger MW, et al. Bosutinib versus Imatinib for newly diagnosed chronic myeloid leukemia: results from the randomized BEFORE trial. *JCO.* 2018;36(30):231–237.
3. Cortes JE, Saglio G, Kantarjian HM, et al. Final 5-year study results of DASISION: the dasatinib versus imatinib study in treatment-naïve chronic myeloid leukemia patients trial. *JCO.* 2016;34(20):2333–2340.
4. Hijiya N, Suttorp M. How I treat chronic myeloid leukemia In children and adolescents. *Blood.* 2019;133(22):2374–2384.
5. Hochhaus A, Baccarani M, Silver RT, et al. European LeukemiaNet 2020 recommendations for treating chronic myeloid leukemia. *Leukemia.* 2020;34:966–984.
6. Hochhaus A, Saglio G, Hughes TP, et al. Long-term benefits and risks of frontline nilotinib vs imatinib for chronic myeloid leukemia in chronic phase: 5-year update of the randomized ENESTnd trial. *Leukemia.* 2016;30(5):1044–1054.
7. Kucine N. Myeloproliferative neoplasms in children, adolescents, and young adults. *Current Hematologic Malignancy Reports.* 2020;15:141–148.
8. Vardiman JW, Melo JV, Baccarani, et al. Chronic myeloid leukemia, BCR-ABL1 positive. In Swerdlow SH, Campo E, Lee-Harris N, et al (eds). *WHO Classification of Tumors of Haematopoietic and Lymphoid Tissues.* World Health Organization, 2017:30–36.

CHAPTER 33

SOFT TISSUE SARCOMAS

Filemon S. Dela Cruz, MD and Michael D. Kinnaman, MD

1. What is a soft tissue sarcoma?
Soft tissue sarcomas (STS) are a diverse group of malignant tumors believed to originate from developing mesenchyme, which normally give rise to components of connective tissue (muscle, bone, fat, cartilage, blood vessels). The subtypes of STS have classically been named based on the normal tissue type that any given STS most closely resembles.

2. What are the key recurrent molecular alterations associated with soft tissue sarcomas encountered in children and young adults?
A. See Table 33.1.
B. Loss of heterozygosity (LOH).

3. Describe the prevalence of STS in children.
STS represent approximately 7% of all cancers diagnosed in patients less than 20 years of age. The incidence of specific STS subtypes varies by age with rhabdomyosarcoma (RMS) representing 50% to 60% of STS diagnoses in children. Although RMS makes up 60% of STS diagnosed in children less than 5 years of age, its incidence in patients 15 to 19 years of age consists of only 23% of STS diagnoses. Nonrhabdomyosarcoma STS (NRSTS) is more prevalent in older children and young adults, making up more than 75% of STS in patients 15 to 19 years of age.

4. Describe the general approach for the work-up of STS.
As the foundation for the work-up of any suspected malignancy, a comprehensive history and physical exam is critical during the initial intake for patients with STS. Salient elements of the history should include presenting signs, history of constitutional symptoms (e.g., fever, weight loss), prior history and extent of radiation exposure or therapy with cytotoxic chemotherapy, family history of malignancy, immune deficiency or congenital anomalies, and a thorough physical examination with particular attention to draining lymph nodes.

Diagnostic imaging is also important in determining the extent and size of tumor and the presence of metastatic disease, which will help determine the feasibility of surgical resection for localized tumors, provide planning for radiation therapy, and enable prognostic information that will be used in the development of a treatment plan.

Table 33.1 Molecular Alterations in Soft Tissue Sarcoma

TUMOR TYPE	MOLECULAR ALTERATION
Alveolar/fusion-positive rhabdomyosarcoma	*PAX3-FOXO1, PAX7-FOXO1, MYOD1*
Alveolar soft part sarcoma	*TFE3-APSL*
Congenital or infantile fibrosarcoma	*ETV6-NTRK3*
Dermatofibrosarcoma protuberans	*COL1A1-PDGFB*
Desmoid tumor	*APC, CTNNB1* (Beta-catenin)
Desmoplastic small round cell tumor	*ESWR1-WT1*
Epithelioid sarcoma	*SMARCB1* (INI1) loss
Inflammatory myofibroblastic tumor	*ALK, ROS1,* or *PDGFRbeta* fusions
Leiomyosarcoma	LOH in chromosomes 11 and 13
Liposarcoma	*FUS* (TLS) *-DDIT3* (CHOP), *EWSR1-DDIT3*
Malignant peripheral nerve sheath tumor	*NF1,* 17q11.2
Clear cell sarcoma of soft tissue (melanoma of soft tissue)	*EWSR1-ATF1*
PEComa (perivascular epithelioid cell tumor)	*TSC1, TSC2*
Synovial sarcoma	*SS18* (SYT)-*SSX1, SS18-SSX2, SS18-SSX4*
Undifferentiated sarcoma of the liver	*MALAT1*-MHLB1 locus, *TP53*

- Magnetic resonance imaging (MRI) is generally preferred for imaging of soft tissue tumors given its ability to provide higher resolution images and delineation of tissue layers important for surgical planning and evaluation of tumor extent and infiltration of surrounding tissues.
- Given the proclivity of STS to disseminate to the lungs and present as metastatic disease, a dedicated computed tomography (CT) of the chest is generally included in the battery of diagnostic imaging and is preferred over MRI given the ability of CT to detect calcifications associated with some pulmonary metastases and lower image acquisition times.
- Positron emission tomography (PET) has become increasingly used in diagnostic imaging given its ability to provide baseline metabolic activity of tumors, which can be used to monitor biologic response to therapy over time.
- Bone scintigraphy with technetium-99m diphosphonate (bone scan) is used to evaluate for osseous metastatic disease, particularly for bone sarcomas, but has been substituted with PET in some centers given the increasing availability of PET scanners and the ability of PET to visualize both osseous and soft tissue disease.
- For patients with RMS or undifferentiated sarcoma, bilateral bone marrow biopsies are performed as a component of disease staging and to evaluate for bone marrow involvement.
- Patients with parameningeal RMS also have lumbar puncture performed to evaluate for metastasis into cerebrospinal fluid.
- An echocardiogram and electrocardiogram (ECG) are also performed for patients likely to require treatment with chemotherapy given the use of anthracyclines for a majority of STS cases.
- Routine laboratory studies are done to evaluate baseline organ function and in anticipation of procedures and chemotherapy.
- Lastly, coordination with surgery, radiation oncology, if applicable, and additional support services (rehabilitation, nutrition, psychosocial services) should be initiated if not already involved in the clinical management of the patient given the complexities of therapy for STS.

5. **What factors predispose to the development of STS?**
   Although the majority of patients with STS will have no underlying genetic predisposition, the following instances have been associated with the development of STS (Table 33.2).
   - Li-Fraumeni syndrome (LFS) is an autosomal-dominant cancer predisposition syndrome resulting from germline mutations of the *TP53* gene. In addition to an increased risk for STS, patients with LFS are also at risk for developing bone sarcoma (osteosarcoma), brain tumors, adrenocortical carcinomas, leukemia, early-onset breast carcinoma in affected females, and radiation-associated malignancies.
   - RB1 germline mutations encountered in children with hereditary retinoblastoma are also at increased risk for subsequently developing STS, particularly leiomyosarcoma.
   - Neurofibromatosis type 1 (NF1 or von Recklinghausen disease) is an autosomal-dominant disorder resulting from mutational loss or reduced function of NF1 (neurofibromin) and is characterized by café-au-lait macules and neurofibromas. Individuals with NF1 have significantly increased risk for developing RMS, malignant peripheral nerve sheath tumor (MPNST), and gastrointestinal stromal tumor (GIST), in addition to other cancers including brain tumor, leukemia, Wilms tumor (nephroblastoma), and pheochromocytoma.
   - Beckwith-Wiedemann syndrome (BWS) is an overgrowth disorder that results from mutations localized to the chromosomal locus 11p15. BWS is associated with an increased risk for developing embryonal tumors including Wilms tumor, hepatoblastoma, neuroblastoma, and RMS.
   - Radiation or alkylator exposure has been associated with increased risk for developing secondary malignancies including STS, particularly in individuals with cancer predisposition syndrome including LFS, NF1, and hereditary retinoblastoma.
   - Familial adenomatous polyposis (FAP) is an inherited colorectal cancer syndrome caused by germline mutations in the *APC* gene. Individuals with FAP are also at increased risk for developing desmoid fibromatosis (a sarcoma of intermediate malignant potential) or aggressive fibromatosis.
   - RMS is associated with a variety of hereditary syndromes summarized in Table 33.2.
   - Children with acquired immunodeficiency syndrome (AIDS) or Epstein-Barr virus (EBV) infection in immunosuppressed children or other conditions resulting in immunosuppression (leukemia, solid organ transplantation) have developed leiomyosarcoma.

6. **Describe the variants of RMS and the clinical and molecular alterations that characterize each subtype.**
   RMS is the most common STS of childhood and the third most prevalent extracranial solid tumor diagnosed in children. There are two major variants of RMS, embryonal (eRMS or fusion-negative RMS) and alveolar (aRMS or fusion-positive RMS). Other described variants of RMS include pleomorphic and sclerosing/spindle cell subtypes. The major variants (eRMS and aRMS) are biologically distinct and differ in terms of age at diagnosis, presenting tumor site, metastatic potential, and long-term outcome. eRMS accounts for approximately 60% of all RMS and is also composed of botryoid and spindle cell variants, which make up 6% and 3% of RMS cases, respectively. Classical eRMS bears the histologic appearance of developing embryonic rhabdomyoblasts, whereas the botryoidal variant references the clinical appearance of grape-like polypoid masses reminiscent of a cluster of grapes (botryoid is derived from the Greek "botrus" or cluster of grapes). The spindle cell variant has a characteristic elongated, spindle appearance arranged in a

Table 33.2 Genetic Predispositions Associated With STS

INHERITED SYNDROME	INHERITANCE	INVOLVED GENES	CLINICAL FEATURES
Li-Fraumeni syndrome	AD	TP53	Predisposition and early-onset cancers
Beckwith-Wiedemann syndrome	Sporadic/AD	CDKN1C, KCNQ1OT1, LIT1, IGF2, H19	Overgrowth syndrome
Hereditary retinoblastoma	AD	RB1	Retinoblastoma in early childhood
Bloom syndrome	AR	RECQL3	Progeroid syndrome
Constitutional mismatch repair syndrome	AR	PSM2	Predisposition to hematologic, CNS, and other embryonic tumors
Costello syndrome	AD	HRAS	RASopathy and characterized by short stature, developmental delay, coarse facies, and cardiac anomalies
Familial pleuropulmonary blastoma (DICER1 syndrome)	AD	DICER1	Predisposition to pleuropulmonary blastoma and other malignancies
Gorlin syndrome/ Nevoid basal cell carcinoma syndrome	AD	PTCH	Multiple basal cell carcinomas, rib abnormalities
Nijmegen breakage syndrome	AR	NBS1	Chromosomal instability, microcephaly, immune deficiency, tumor predisposition
Noonan syndrome	AD	PTPN11, SOS1	RASopathy characterized by facial dysmorphism, short statue, webbed neck, cardiac anomalies, hearing loss, and bleeding disorders
Rubinstein-Taybi syndrome	AD	CREBBP	Multiple congenital anomalies, developmental delay, microcephaly
Werner syndrome	AR	WRN	Progeroid syndrome

AD, Autosomal dominant; AR, autosomal recessive; CNS, central nervous system.

whorl/star-like pattern (storiform) or as bundles and often harbor recurrent mutations in MYOD1. Pleomorphic RMS demonstrates intersecting bundles of large myogenic spindle cells, whereas aRMS bears a vague resemblance to fetal alveoli and is characterized by the presence of recurrent chromosomal translocations fusing the PAX3 or PAX7 gene with FOXO1 [t(2;13)(q35;q14) or t(1;13)(p36;q14) respectively]. However, current practice emphasizes classification based on fusion oncogene status rather than by histology.

eRMS is more common in younger children (<8 years) with primaries in the head and neck or genitourinary regions. Orbital tumors arising in younger children are almost always of the embryonal variant, and tumors arising from the bladder and vagina represent the majority of the botryoidal variant, which is encountered almost exclusively in younger children. In contrast, aRMS tends to occur in older patients (adolescents and young adults) and to present as extremity tumors. The alveolar variant tends to be more clinically aggressive with a higher likelihood of presenting with metastatic disease and an overall worse prognosis despite intensive chemotherapy compared with eRMS. Pleomorphic variants tend to present as extremity tumors and primarily occur in adults. MYOD1-mutant, spindle/sclerosing cell variants generally occur in older individuals with a predilection for distant recurrence and overall poor prognosis (estimated 4-year overall survival [OS] of 18%).

7. **What are the more common types of NRSTS encountered in children and young adults?**
The distribution of STS subtypes differs between children and adults. Table 33.3 lists the top 10 most common STS subtypes encountered in children and young adults (less than 20 years of age) based on data from the Surveillance, Epidemiology, and End Results Database (SEER) between 1993 and 2002.

Table 33.3 Soft Tissue Sarcoma Subtypes	
SARCOMA SUBTYPE	**% OF STS**
Rhabdomyosarcoma	41.3
Dermatofibrosarcoma protuberans	8.4
Synovial sarcoma	7.7
Sarcoma NOS	5.4
Malignant fibrous histiocytoma/Undifferentiated pleomorphic sarcoma	4.9
Fibrosarcoma	4.5
Malignant peripheral nerve sheath tumor (MPNST)	3.4
Liposarcoma	2.8
Epithelioid sarcoma	2
Leiomyosarcoma	1.8

NOS, Not otherwise specified; *STS,* soft tissue sarcoma.

8. **Describe the clinical staging system for RMS and undifferentiated sarcomas and its utility in predicting prognosis.**
   - The staging of RMS and undifferentiated sarcoma is based on a pretreatment TNM (tumor, nodes, metastasis) staging system. The TNM staging system is used in conjunction with a surgical/pathologic grouping system established in 1972 by the Intergroup Rhabdomyosarcoma Study (IRS) Group (IRSG) to risk stratify patients. Pretherapy staging takes into account tumor size, invasiveness, nodal involvement, and primary tumor site.
   - Clinical group is determined after initial surgery, if appropriate, and before initiation of systemic therapy and is primarily based on the extent of residual tumor after surgical resection along with involvement of regional lymph nodes. Since its development, the IRS staging and grouping system remains highly predictive of outcome (eventual disease-free/failure-free survival). Furthermore, the dosage and extent of radiotherapy is largely guided by the Clinical Group staging system.
   - Two other prognostic factors in RMS include age at diagnosis and fusion oncogene status and have been incorporated into a prognostic stratification system for RMS categorizing patients into low-, intermediate-, and high-risk groups, which subsequently can guide therapy determination. Children younger than 1 year old or older than 10 years have less favorable outcomes.
   - See Tables 33.4 to 33.6.

9. **Describe the upfront treatment approach for children with RMS.**
   The treatment of RMS and undifferentiated sarcoma involves a multimodality approach including surgery, radiation therapy, and chemotherapy with the goal of optimizing control of locoregional disease and treatment of micrometastatic disease. The timing and sequence of therapy is guided by the primary tumor site and extent of disease, in addition to other risk factors that are taken into account in the clinical TNM and group staging for RMS. Ultimate assignment of patients into risk groups (low, intermediate, or high risk) determine the specific chemotherapy agents to be used, timing of surgery and radiation therapies, and duration of therapy.

   All patients, regardless of risk group, will require systemic chemotherapy. Surgical intervention involves complete resection with adequate surgical margins of normal tissue and is the preferred approach for localized tumors if deemed feasible (e.g., extremity and truncal tumors). Nevertheless, tumors of the orbit, head and neck, or genitourinary system are not generally deemed to be resectable without considerable morbidity. Parameningeal tumors, particularly those demonstrating intracranial extracranial extension, may require initiation of upfront radiotherapy. For unresectable tumors, neoadjuvant chemotherapy is administered followed by local control at the primary site using radiation with or without subsequent surgery. Tumors amenable to surgical resection after neoadjuvant chemotherapy may enable a reduction of radiotherapy dose.

10. **Describe the clinical staging for NRSTS.**
    NRSTS have traditionally been staged using the IRSG grouping system and the International Union Against Cancer staging systems; however, a Children's Oncology Group (COG) clinical trial initiated in 2007 (ARST0332) evaluated a risk-based treatment approach for patients with all stages of NRSTS. Tumor resectability or resection status (unresected vs. grossly resected), tumor grade, size (≤5 or >5 cm), surgical margin status if resected (positive microscopic margin vs. negative), and presence of metastatic disease was used to risk stratify patients and dictated treatment assignment.

Table 33.4 IRS TNM Pretreatment Staging

STAGE	ANATOMIC SITE	INVASIVENESS	SIZE	NODAL STATUS	METASTASIS
I	Orbit	T1 or T2	Any	Any	Absent
	Head and neck (not parameningeal)	T1 or T2	Any	Any	Absent
	Genitourinary (nonbladder, nonprostate)	T1 or T2	Any	Any	Absent
II	Bladder/prostate	T1 or T2	≤5 cm	N0 or Nx	Absent
	Extremity	T1 or T2	≤5 cm	N0 or Nx	Absent
	Cranial parameningeal	T1 or T2	≤5 cm	N0 or Nx	Absent
	Other[a]	T1 or T2	≤5 cm	N0 or Nx	Absent
III	Bladder/prostate	T1 or T2	≤5 cm	N1	Absent
	Extremity	T1 or T2	>5 cm	Any	Absent
	Cranial parameningeal	T1 or T2	>5 cm	Any	Absent
	Other[a]	T1 or T2	>5 cm	Any	Absent
IV	All	T1 or T2	Any	Any	Present

[a]Trunk, retroperitoneum, etc.

IRS, Intergroup Rhabdomyosarcoma Study; *N0*, no clinical involvement; *N1*, clinically involved; *Nx*, status unknown; *T1*, confined to anatomic site of origin; *T2*, extension beyond site of origin; *TNM*, tumor, nodes, metastasis.

Table 33.5 IRS Clinical Group System

CLINICAL GROUP	DISEASE EXTENT AND SURGICAL RESULT
I	Localized disease, completely resected
II	Total gross resection with evidence of regional lymph node involvement
A	Grossly resected tumor with microscopic residual disease
B	Involved regional nodes are completely resected with no microscopic residual disease
C	Involved regional nodes grossly resected with evidence of microscopic residual disease
III	Biopsy only or incomplete resection with gross residual disease
IV	Distant metastatic disease, excludes regional nodal spread or adjacent organ infiltration

IRS, Intergroup Rhabdomyosarcoma Study.

11. **What is the upfront treatment strategy employed for NRSTS?**
    Similar to the risk-based treatment strategy employed in RMS, the general approach for NRSTS is wide surgical resection with negative surgical margins (R0 resection). For large tumors or those deemed unresectable at presentation, neoadjuvant chemoradiotherapy is employed to enable future resection with less morbidity. For grossly resected disease and for microscopic residual tumor after resection, adjuvant radiotherapy has been employed to maximize local control. For patients with metastatic disease, high-grade, and large (>5 cm) tumors, chemotherapy is used in a neoadjuvant and adjuvant manner.

12. **Which chemotherapy agents are used in the treatment of RMS and other STS?**
    Newly diagnosed RMS and undifferentiated sarcoma are treated using a standard regimen consisting of vincristine, actinomycin D (dactinomycin), and cyclophosphamide (VAC). In Europe, ifosfamide is used in combination with vincristine and actinomycin D (IVA) for initial therapy followed by VAC with similar outcomes in patients with nonmetastatic RMS. The utility of camptothecin derivates, topotecan and irinotecan, inhibitors of topoisomerase I, were evaluated in combination with VAC in patients with intermediate-risk disease given promising preclinical and early-phase clinical studies. Doxorubicin in combination with vincristine and cyclophosphamide (VDC), ifosfamide and etoposide (IE), temozolomide and irinotecan, and cixutumumab (IGF1 receptor antibody) have also been used in the treatment of high-risk disease. Nevertheless, inclusion of additional agents does not appear to significantly improve overall outcomes, which remain poor for patients with high-risk disease. Treatment with vinorelbine and continuous low-dose (metronomic dosing) cyclophosphamide administered to patients with high-risk disease (RMS 2005 trial)

Table 33.6 Risk Stratification in Rhabdomyosarcoma

RISK GROUP (EFS)	STAGE	GROUP	SITE	SIZE	AGE (YR)	HISTOLOGY	METASTASIS	NODAL STATUS
Low Risk / Excellent (≥85%)	1	I	Favorable	Any	<21	eRMS	Absent	N0
	1	II	Favorable	Any	<21	eRMS	Absent	N0
	1	III	Orbit only	Any	<21	eRMS	Absent	N0
	2	I	Unfavorable	≤5 cm	<21	eRMS	Absent	N0 or Nx
Low Risk / Very Good (70%–85%)	1	II	Favorable	Any	<21	eRMS	Absent	N1
	1	III	Orbit only	Any	<21	eRMS	Absent	N1
	1	III	Favorable excluding orbit	Any	<21	eRMS	Absent	Any
	2	II	Unfavorable	≤5 cm	<21	eRMS	Absent	N0 or Nx
	3	I or II	Unfavorable	≤5 cm	<21	eRMS	Absent	N1
	3	I or II	Unfavorable	> 5 cm	<21	eRMS	Absent	Any
Intermediate Risk / Good (50%–70%)	2	III	Unfavorable	≤5 cm	<21	eRMS	Absent	N0 or Nx
	3	III	Unfavorable	≤5 cm	<21	eRMS	Absent	N1
	3	III	Unfavorable	≤5 cm	<21	eRMS	Absent	Any
	1, 2, 3	I, II, III	Any	Any	<21	aRMS	Absent	Any
High Risk / Poor (≤30%)	4	IV	Any	Any	Any	eRMS	Present	N0 or N1
	4	IV	Any	Any	Any	aRMS	Present	N0 or N1

aRMS, Alveolar RMS; EFS, event-free survival; eRMS, embryonal RMS; N0, no clinical involvement; N1, clinically involved Nx, status unknown; RMS, rhabdomyosarcoma; Yr, years.

was recently shown to improve survival and is being explored as a maintenance therapy regimen after treatment with VAC. Doxorubicin, with or without ifosfamide, is a standard backbone regimen in patients requiring systemic therapy for NRSTS.

13. **Describe the clinical outcomes based on risk group for patients with RMS and NRSTS.**
Patients with low-risk RMS receiving vincristine and actinomycin D (VA) or inclusion of cyclophosphamide (VAC) and radiation therapy have generally excellent outcomes and overall treatment duration of 24 weeks. Low-risk patients had failure-free survival (FFS) of 89% and OS of 98%.

The inclusion of topoisomerase I inhibitors to VAC has been explored in a series of trials, but the inclusion of either topotecan or irinotecan did not appear to be superior to "standard" VAC therapy. Thus VAC remains the standard backbone of therapy for intermediate-risk patients. The 4-year FFS for intermediate risk patients is 68% to 73% and 5-year OS is 79%.

Despite the addition of drugs to the standard VAC backbone and interval compressed therapy (shorter time intervals between therapy administrations), the outcomes for patients with high-risk disease remain poor with an overall 3-year EFS of 38% and OS of 56%. The addition of vinorelbine and low-dose, continuous cyclophosphamide as "maintenance" therapy to RMS patients at high risk of relapse (e.g., Group III or nonmetastatic aRMS) had improvements in 5-year disease-free survival (78% vs. 70% without maintenance therapy) and 5-year OS (87% vs. 74% with maintenance therapy; Table 33.7).

Results from a risk-based treatment approach for children and young adults with NRSTS (ARST0332) demonstrated that most low-risk patients can be cured with surgery alone and without use of adjuvant therapy. For low-risk patients, 5-year EFS and OS were 89% and 96%, respectively. Intermediate-risk patients did require chemoradiotherapy and had 5-year EFS and OS of 65% and 79%, respectively. The high-risk group continue to do poorly with 5-year EFS and OS of 21% and 36%, respectively.

14. **Are there differences in outcomes for patients with fusion-negative and fusion-positive RMS?**
In general, eRMS cases have better outcomes compared with patients with aRMS. Although clinical risk factors remain highly prognostic, the presence of either the *PAX3-* or *PAX7-FOXO1* gene fusions in aRMS appear to have prognostic significance. Patients with fusion-positive RMS (RMSp) have poorer outcomes compared with fusion-negative (RMSn) disease with 5-year EFS of 9% (RMSp) versus 40% (RMSn) and 5-year OS of 20% (RMSp) versus 50% (RMSn). Some studies suggest that fusion-negative aRMS and *PAX7-FOXO1* positive aRMS have slightly improved outcomes compared with patients with *PAX3-FOXO1* fusions, but small sample sizes for these patients have hampered a more definitive conclusion.

15. **Aside from fusion oncogene status, what additional molecular alterations have been associated with clinical behavior and outcome in RMS?**
Although the *PAX3/7-FOXO1* fusion status characteristic of aRMS currently remains the only molecular alteration shown to have prognostic significance in RMS, genomic studies have identified potential recurrent mutations that may also be prognostic. Amplifications of the 12q13-q14 locus, which includes the *CDK4* gene, and seen in aRMS cases, have been associated with worse FFS and OS independent of *PAX/FOXO1* fusion status. Although 2p24 amplifications, harboring the *MYCN* gene, have been observed in RMS, it remains unclear if their presence is prognostic of outcome or therapy response. Recurrent mutations in Ras genes *(NRAS, KRAS, HRAS)* may also play a role in treatment response given the association of Ras mutations with high- and intermediate-risk RMS. Recurrent mutations in MYOD1, which characterize a rare RMS variant, spindle cell/sclerosing RMS, have also been shown to have significantly poorer outcomes compared with other types of RMS with higher rates of treatment failure and recurrence.

Table 33.7 Outcomes by Risk Stratification

RISK GROUP	STAGE	GROUP	HISTOLOGY	FFS	OS	STUDY
Low Risk	1–3	I, II, III	eRMS	85%[a]	95%[a]	D9602
			eRMS	89%[b]	98%[b]	ARST0331
Intermediate Risk	2 or 3	III	eRMS	68%–73%	79%	D9803
	1, 2, or 3	I, II, or III	aRMS			ARST0531
High Risk	4	IV	Any	15%–38%	50%–56%	D9802
				69%[c]	79%[c]	ARST0431

[a]Five-year FFS and OS from D9602 study.
[b]Three-year FFS and OS from ARST0331 subset 1 patients.
[c]Three-year FFS and OS for patients with 1 or no Oberlin risk factors on ARST0431.
aRMS, Alveolar RMS; *eRMS*, embryonal RMS; *FFS*, failure-free survival; *OS*, overall survival; *RMS,* rhabdomyosarcoma.

BIBLIOGRAPHY

1. Casey DL, Chi YY, Donaldson SS, et al. Increased local failure for patients with intermediate-risk rhabdomyosarcoma on ARST0531: a report from the Children's Oncology Group. *Cancer.* 2019;125(18):3242–3248.
2. Malempati S, Hawkins DS. Rhabdomyosarcoma: review of the Children's Oncology Group (COG) Soft-Tissue Sarcoma Committee experience and rationale for current COG studies. *Pediatr Blood Cancer.* 2012;59(1):5–10.
3. Minn AY, Lyden ER, Anderson JR, et al. Early treatment failure in intermediate-risk rhabdomyosarcoma: results from IRS-IV and D9803–a report from the Children's Oncology Group. *J Clin Oncol.* 2010;28(27):4228–4232.
4. Parham DM, Barr FG. Classification of rhabdomyosarcoma and its molecular basis. *Adv Anat Pathol.* 2013;20(6):387–397.
5. Pizzo PA, Poplack DG. *Principles and Practice of Pediatric Oncology.* 6th ed. Wolters Kluwer/Lippincott Williams: Wilkins Health, 2011:923–986.
6. Rudzinski ER, Anderson JR, Chi YY, et al. Histology, fusion status, and outcome in metastatic rhabdomyosarcoma: a report from the Children's Oncology Group. *Pediatr Blood Cancer.* 2017;64(12).
7. Spunt SL, Million L, Chi YY, et al. A risk-based treatment strategy for nonrhabdomyosarcoma soft-tissue sarcomas in patients younger than 30 years (ARST0332): a Children's Oncology Group prospective study. *Lancet Oncol.* 2020;21(1):145–161.
8. Walterhouse DO, Pappo AS, Meza JL, et al. Shorter-duration therapy using vincristine, dactinomycin, and lower-dose cyclophosphamide with or without radiotherapy for patients with newly diagnosed low-risk rhabdomyosarcoma: a report from the Soft Tissue Sarcoma Committee of the Children's Oncology Group. *J Clin Oncol.* 2014;32(31):3547–3552.
9. Weigel BJ, Lyden E, Anderson JR, et al. Intensive multiagent therapy, including dose-compressed cycles of ifosfamide/etoposide and vincristine/doxorubicin/cyclophosphamide, irinotecan, and radiation, in patients with high-risk rhabdomyosarcoma: a report from the Children's Oncology Group. *J Clin Oncol.* 2016;34(2):117–122.

CHAPTER 34

BONE TUMORS

Michael D. Kinnaman, MD and Filemon S. Dela Cruz, MD

1. **What are the most common malignant bone tumors in children, adolescents, and young adults?**
   - Malignant bone tumors account for 6% of all childhood malignancies.
     - Osteosarcoma (OS) represents 56% of new malignant bone tumor diagnosis, followed by Ewing sarcoma (ES) with 34% of new diagnosis.
   - OS is the most common malignant bone tumor in this patient population, with approximately 400 to 450 new diagnoses each year in the United States.
   - ES is the second most common malignant bone tumor in this patient population with approximately 200 to 250 new diagnoses each year in the United States.

2. **What are the presenting signs and symptoms of OS and ES?**
   - The most common presenting symptom for both OS and ES is pain at the primary site (90% vs. 96%, respectively).
     - Pain can often be misattributed to "bone growth."
   - The second most common presenting symptom for both OS and ES is local swelling or a palpable mass at the primary site of disease (50% vs. 61%, respectively).
   - Pathologic fracture, although rare, can be seen in both OS (8%) and ES (16%).
   - Although fever can be seen in about 20% of patients with ES, it is a rare presenting symptom in OS.
   - The average lag time from start of initial symptoms to diagnosis is about 2 to 4 months in OS and 3 to 6 months in ES.

3. **How does the incidence of OS and ES compare with regards to age, race, and sex?**
   - The peak incidence for OS is correlated with increased growth velocity as suggested by the fact that the age peak for females is 12 years and for males is 16 years, correlating with the different average ages of pubertal development.
   - The peak incidence of ES is between 10 to 15 years of age, with 30% of cases arising in patients under the age of 10 and another 30% of cases presenting in adults over the age of 20.
   - Both OS and ES have a slight male predominance.
   - Age-adjusted incidence rates for OS are higher among Blacks compared with other racial groups, whereas the incidence of ES in Whites is about nine times greater than in Blacks.

4. **What are the most common skeletal locations for primary OS and ES?**
   - A majority of primary OS presents in the metaphysis of long bones in skeletal regions affected by the greatest growth rate, with the most common sites being the distal femur, proximal tibia, and proximal humerus in descending order.
   - ES often arises in the long bones of extremities and the bones of the pelvis.
     - ES cases are more likely to present in the axial skeleton versus the appendicular skeleton (54% vs. 42%).
     - The most common site of presentation is the pelvis (25%) followed by the femur (16.4%).

5. **What are the most common metastatic sites in OS and ES?**
   - In OS, 20% of patients will have metastatic disease at the time of diagnosis.
     - 90% of these patients will have metastatic disease present in their lungs.
     - The second most common site of metastatic disease is another bone.
   - In ES, 25% of patients will have metastatic disease at the time of diagnosis.
     - The most common sites of metastatic disease are lungs (38%), bones (31%), bone marrow (11%), or a combination of these different sites.

6. **How do you adequately stage a patient suspected to have a malignant bone tumor? Are there differences in how you would stage a patient suspected to have OS versus ES?**
   - **Plain film of the primary site:**
     - The typical radiographic findings for OS are a radial or "sunburst" pattern, whereas ES can have a "permeative or "moth-eaten" pattern and the bone deposited may have an "onion peel" appearance.
     - Both OS and ES can have Codman triangle appearance, which occurs when a tumor raises the periosteum away from the bone.
   - If the plain film is concerning for a malignant bone tumor, the next best study to order to more fully characterize the primary site is a magnetic resonance image (MRI) of the entire length of the involved bone.
     - MRI is thought to be superior to computed tomography (CT) for malignant bone tumors because it provides a more accurate measurement of tumor size and better definition of soft tissue extension.

- To rule out additional bone metastasis in both OS and ES, a bone scan or positron emission tomography (PET) scan should be obtained.
  - Recent studies have shown PET to be more sensitive in finding bone metastases in ES and may allow for a better assessment of response to preoperative chemotherapy in OS.
    - Regardless of whether a bone scan or PET scan is chosen, the same imaging modality should be used throughout treatment.
  - To rule out pulmonary metastases, a diagnostic noncontrast chest CT should be obtained at initial diagnosis for both OS and ES.
- **Tumor biopsy:**
  - Open biopsy by an experienced orthopedic surgeon is preferable over core needle biopsy in obtaining a high-quality diagnostic specimen.
  - The major difference in staging between OS and ES is the role of bone marrow biopsy.
  - There is no role for bone marrow biopsy for staging in OS.
  - For ES, because there is a predilection for potential spread to the bone marrow, bone marrow biopsies at initial diagnosis (two sites if feasible) have been traditionally performed for complete staging.

7. **What are the cytogenetic and molecular genetic abnormalities associated with OS?**
   - No characteristic translocation or other molecular genetic abnormality compared with other pediatric sarcomas.
   - OS genomes are characterized by complex karyotypic abnormalities, with 200 to 300 structural variants on average per genome.
   - Genomic alterations in *TP53*, either through point mutations or structural alterations, are thought to be present in most OS genomes.
   - *RB1* is the second most commonly mutated gene in OS either through point mutation or, more commonly, deletion events.
   - Although point mutations in OS often involve tumor suppressor genes such as *TP53, RB1, PTEN*, and thus are not currently targetable, many of the recurrent copy number alterations are seen in known oncogenes (*CDK4, CCNE1, MYC, AKT1, AURKB, VEGFR*), making them potentially targetable

8. **What are the genetic predisposition syndromes associated with increased risk of developing OS?**

Genetic Predisposition Syndrome	Description	Chromosome involved	Gene	Function	% of Malignancies that are Osteosarcoma
Li-Fraumeni Syndrome	Autosomal dominant, germline inactivating mutation of *TP53*. Affected patients may develop a spectrum of cancers including breast cancer, brain tumors, leukemia, and sarcomas.	17p13.1	*P53*	DNA damage response	10
Retinoblastoma	Germline mutation of *RB1* gene. In addition to retinoblastoma, these patients have an increased risk of developing second primary cancers, with 60% being osteosarcoma or soft-tissue sarcoma.	13q14.2	*RB1*	Cell cycle regulation	50%
Bloom syndrome	Inherited disorder characterized by short stature and sun-sensitive skin changes. Patients typically have a long, narrow face with a small lower jaw, large nose, and prominent ears.	15q26.1	*BLM*	DNA helicase	<10%

Rothmund-Thomson Syndrome	Autosomal recessive syndrome with characteristic features including sparse hair, small stature, skeletal anomalies, cataracts, and skin findings, such as atrophy, pigmentation, and telangiectasias. Increased incidence of osteosarcoma at young age	18q24.3	*RECQL4*	DNA helicase	30%
Werner syndrome	Inherited disorder characterized by patients with short stature that develop signs of early aging In their twenties. These patients develop cataracts, skin ulcers, and atherosclerosis at an early age.	15q26.1	*WRN*	DNA helicase; exonuclease activity	<10%

9. **What is the overall prognosis for patients diagnosed with localized and metastatic OS with regards to 5-year event-free and overall survival? What are some prognostic factors that influence these numbers?**
   - The 5-year event-free survival (EFS) for patients with localized osteosarcoma is 59%, whereas the 5-year overall survival is 75%.
   - The 5-year EFS for patients with metastatic disease is 29%, whereas the 5-year overall survival is 46%.

Prognostic Factor	*Influence*
Primary Tumor Site	• Extremity tumors have more favorable outcomes than axial tumors. • Distal tumors have more favorable outcomes than proximal tumors. • Craniofacial/head and neck tumors have better outcomes than other primary sites.
Size	Larger tumors have worse prognosis.
Presence of Metastatic Disease	**Most important prognostic factor** • Patients with unilateral lung nodules have better prognosis than those with bilateral pulmonary metastases. • Patients with skip metastases (two distinct lesions in same primary) have worse outcomes. • Patients with multifocal osteosarcoma have a dismal prognosis. • Patients whose metastases are surgically resectable have better outcomes.
Age	Older patients (18–40) have worse outcomes than younger patients.
Sex	Male sex is associated with worse outcomes.
Lactate Dehydrogenase (LDH) and Alkaline Phosphatase	Increased levels of these serum biomarkers at diagnosis have been associated with worse outcomes.
% Necrosis after Neoadjuvant Chemotherapy	Patients with >90% necrosis have more favorable outcomes.

10. **What are the cytogenetic and molecular genetic abnormalities associated with ES?**
    - Chromosomal translocations are the defining molecular feature for many sarcomas, and ES is a prototypical example characterized most commonly (85%) by the t (11; 22) (q24; q12) chromosomal translocation that leads to the expression of the EWSR1-FLI1 transcription factor.

- The second most common translocation occurring in about 10% of ES is the t(21; 22) (q22; q12) that generates the EWSR1-ERG transcription factor.
  - In rarer circumstances, *EWSR1* is fused to other ETS-family members including *ETV1, ETV4,* and *FEV.*
    - Together with EWSR1-FLI1 and EWRS1-ERG, these fusions represent what is now called FET-ETS translocation ES.
- *EWSR1* is a promiscuous fusion partner and has also been described to partner with rare non-ETS genes such as *PATZ1, SMARCA5,* and *NFATc2a.*
  - There are now considered EWSR1 round cell sarcomas with non-ETS partners (Figure 34.1A–B).

11. **What are the different molecular assays used in the diagnosis of ES?**
- Fluorescence in situ hybridization (FISH) using the *EWSR1* gene break-apart probe has been the established molecular diagnostic test for ES.
  - This method has limitations because *EWSR1* has at least 17 other potential fusion partners across various soft tissue sarcomas, which could potentially lead to an erroneous diagnosis of ES.
- When feasible, specific FISH rearrangement probes for all potential partners genes, reverse transcription polymerase chain reaction (RT-PCR), or next-generation sequencing techniques should be employed to establish a definitive molecular diagnosis.

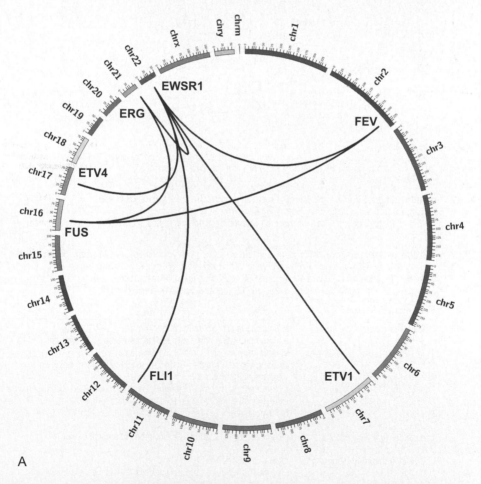

A

Figure 34.1 World Health Organization (WHO) Classification of Tumors of Soft Tissue and Bone for Ewing and Ewing-Like Sarcoma. (A) Circos plot of Ewing sarcoma with all FET-ETS variants.

(Continued)

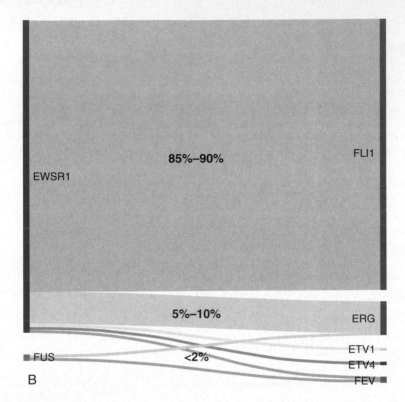

Figure 34.1, **Cont'd** (B) Sankey plot of FET-ETS translocation Ewing sarcoma scaled to represent the percentage of total cases. (Adapted from Kinnaman MD, Zhu C, Weiser DA, et al. Survey of paediatric oncologists and pathologists regarding their views and experiences with variant translocations in Ewing and Ewing-like sarcoma: a report of the Children's Oncology Group. *Sarcoma*. 2020:3498549.)

12. **What is the differential diagnosis of a small round blue cell tumor of bone?**
    - Common: ES and eosinophilic granuloma
    - Uncommon: Primary and metastatic lymphoma, rhabdomyosarcoma, metastatic neuroblastoma, mesenchymal chondrosarcoma, small cell OS

13. **What is the overall prognosis for patients diagnosed with localized and metastatic ES with regards to 5-year EFS and overall survival? What are the prognostic variables in ES?**
    - The 5-year EFS and overall survival for localized ES are 73% and 82%, respectively.
    - The 5-year EFS and overall survival for metastatic ES are 22% and 39%, respectively.

Prognostic Factor	Influence
Presence of metastatic disease	Most important prognostic factor
	• Combined bone and lung metastases worse than bone only
	• Bone only worse than lung only metastases
Tumor size	Larger primary tumors (>8 cm in a single dimension) have worse prognosis than smaller
Tumor site	Axial primary worse than extremity primary in localized Ewing sarcoma
Skeletal vs extraskeletal	Extraskeletal primary fare better than skeletal primary
Age	Older patients (>15) fare worse than younger patients
Sex	Males fare worse the females
Lactate dehydrogenase (LDH) at diagnosis	Increased LDH at diagnosis associated with worse outcome
Pathologic fracture at diagnosis	Worse outcomes
Histology	Presence of neural differentiation does NOT influence survival
EWSR1-ETS translocation breakpoint site	No impact

14. **Describe the concepts of neoadjuvant chemotherapy and local control and how they apply to OS and ES.**
    - *Neoadjuvant chemotherapy:* Chemotherapy given before the resection of the primary tumor
      - Allows for immediate treatment of micrometastases
      - Provides time for surgical planning if warranted
      - Permits assessment of how chemo-sensitive tumor as determined by degree of necrosis at time of primary resection
      - In both OS and ES, the duration of neoadjuvant chemotherapy is 2 to 3 months.
    - *Local control:* The eradication of the primary tumor
      - Surgery is the preferred method of local control in OS because it is thought to be a relatively radio-insensitive tumor.
      - In ES, local control can be achieved via surgery, radiation, or a combination of the two.
        - Depends on the tumor's location, size, and response to treatment and patient's age and growth potential
        - Decisions regarding local control in ES should be made through consensus of a multidisciplinary team of oncologists, surgeons, pathologists, radiologists, and radiation oncologists.

15. **What chemotherapy is used to treat OS and ES?**
    - OS:
      - In most centers, patients receive high-dose methotrexate, doxorubicin, and cisplatin (MAP).
      - Patients typically receive 10 weeks of neoadjuvant or induction chemotherapy followed by 19 weeks of adjuvant or maintenance chemotherapy.
      - Attempts at augmenting therapy for patients who have less than 90% necrosis at time of resection have failed to improve outcomes.
    - ES:
      - Standard therapy consists of alternating cycles of vincristine, doxorubicin, and cyclophosphamide with ifosfamide and etoposide (VDC/IE).
      - Administering these agents in an interval dose–compressed fashion, meaning every 14 days or as soon as blood counts have sufficiently recovered, has been shown to be superior to the standard every 3-week dosing schedule in patients with localized disease.

16. **What is the optimal management of metastatic lung metastases in OS?**
    - For the patient with lung-only metastases at diagnosis, complete resection of all sites of pulmonary disease should be attempted if feasible.
    - Timing of resection is typically after patient has had the primary resection and has resumed postoperative chemotherapy.
      - Staged thoracotomies are typically performed for patients with bilateral disease at diagnosis.
    - For patients with unilateral pulmonary–only metastases at diagnosis, there is debate regarding the role of contralateral exploratory thoracotomy to look for lung metastases that may not be radiographically evident.
    - For patients with lung-only relapse, thoracotomy or repeat thoracotomy to remove all sites of relapsed disease is considered to be an essential aspect of management for any chance of long-term survival.

17. **What are the complications and late effects of treatment of OS and ES?**
    - Late effects secondary to chemotherapy:
      - Alkylators (cyclophosphamide/ifosfamide) used in ES treatment may result in infertility in male patients and early menopause and decreased fertility in females.
        - Males are advised to sperm bank before initiation of therapy, and females should be considered for ovarian harvest if appropriate.
      - Doxorubicin may affect cardiac function.
        - Patients should be followed with echocardiograms while on therapy and periodically while off therapy to monitor function.
      - Cisplatin may cause renal dysfunction, including magnesium wasting.
      - Cisplatin may cause high-frequency hearing loss.
        - An audiogram should be obtained before each cycle of cisplatin.
      - Methotrexate may cause kidney or liver damage, usually transient.
    - Orthopedic complications:
      - Complications involving their endoprosthesis such as infection of hardware or malfunction
    - Secondary malignancies:
      - Two percent to three percent of survivors of OS and 5% of survivors of ES develop secondary malignancies.

BIBLIOGRAPHY

1. Duong LM, Richardson LC. Descriptive epidemiology of malignant primary osteosarcoma using population-based registries, United States, 1999-2008. *Journal of Registry Management.* 2013;40(2):59–64. http://www.ncbi.nlm.nih.gov/pubmed/24002129.
2. Fuchs B, Valenzuela RG, Petersen IA, Arndt CA, Sim FH. Ewing's sarcoma and the development of secondary malignancies. *Clin Orthop Relat Res.* 2003;415:82–89.

3. Hawkins DS, Brennan B, Bölling T, et al. Ewing sarcoma. In Pizzo PA, Poplack DG (eds). *Principles and Practice of Pediatric Oncology.* 7th ed. LWW, 2015:854–875.

4. Gorlick R, Bielack SS, Teot L, Meyer J, Randall RL, Marina N. Osteosarcoma: biology, diagnosis, treatment, and remaining challenges. In Pizzo PA, Poplack DG (eds). *Principles and Practice of Pediatric Oncology.* 7th ed. LWW, 2015.

5. Kinnaman MD, Zhu C, Weiser DA, et al. Survey of paediatric oncologists and pathologists regarding their views and experiences with variant translocations in Ewing and Ewing-like sarcoma: a report of the Children's Oncology Group. *Sarcoma.* 2020;2020:3498549.

6. PDQ Pediatric Treatment Editorial Board. Ewing Sarcoma Treatment (PDQ®): Health Professional Version. In *PDQ Cancer Information Summaries.* National Cancer Institute, 2002. http://www.ncbi.nlm.nih.gov/pubmed/26389480.

7. PDQ Pediatric Treatment Editorial Board. Osteosarcoma and Undifferentiated Pleomorphic Sarcoma of Bone Treatment (PDQ®): Health Professional Version. In *PDQ Cancer Information Summaries.* National Cancer Institute, 2002. http://www.ncbi.nlm.nih.gov/pubmed/26389179.

8. Smeland S, Bielack SS, Whelan J, et al. Survival and prognosis with osteosarcoma: outcomes in more than 2000 patients in the EURAMOS-1 (European and American Osteosarcoma Study) cohort. *Eur J Cancer.* 2019;109:36–50.

9. Womer RB, West DC, Krailo MD, et al. Randomized controlled trial of interval-compressed chemotherapy for the treatment of localized Ewing sarcoma: a report from the Children's Oncology Group [published correction appears in J Clin Oncol. 2015 Mar 1;33(7):814. Dosage error in article text]. *J Clin Oncol.* 2012;30(33):4148–4154.

CHAPTER 35

NEUROBLASTOMA

David Gass, MD, MS and Darrell J. Yamashiro, MD, PhD

1. **What is neuroblastoma?**

   Neuroblastoma is the most common extracranial malignant tumor of infants and children. It originates from neural crest cells that normally give rise to the adrenal gland and the sympathetic nervous system. It can have widely varying outcomes: tumors can spontaneously regress, differentiate into benign ganglioneuromas, or metastasize with high mortality rate.

2. **What is the incidence of neuroblastoma in the United States?**

   In the United States, more than 650 cases are diagnosed with neuroblastoma annually.[1] Neuroblastoma accounts for 7.6% of all cancers in children younger than 15 years of age with average age-adjusted incidence rate of 10.54 cases per million children. There is a marked age dependence in the incidence rate, making neuroblastoma truly a disease of infancy (patients younger than 1 year). The incidence rate for infants is 64 per million and drops to 29 per million during the second year of life. Sixteen percent of infant neuroblastomas are diagnosed during the first month after birth and 41% are diagnosed in the first 3 months of life; 90% of cases will occur before age 5.[2] The increased incidence rate among infants may be the result of the identification of previous undetected tumors in minimally symptomatic infants by noninvasive diagnostic tests and routine use of prenatal ultrasound.

3. **In neuroblastoma, what is the utility of screening with urine catecholamines?**

   About 90% to 95% of patients with neuroblastoma secrete one or both of the urinary catecholamine metabolites, homovanillic (HVA) or vanillylmandelic acid (VMA). Screening of urinary VMA/HVA was conducted with the hope that earlier detection would lead to more localized disease and increase possibility of cure. Nevertheless, although screening of infants at 6 months of age or earlier leads to a marked increase in overall incidence of neuroblastoma, it does not reduce the incidence of advanced stage patients with poor prognosis. Screening results in the overdiagnosis of tumors that would otherwise spontaneously regress.[3]

4. **What are the common cytogenetic and molecular abnormalities found in neuroblastoma?**

   Increased DNA index: Tumors of infants often demonstrate a hyperdiploid content (DNA index >1). These infants are more likely to have lower states of disease, improved response to chemotherapy, and an overall improved outcome. Cytogenetically, the hyperdiploid tumors have whole-chromosome gains with few structural rearrangements.

   Loss at 1p: Deletion of the short arm of chromosome 1 is a common cytogenetic feature of neuroblastoma, occurring in 30% to 50% of tumors. The common region of loss is at the distal end in an area of 1p36 and is thought to contain a tumor suppressor gene for neuroblastoma. Chromosome 1p loss is a risk factor for relapse but not for diminished overall survival (OS) in patients younger than 18 months.[4]

   Gain of 17q: Gain of genetic material on chromosome 17 is the most common genetic abnormality in neuroblastoma, occurring in 54% to 72% of cases. Gain at 17q is characteristic of tumors in children older than 1 year and advanced stage tumors and is strongly associated with deletion of 1p and amplification of *MYCN*. The finding of recurring gains on chromosome 17 suggests the presence of one or more oncogenes that may contribute to neuroblastoma pathogenesis.

   Loss of 11q: Loss of genetic material on the long arm of chromosome 11 has been associated with reduced survival and with an increased risk of relapse in both the patients older than 18 months and younger than 18 months.

   ***MYCN* amplification:** Genomic amplification of the proto-oncogene *MYCN* (also known as N-myc) occurs in about 25% of patients with neuroblastoma. Amplification may result in 30 to 400 copies of *MYCN* per cell. Amplification of *MYCN* (defined as >10 copies) is at all stages a predictor of poorer prognosis both in time to progression and overall survival. Patients whose outcome was most impacted by MYCN status were those with otherwise favorable features, including age younger than 18 months, high DNA index, and low ferritin.[5]

5. **What are the most common sites at which neuroblastoma originates and metastasizes?**

   Neuroblastoma can originate from any site in the sympathetic nervous system. Most primary tumors arise in the abdomen (65%), with the primary site being the adrenal gland occurring more frequently in children older than 1 year (40%) than in infants younger than 1 year (25%). Cervical and thoracic tumors occur more frequently in infants (33%) than older children (15%).

   At presentation, about half of the patients will have metastatic disease. The most common sites of metastases include:

   Bone marrow: 70%
   Bone: 56%
   Lymph node: 31%

Liver: 30%

Intracranial/Orbit: 18%

Infants are much more likely to have liver metastases than children older than 1 year.

6. **What are the signs and symptoms of a child with neuroblastoma?**

The signs and symptoms of neuroblastoma depend on the location and extent of the primary tumor and the presence of metastases. Large abdominal masses can cause discomfort, vomiting, and anorexia. High thoracic or cervical masses can present with Horner's syndrome (unilateral ptosis, miosis, and anhidrosis). Neuroblastoma originating in paraspinal ganglia may have epidural or intradural extension and compress the spinal cord extradurally. Symptoms of spinal cord compression could be pain, bladder and bowel dysfunction, paraparesis, or paraplegia.

Metastatic neuroblastoma classically presents with proptosis and periorbital ecchymoses, as well as bone pain, pancytopenia, irritability, limp, or refusal to walk. Infants can have rapidly enlarging liver metastases, leading to abdominal distension that can cause respiratory compromise and renal and hepatic failure. Infants may have "blueberry muffin" lesions because of neuroblastoma metastasizing to the skin

Patients may also have paraneoplastic syndromes because of neuroblastoma. Excessive secretion of catecholamines may rarely lead to attacks of sweating, flushing, pallor, headaches, palpitation, and hypertension. Excretion of vasoactive intestinal peptide (VIP) can cause intractable watery diarrhea. Infrequently, patients may have opsoclonus myoclonus ataxia syndrome (OMAS) with bursts of rapid chaotic eye movements along with frequent irregular jerking movements of muscles with imbalance with walking. Patients with OMAS have a favorable outcome with respect to survival. Nevertheless, even when no tumor is present, patients may remain symptomatic, with long-term neurological deficits that include learning disabilities, motor and language delay, and behavioral abnormalities.

7. **Discuss the work-up for a child with suspected neuroblastoma.**

Laboratory evaluation should include a complete blood count (CBC), complete metabolic panel (including liver function tests, renal function tests, calcium), and urinalysis. Serum ferritin and lactate dehydrogenase (LDH) should be measured because higher levels have been associated with poorer prognosis. Prothrombin time (PT), partial thromboplastin time (PTT), and fibrinogen should be obtained because of the increased risk of disseminated intravascular coagulation in patients with metastatic disease and can help guide management of coagulopathy. Urine should be tested for urinary catecholamines, HVA, and VMA.

Diagnostic imaging should include a computed tomography (CT) scan and/or a magnetic resonance imaging (MRI) to evaluate the primary tumor and liver and lymph node metastases. Bilateral bone marrow biopsies and aspirates are required to determine the presence of bone marrow metastases. For cortical bone involvement, a metaiodobenzylguanidine (MIBG) scan is a standard part of evaluation for neuroblastoma because about 90% of cases are MIBG-avid. For non-MIBG-avid scans, a fluorine F 18-fludeoxyglucose positron emission tomography (PET) scan is used.

Biopsy of primary tumor tissue is crucial to obtain all the biological data required for risk-group assignment and subsequent treatment stratification in current clinical trials. Additionally, a significant number of tumor cells are needed to determine *MYCN* copy number, DNA index, and the presence of segmental chromosomal aberrations. Tissue from several core biopsies, or approximately 1 cm^3 of tissue from an open biopsy, is needed for adequate biologic staging.

8. **How is neuroblastoma staged?**

To facilitate the comparison of clinical trials and biological studies, an international consensus regarding the criteria for diagnosis of neuroblastoma, staging system, and response criteria was published in 1998 and revised multiple times with the last in 2009.[6] The staging system is termed the International Neuroblastoma Staging system (INSS) and is described in the following table. The INSS takes into account the extent of tumor resection and also retains the "special" category of 4S for infants younger than 1 year with a localized primary tumor who have metastases to the liver and skin and minimal amount in the bone marrow.

International Neuroblastoma Staging System (INSS)

Stage	Definition
1	Localized tumor with complete gross excision, with or without microscopic residual disease; representative ipsilateral lymph nodes negative for tumor microscopically (i.e., nodes attached to and removed with the primary tumor may be positive).
2a	Localized tumor with incomplete gross excision; representative ipsilateral nonadherent lymph nodes negative for tumor microscopically.
2b	Localized tumor with or without complete gross excision, with ipsilateral nonadherent lymph nodes positive for tumor. Enlarged contralateral lymph nodes must be negative microscopically.
3	Unresectable unilateral tumor infiltrating across the midline, with or without regional lymph node involvement; or localized unilateral tumor with contralateral regional lymph node involvement; or midline tumor with bilateral extension by infiltration (unresectable) or by lymph node involvement. The midline is defined as the vertebral column. Tumors originating on one side and crossing the midline must infiltrate to or beyond the opposite side of the vertebral column.
4	Any primary tumor with dissemination to distant lymph nodes, bone, bone marrow, liver, skin, and/or other organs, except as defined for stage 4S.

4s	Localized primary tumor, as defined for stage 1, 2A, or 2B, with dissemination limited to skin, liver, and/or bone marrow (by definition limited to infants younger than 12 months). Marrow involvement should be minimal (i.e., <10% of total nucleated cells identified as malignant by bone biopsy or by bone marrow aspirate). More extensive bone marrow involvement would be considered stage 4 disease. The results of the metaiodobenzylguanidine (MIBG) scan, if performed, should be negative for disease in the bone marrow.

9. **Discuss the criteria necessary to make the diagnosis of neuroblastoma.**
   According to the INSS criteria, a diagnosis of neuroblastoma is established by one of the following:
   - Unequivocal tumor histopathology
   - Unequivocal tumor cells by bone marrow aspirate or biopsy and increased urinary catecholamines (VMA and/or HVA)
   - If tumor histology is equivocal, then genetic features such as *MYCN* amplification or 1p LOH can be used to support the diagnosis of neuroblastoma

10. **Describe the pathological classification of neuroblastoma.**
    The histopathologic appearance of neuroblastoma ranges from undifferentiated neuroblasts to more mature ganglioneuroblastoma to fully differentiated and benign ganglioneuroma. The morphologic system originally proposed by Shimada classified tumors into favorable histology or unfavorable histology and is dependent on age, the degree of neuronal differentiation, the mitotic rate, and the presence or absence of schwannian stromal development. The International Neuroblastoma Pathology Committee (INPC) has devised a morphologic classification of neuroblastoma tumors that is modeled on the one proposed by Shimada and colleagues.

11. **What are image-defined risk factors (IDRFs), and how do the factor into the most current Risk Group Staging System?**
    Since 2011, a new International Neuroblastoma Risk Group Staging System (INRGSS) replaced the INSS in active clinical trials. This new staging system incorporates the presence or absence of IDRFs and/or metastatic tumor at the time of diagnosis before treatment and/or surgery. IDRFs are surgical risk factors, detected by imaging, which could potentially make total tumor excision risky or difficult at the time of diagnosis and increase the risk of surgical complications and possibly inability to perform successful gross total resection or primary mass.[6]

Stage	Description
L1	Localized tumor not involving vital structures as defined by the list of IDRFs and confined to one body compartment.
L2	Locoregional tumor with presence of one or more IDRFs.
M	Distant metastatic disease (except stage MS).
MS	Metastatic disease in children younger than 18 months with metastases confined to skin, liver, and/or bone marrow. The primary tumor can be INSS stage 1, 2, or 3.

Note that the INSS allows patients up to age 12 months to be classified as stage 4S, whereas the INRGSS allows patients up to age 18 months to be staged as MS. The primary tumor in INSS stage 4S must be INSS stage 1 or 2, whereas the primary tumor in MS can be INSS stage 3.

IDRF, Image-defined risk factors; *INRGSS*, International Neuroblastoma Risk Group Staging System; *INSS*, International Neuroblastoma Staging System.

IDRFs are determined through a multidisciplinary discussion between radiology, oncology, and surgery but generally include the following:
- Ipsilateral tumor extension within two body compartments: neck and chest, chest and abdomen, or abdomen and pelvis.
- Infiltration of adjacent organs or structures including but not limited to pericardium, diaphragm, kidney, liver, intestine, pancreas, or mesentery.
- Infiltration of portohepatic or hepatoduodenal ligament.
- Encasement of major vessels by tumor.
- Compression of trachea or central bronchi.
- Encasement of brachial plexus.
- Infiltration of the costovertebral junction between T9 and T12.
- Tumor crossing the sciatic notch.
- Tumor invading renal pedicle.
- Extension of tumor to base of skull.
- Intraspinal tumor extension such that more than one-third of the spinal canal is invaded, leptomeningeal space is obliterated, or spinal cord MRI signal is abnormal.

12. **What prognostic factors are used to stratify patients into different risk groups?**

Historically, numerous prognostic factors have been described in neuroblastoma. Poor prognosis has been associated with the following parameters: advanced stage, unfavorable histology elevated serum ferritin or LDH, VMA/HVA ratio of less than 1, diploid tumors in infants (DNA index = 1), amplification of *MYCN,* Loss at chromosome 1p, gain at chromosome 17q, or age greater than 1 year.

Nevertheless, in an effort to unify multiple international consortia, mainly INRGSS stage, patient age (days), histology, *MYCN* status, and ploidy are used to risk-stratify patients into low-, intermediate-, and high-risk groups. In addition, in recent low-risk protocols, whether patient symptoms are present or absent has been incorporated into treatment decisions to whether patients undergo surgical resection or observation in some cases.

13. **What is the treatment and prognosis for patients with low-risk neuroblastoma?**

INRG stage	Histology	MYCN	11q aberration	Ploidy	Risk Group
L1/L2	GN maturing or GNB	Nonamplified	None		Very low
L1	Any	Nonamplified	None		Very low
L2 Age <18 months	Any	Nonamplified	None		Low
L2, Age >18 months	GNB	Nonamplified	None		Low
M (<18 months)	Any	Nonamplified	None	Hyperdiploid	Low
MS (<18 months)	Any	Nonamplified	None		Very Low

GN, Ganglioneuroma; *GNB*, ganglioneuroblastoma; *INRG,* International Neuroblastoma Risk Group; *NA*, not amplified.

Low-risk patients are those with localized tumors (L1 INRGSS stage) and L2, M, and MS stages with various biological and histological characteristics (see previous table).[7] These patients have an excellent survival estimated at 5-year survival of more than 95% with primarily surgery and supportive care. Chemotherapy is reserved for the few patients with symptomatic disease because of paraspinal tumors resulting in spinal cord compression. Patients who do have a local recurrence of tumor after surgery are usually easily treated with either further surgery or with moderate chemotherapy or local radiation. Additionally, with the increase in diagnosis of L1 and L2 stage tumors with prenatal ultrasound, there are multiple active efforts at treating asymptomatic incidental masses that are consistent with likely neuroblastoma with observation alone without biopsy.

Infants with M or MS disease and favorable biological features also have excellent 5-year survival of 85% to 90%, and treatment has ranged from supportive care alone to modest chemotherapy for 4 to 5 months. For patients with M or MS stage disease to be considered for low-risk therapy, they need to be *MYCN* nonamplified and without 11q aberrations and hyperdiploidy. Because age greater than 18 months carries poorer outcome, older patients with M or MS disease will not be considered low-risk disease.[7]

Infants with MS disease who have a poor outcome are generally those with very extensive hepatic infiltration causing respiratory compromise and occasionally renal and venous obstruction. These infants receive emergency abdominal decompression, mechanical ventilation, chemotherapy, and hepatic radiotherapy and often die of sepsis or respiratory, renal, or hepatic failure.

14. **Describe treatment and prognosis for patients with intermediate-risk neuroblastoma.**

INRG stage	Histology	MYCN	11q aberration	Ploidy	Risk Group
L2 (<18 months)	Any, not GN or GNB	Nonamplified	Yes		Intermediate
L2 (>18 months)	GNB differentiating	Nonamplified	Yes		Intermediate
L2 (>18 months)	GNB, poorly differentiated	Nonamplified	None		Intermediate
M <18 months	Any	Nonamplified	None	Diploid	Intermediate

GN, Ganglioneuroma; *GN*, ganglioneuroblastoma; *INRG,* International Neuroblastoma Risk Group; *NA*, not amplified.

The intermediate-risk group involves patients who have an excellent prognosis, with 80% to 90% survival. These patients include those with L2 disease and generally 1 unfavorable risk feature but not including *MYCN* amplification. *MYCN* amplification continues to upstage almost every patient into the high-risk group.

Treatment has consisted of surgery and moderately intensive combination chemotherapy (four or eight cycles). Intermediate risk-patients with favorable biology receive four cycles of chemotherapy, using a combination of carboplatin, etoposide, doxorubicin, and cyclophosphamide. Patients with less favorable biology, such as infants with either unfavorable histology or diploid tumors, receive eight cycles of chemotherapy. At this time, radiation in this risk group is only used for progressive disease or emergency situations like spinal compression.

15. Describe the treatment and prognosis for patients with high-risk neuroblastoma.

INRG stage	Histology	MYCN	11q aberration	Ploidy	Risk Group
L1 (Any age)	Any, not GN or GNB	Amplified	Any		High
L2 (>18 months)	GNB, poorly differentiating	Amplified	Any		High
M <18 months	Any	Amplified	Any		High
M >18 months	Any	Any	Any		High
MS <18 months	Any	Amplified			High
MS <18 months	Any	Nonamplified	Present		High

GN, Ganglioneuroma; *GN*, ganglioneuroblastoma; *INRG*, International Neuroblastoma Risk Group; *NA*, not amplified.

The high-risk group of patients with neuroblastoma consists primarily of patients with patients with hallmark high-risk features, which include *MYCN* amplification in any INRGSS stage and metastatic disease patients older than 18 months of age. Additionally, MS stage patients with an additionally poor risk feature are included in this risk group. These characteristics have outweighed any other influences from ploidy, and this feature is not factored into this risk group.

Modern treatment for high-risk neuroblastoma features multimodal therapy including five to six cycles of induction chemotherapy with surgical resection of primary mass. This is followed by consolidation high-dose chemotherapy with autologous stem cell rescue, followed by radiotherapy to the primary mass. Postconsolidation therapy with immunotherapy with cytokine stimulation (GM-CSF) and retinoic acid have become the new standard care based on recent large scale randomized studies. With this combination regiment, EFS has reached a peak of 66%.[8]

16. How is the MIBG scan used to predict more advanced disease and risk of progression, and what are treatment approaches to relapsed neuroblastoma?

For MIBG-avid disease, the MIBG scan has been an integral part of disease monitoring after completion of portions of a treatment regimen. The scan is highly sensitive in recognizing sites of disease in abdomen, soft tissue, and bones and cooperative groups have tried to use this technology to develop scores to evaluate disease extent and prognostic value. One of the most common scoring methods is the Curie score method, which has successfully been used as a prognostic marker for response and survival with MIBG-avid, stage 4, newly diagnosed, high-risk neuroblastoma.

For patients with *MYCN*-nonamplified neuroblastoma, a postinduction chemotherapy Curie score greater than 2 was associated with a higher risk of an event, independent of other known neuroblastoma clinical and biological factors. For patients with *MYCN*-amplified tumors, a postinduction Curie score greater than 0 was associated with worse outcomes.[9]

For patients with relapsed high-risk neuroblastoma more options exist, including chemoimmunotherapy, immunotherapy targeted against GD2, and MIBG therapy. MIBG therapy is a high-dose radioimmunotherapy approach using 131I-MIBG followed by autologous stem cell support if needed.

REFERENCES

1. Howlader N, Noone AM, Krapcho M, et al, eds. *SEER Cancer Statistics Review, 1975-2009 (Vintage 2009 Populations)*. National Cancer Institute, 2012.
2. London WB, Castleberry RP, Matthay KK, et al. Evidence for an age cutoff greater than 365 days for neuroblastoma risk group stratification in the Children's Oncology Group. *J Clin Oncol*. 2005;23(27):6459–6465.
3. Woods WG, Gao RN, Shuster JJ, et al. Screening of infants and mortality due to neuroblastoma. *N Engl J Med*. 2002;346(14):1041–1046.
4. Ambros IM, Tonini GP, Pötschger U, et al. Age dependency of the prognostic impact of tumor genomics in localized resectable MYCN-nonamplified neuroblastomas. Report From the SIOPEN Biology Group on the LNESG Trials and a COG Validation Group. *J Clin Oncol*. 2020;38(31):3685–3697.
5. Campbell K, Shyr D, Bagatell R, et al. Comprehensive evaluation of context dependence of the prognostic impact of MYCN amplification in neuroblastoma: a report from the International Neuroblastoma Risk Group (INRG) project. *Pediatr Blood Cancer*. 2019;66(8), e27819.
6. Monclair T, Brodeur GM, Ambros PF, et al. The International Neuroblastoma Risk Group (INRG) staging system: an INRG Task Force report. *J Clin Oncol*. 2009;27(2):298–303.
7. Pinto N, et al. Advanced in risk classification and treatment strategies for neuroblastoma. *J Clin Oncol*. 2015;33(27):3008–3017.
8. Yu AL, Gilman AL, Ozkaynak MF, et al. Anti-GD2 antibody with GM-CSF, interleukin-2, and isotretinoin for neuroblastoma. *N Engl J Med*. 2010;363(14):1324–1334.
9. Yanik GA, Parisi MT, Shulkin BL, et al. Semiquantitative mIBG scoring as a prognostic indicator in patients with stage 4 neuroblastoma: a report from the Children's oncology group. *J Nucl Med*. 2013;54(4):541–548.

CHAPTER 36

HEPATIC TUMORS

Hanna Moisander Joyce, MD, MSc and Darrell J. Yamashiro, MD, PhD

1. **What is the differential diagnosis of a liver mass in a child?**

   Liver tumors in children are rare but mostly malignant. Differential diagnosis varies by age. In infants and toddlers, the most common malignant liver mass is hepatoblastoma (HB; 43%). Rhabdoid tumors (1%) and malignant germ cell tumors (1%) are less likely. The most common benign liver masses in this age group are vascular tumors/hemangiomas (14%) and mesenchymal hamartomas (6%).

   In school-aged children and adolescents, most malignant liver masses are either hepatocellular carcinomas (HCC; 23%) or undifferentiated sarcomas (7%). Focal nodular hyperplasia (3%) and hepatic adenoma (1%) are the most common benign liver masses.

   In children, especially in infants, liver metastases are also common. Occasionally, metastases or contiguous invasion from primary extrahepatic tumors, such as neuroblastoma (4S in particular) or Wilms tumor, may be the presenting feature.

2. **Describe the initial work-up for a liver mass.**

   Laboratory evaluation should include a complete blood count, liver function tests, and coagulation studies, as well as alpha-fetoprotein (AFP) and β-HCG tumor marker levels. Ultrasonography is frequently used in the initial assessment, but computed tomography (CT) or magnetic resonance imaging (MRI) will allow for a more accurate evaluation. Chest CT is required for evaluation for metastatic disease. It is recommended that all patients undergo biopsy, which needs to be carried out in close communication between the surgeon and radiologist to avoid seeding.

3. **What are the differences in the clinical presentation of hepatoblastoma and hepatocellular carcinoma?**

   Clinical Presentations of Hepatoblastoma and Hepatocellular Carcinoma

Hepatoblastoma	Hepatocellular Carcinoma
Median age at diagnosis: 1 year	Median age at diagnosis: 12 years
Usually an asymptomatic abdominal mass	Usually symptomatic (anorexia, weight loss, emesis, fever, abdominal pain/distention)
Thrombocytosis	Polycythemia
Acute abdomen because of tumor rupture rare	Acute abdomen because of tumor rupture more common
Jaundice in 5%	Jaundice in 25%
Alpha-fetoprotein (AFP) elevation in 90%	AFP elevation in 50%

4. **Describe the appearance of the most common malignant liver tumors.**

   HB makes up 80% of all pediatric liver tumors. It typically presents as a single, well-circumscribed mass arising in an otherwise normal liver; 60% are in the right lobe. Histologically, HB is an embryonal tumor consisting of epithelial cells that resemble different stages of developing liver.

   More than two-thirds of pediatric HCC occur during the second decade of life. It can be sporadic without preceding liver disease or occur in the context of liver disease. The former usually happens later and has poorer outcomes. Histologically, HCC can be divided into classic or "adult-type" and fibrolamellar (FL-HCC). Classic HCC is typically multicentric and consists of well-differentiated cells that resemble normal hepatocytes. The adjacent liver tissue is often marked by cirrhosis.

   FL-HCC represents 10% to 25% of HCC in adolescents and usually presents without underlying severe liver disease or cirrhosis. FL-HCC is typically a well-circumscribed and solitary tumor. It is composed of sheets of polygonal tumor cells, which are larger than normal hepatocytes, mixed with fibrous stroma.

   In addition, a transitional tumor variant (HCC-NOS) has been described. It has cells with features of hepatoblasts and mature hepatocytes.

   Undifferentiated embryonal sarcoma of the liver is the third most common pediatric liver malignancy. This mesenchymal tumor is usually uniform and large (>10 cm) but well demarcated from liver. The mass appears as a hypodense mixture of cystic and solid components.

5. **What are the most common benign liver tumors?**

   The most common benign hepatic tumors are classified as hemangioendotheliomas, either infantile/juvenile hepatic hemangiomas or congenital vascular malformations. The former can be focal, multifocal, or diffuse and usually involute and regress. Vascular malformations are associated with capillary proliferation, involving a single mass that does not regress. They can be associated with consumption coagulopathy.

Hepatic mesenchymal hamartomas (HMHs) have an age distribution and clinical presentation similar to HB, apart from elevated AFP level. HMHs are characterized by cystic appearance in imaging and massive growth, which can cause morbidity by compressing adjacent structures.

6. **What are some genetic syndromes that predispose to liver tumors?**

Genetic Syndromes Predisposing to Liver Tumors

Disease	Tumor Type	Gene
Familial adenomatous polyposis	Hepatoblastoma (HB), hepatocellular carcinoma (HCC), adenoma	APC
Beckwith-Wiedemann syndrome	HB, hemangioendothelioma	Multiple candidates
Simpson-Golabi-Behmel syndrome	HB	GPC3
Trisomy 18	HB	No single gene
Li-Fraumeni Syndrome	HB, undifferentiated sarcoma	TP53
Glycogen Storage disease types I–IV	HB, HCC, adenoma	G6PC
Alagille syndrome	HCC	JAG1, NOTCH2
Neurofibromatosis	HCC, angiosarcoma	NF-1
Ataxia-telangiectasia	HCC	ATM
Fanconi anemia	HCC, fibrolamellar cancer, adenoma	FAA, FAC
Tuberous sclerosis	Angiomyolipoma	TSC1, TSC2

7. **Describe the most common molecular aberration in hepatoblastoma.**

Most patients have an aberration in the Wnt/β-catenin signaling pathway, leading to accumulation of β-catenin, whose oncogenic mutations cause chromosomal instability.

8. **How are hepatic tumors are staged?**

The currently accepted staging system, called PRETEXT stage, describes tumor extension before any chemotherapy or surgical treatment based on the number of involved Couinaud liver segments, vascular extension, and the presence of metastatic and extrahepatic disease. POSTTEXT stage is defined after any neoadjuvant (preoperative) chemotherapy and before resection.

9. **What factors affect the prognosis in hepatoblastoma?**

PRETEXT stage, resectability, age, AFP level, and metastases at diagnosis are important prognostic factors. In completely resected tumors, pure fetal histology confers the best prognosis, whereas small cell undifferentiated histology is associated with poor prognosis.

10. **What are the most effective chemotherapy agents in the treatment of hepatoblastoma?**

Cisplatin and doxorubicin have shown excellent effects in the treatment of HB.

11. **Discuss the role of liver transplantation in the treatment of malignant liver tumors.**

Liver transplantation can cure patients whose tumors are unresectable after neoadjuvant chemotherapy. Active metastatic disease will preclude liver transplantation.

BIBLIOGRAPHY

1. Myers RL, Trobaugh-Lotrario AD, Malogolowkin MH, et al. Liver tumors. In Pizzo PA, Poplack DG (eds). *Principles and Practice of Pediatric Oncology.* 7th ed. Lippincott-Raven, 2016:726–752.
2. Ng, K, Mogul, DB. Pediatric liver tumors. *Clin Liver Dis.* 2018;22:753–772.
3. Tomlinson GE. Hepatoblastoma and other liver tumors in children. In Orkin SH, Fischer DE, et al. (eds). *Nathan and Oski's Hematology and Oncology of Infancy and Childhood.* Vol 2. 8th ed. Saunders, 2015:1186–1905.

CHAPTER 37

KIDNEY TUMORS IN CHILDREN AND ADOLESCENTS

Hanna Moisander Joyce, MD, MSc and Darrell J. Yamashiro, MD, PhD

1. What is the differential diagnosis of a child with an abdominal mass?

The most likely diagnoses in a child with an abdominal mass are neuroblastoma and Wilms tumor or nephroblastoma. Clinically, children with advanced stage neuroblastoma appear ill, often having signs or symptoms of metastatic disease such as periorbital ecchymoses or pain from skeletal lesions. Patients with Wilms tumor are often asymptomatic, and the mass may be discovered incidentally. Computer tomography (CT) scan of the abdomen can usually distinguish between the two cancers because neuroblastoma arises from the adrenal gland and compresses and displaces the kidney, whereas Wilms tumor is intrarenal and distorts the kidney.

2. What is the most common renal cancer in children?

Renal cancers represent about 7% of cancer diagnoses among children. Wilms tumor is by far the most common primary renal tumor in children younger than 15 years old, representing approximately 95% of diagnoses. In the United States, approximately 600 children are diagnosed with Wilms tumors each year. Renal cell carcinoma (RCC), the most common form of renal cancer in adults, represents only 2.5% of renal cancers in children younger than 15 years old, but in the 15- to 19-year age group, it surpasses Wilms tumor as the most common renal malignancy. Rhabdoid tumors and clear cell sarcoma of the kidney represent 1% and 1.6% of renal cancers, respectively.

3. What are the most common sites for metastatic spread of renal tumors?

The most common sites of metastases in Wilms tumor are the lungs, regional lymph nodes, and liver. In patients with stage IV disease, the lungs are the only site of metastases in 80% of cases. Metastases to the liver, with or without lung metastases, are diagnosed in 15% of cases. Other sites of metastases in Wilms tumor are uncommon. Metastases to the brain can occur in rhabdoid tumors and clear cell sarcoma of the kidney. Bone lesions can be found in RCC.

4. At what age is a child most commonly diagnosed with Wilms tumor?

Wilms tumor occurs most commonly in children between 1 and 5 years old, with a mean age at diagnosis of 3.2 years. Wilms tumor incidence is slightly higher in girls and in Black children than in other races in the United States.

5. What is the typical clinical presentation of a child with Wilms tumor?

The most common presentation is an asymptomatic abdominal mass or swelling, often noted by a parent when bathing or dressing the child. Less common symptoms are fever, abdominal pain, gross or microscopic hematuria, and hypertension. Rarely, a child can present with an acute abdomen and uncontrolled bleeding because of tumor rupture. During the physical examination, special attention should be paid to signs of syndromes associated with Wilms tumor, such as aniridia, hemihypertrophy, and genitourinary anomalies.

6. What are the three different clinical scenarios in which Wilms tumor arises?

Most Wilms tumors occur in children with no unusual physical features or positive family history. These cases of Wilms tumor are termed *sporadic*. The second clinical scenario is Wilms tumor arising in children with *congenital anomalies or predisposing syndromes*. About 10% of cases of Wilms tumor have associated congenital anomalies. The third scenario is Wilms tumors arising in more than one person in a family—*familial Wilms tumor*—which occurs in 1% to 2% of cases.

7. List the congenital anomalies and syndromes most commonly associated with Wilms tumor.

The most common congenital anomalies associated with Wilms tumor include:
- Aniridia
- Hemihypertrophy
- Cryptorchidism
- Hypospadias
- Other genitourinary anomalies

There are over 100 syndromes that are associated with Wilms tumor. The diagnosis of a predisposing syndrome is usually made in infancy, but some may not be discovered until a patient develops Wilms tumor. The most common predisposing syndromes are:
- WAGR syndrome: Wilms tumor, Aniridia, Genitourinary malformations, mental Retardation
- Beckwith-Wiedemann syndrome (BWS): visceromegaly, macroglossia, omphalocele, hemihypertrophy, mental retardation

- Denys-Drash syndrome: nephropathy, macrosomia, organomegaly
- Perlman syndrome: macrocephaly, macrosomia, organomegaly, characteristic facies

8. **What genes are associated with the development of Wilms tumor?**
   WT1 at chromosome 11p13 was the first gene found to be specifically mutated in Wilms tumor. Initially, it was classified as a tumor suppressor gene, but more recently it has been identified as an oncogene involved in several malignancies. Its expression is limited to the genitourinary system. *WT1* mutations account for approximately 20% of Wilms tumor cases. Children with the WAGR syndrome have constitutional deletions encompassing chromosome 11p13, resulting in loss of several contiguous genes. These include the aniridia gene *Pax6* and *WT1*. Loss of one copy of *Pax6* is responsible for aniridia, whereas mutations in *WT1* may confer genitourinary defects. Congenital point mutations in WT1 gene are also the basis of Denys-Drash syndrome.
   Cytogenic analyses have long suggested the presence of *WT2 gene* at chromosome 11p15 where there is loss of heterozygosity in a subset of Wilms tumors. The 11p15 locus is also associated with Beckwith-Wiedemann syndrome. Although the exact locus of WT2 is yet to be definitively confirmed, the most likely candidates are H19 and IGF2.
   Activating mutations in *CTNNB1,* coding for the β-catenin protein in the WNT signaling pathway, occur in approximately 15% of Wilms tumors. Many of these cases overlap with WT1 mutations. *WTX gene* is another commonly mutated gene in Wilms tumor.
   Analysis of families with Wilms tumor has indicated that the predisposition is an autosomal dominant trait with incomplete penetrance. Linkage analysis has excluded both *WT1* and *WT2* as the loci for familial Wilms tumor. Instead, two familial Wilms tumor genes, designated *FWT1* and *FWT2,* have been mapped to 17q12-21 and 19q, respectively.

9. **Give the recommendations for screening children who are at increased risk for developing Wilms tumor.**
   Children with sporadic aniridia, WAGR syndrome, hemihypertrophy, and BWS should have an abdominal ultrasound and urine analysis for microscopic hematuria every 3 to 4 months until at least age 7 years.

10. **What are the histologic features that distinguish favorable histology (FH) Wilms tumor from anaplastic Wilms tumor?**
    Classic nephroblastoma is composed of varying proportions of three cell types: blastemal (the cellular component), stromal, and epithelial tubules. Not all Wilms tumors are triphasic, with biphasic blastemal and stromal patterns frequently seen. When anaplastic nuclear changes are not present, the tumor is classified as being an FH Wilms tumor. Anaplasia with extreme nuclear atypia is present in approximately 4% of cases of Wilms tumor. Anaplasia is characterized by gigantic polyploid nuclei within the tumor specimen. The nuclei have diameters at least three times that of nearby cells, and the mitotic figures are multipolar or polyploid. Anaplastic cells are more resistant to chemotherapy.

11. **What is the importance of distinguishing focal from diffuse anaplasia?**
    Anaplastic changes may be either focal or diffuse. To meet the criteria of focal anaplasia, the anaplastic nuclear changes must be confined to a sharply restricted foci within the primary tumor and may not be present outside the kidney parenchyma. Diffuse anaplasia refers to anaplastic cells that are present in more than one region of the primary tumor or in any extrarenal site, including the renal sinus, nodal metastases, or distant metastases. Patients with focal anaplasia Wilms tumor have outcomes similar to those of FH patients. Patients with diffuse anaplasia have high rates of relapse and death.

12. **Describe the diagnostic work-up for a child with suspected Wilms tumor.**
    Laboratory evaluation should include a complete blood count, liver function tests, renal function tests, serum calcium, and urinalysis. Prothrombin time, partial thromboplastin time, and fibrinogen should be obtained because of the increased risk of acquired von Willebrand disease. If abnormal, factor VIII levels, von Willebrand factor antigen level, and factor VIII ristocetin cofactor activity should be obtained.
    Diagnostic imaging should include an abdominal ultrasound and CT/MRI scan to identify the intrarenal origin of the mass and to evaluate the contralateral kidney for bilateral disease. The inferior vena cava should be carefully examined for the presence and extent of tumor. Echocardiogram is useful for detecting the presence of tumor in the right atrium. A CT scan of chest/abdomen/pelvis should be obtained to check for pulmonary and liver metastases. An MRI/CT scan of the brain should be done in the cases of rhabdoid tumors and clear cell sarcoma of the kidney because both tumors are associated with intracranial metastases. A bone scan should be done in cases of clear cell sarcoma of the kidney.

13. **Describe how Wilms tumor is staged.**
    Children's Oncology Group (COG) Staging system for Wilms tumor:
    - Stage I: The tumor is limited to the kidney and was completely resected. The renal capsule is intact.
    - Stage II: The tumor extends beyond the kidney but is completely resected. There is regional extension of tumor with penetration of the renal capsule. The blood vessels outside the renal parenchyma, including those of the renal sinus, contain tumor. The tumor is biopsied only or there is spillage of tumor before or during surgery that is confined to the flank.

- Stage III: Residual nonhematogenous tumor is present and confined to the abdomen. Any one of the following may occur:
  - Lymph nodes within the abdomen or pelvis are found to be involved by tumor.
  - The tumor has penetrated through the peritoneal surface.
  - Tumor implants are found on the peritoneal surface.
  - Gross or microscopic tumor remains postoperatively.
  - The tumor is not completely resected because of local infiltration into vital structures.
  - Tumor spill not confined to the flank occurred either before or during surgery.
- Stage IV: Hematogenous metastases to the lung, liver, bone, brain, or other organ or lymph node metastases outside the abdominal-pelvic region are present.
- Stage V: Bilateral renal involvement is present at diagnosis. An attempt should be made to stage each side according to the aforementioned criteria.

14. **What is the general surgical approach for Wilms tumor in North America?**
The treatment of Wilms tumor in North America has been guided since 1969 by the National Wilms Tumor Study Group (NWTSG), which merged into the Children's Oncology Group (COG) in 2001. The cornerstone of therapy is surgical removal of the primary tumor at diagnosis. Upfront resection provides the necessary biologic information for risk stratification and selection of appropriate therapy. Tailoring therapy according to biologic risk factors can minimize long-term side effects for low-risk patients and improve survival for high-risk patients.
   The surgeon is responsible not only for removing the primary tumor intact but also for accurately accessing tumor spread. A transabdominal, transperitoneal, large incision is recommended for adequate exposure. Complete exploration of the abdomen should be done. The contralateral kidney should be palpated and visualized to rule out bilateral involvement. This should be done before nephrectomy to exclude bilateral Wilms tumor. The surgeon should assign a "local-regional stage" to the tumor based solely on the operative findings. The presence or absence of disease in hilar and regional lymph nodes is an extremely important factor in accurate staging. Involved or suspicious lymph nodes should be excised. The renal vein and inferior vena cava should be palpated carefully before ligation to rule out extension of the tumor into the wall or the lumen of the vein. A tumor biopsy should not be taken before removal of the tumor. A radical nephrectomy should be performed, and care should be taken to avoid rupture of the tumor capsule with spillage of tumor cells. Partial nephrectomy is not indicated in the routine patient with Wilms tumor. Exceptions include children with synchronous or metachronous bilateral disease or solitary kidneys. The recommended treatment approach for these patients is initial biopsy followed by combination chemotherapy before definitive surgical resection.
   This approach differs from the approach taken in Europe by the International Society of Pediatric Oncology (SIOP), where preoperative chemotherapy is advocated before primary resection. Pretreatment biopsy is not routinely recommended, and the initial treatment is based on radiologic and clinical findings. Using the SIOP protocol, there is a risk that chemotherapy will be given to a benign tumor, such as mesoblastic nephroma, or that less-intensive therapy will be given to unfavorable tumors (i.e., rhabdoid tumor and clear cell sarcoma of the kidney).

15. **Describe the role of radiation therapy in the treatment of Wilms tumor.**
Radiation therapy has been used to treat Wilms tumor since 1915. Survival rates rose from 10% to 20% after nephrectomy alone to 25% to 35% when postoperative radiation was added. With the development of effective chemotherapy and to reduce late effects, the use of radiation therapy has been tailored for the stage and histology of the patient. Abdominal radiation is no longer used for treatment of stage I and II patients with favorable histology. Currently, abdominal radiation is given to stage III favorable histology patients and to stage I to IV diffuse anaplasia patients. Lung radiation is reserved for patients with pulmonary metastases that do not respond to initial chemotherapy.

16. **Which chemotherapy drugs are used for the treatment of Wilms tumor?**
Between 1969 and 2002, there were five studies conducted by the NWTSG. The first two studies, NWTS-I (1969–1973) and NWTS-II (1974–1978) demonstrated that postoperative local radiation was unnecessary for stage I patients, that the combination of vincristine and dactinomycin was more effective than either drug alone, and that the addition of doxorubicin improved survival in higher-stage patients. NWTS-III (1979–1986) and NWTS-IV (1986–1994) demonstrated that the addition of cyclophosphamide to the three-drug treatment regimen improved the 4-year relapse-free survival rate of children with stage II to IV diffuse anaplasia. NWTS-V (1995–2002) demonstrated 100% overall survival (86% 2-year relapse free survival) without chemotherapy for children aged younger than 2 years with stage I FH tumor less than 550 g. Additionally, for patients with stage II to IV diffuse anaplasia, the best reported outcomes to date were achieved with chemotherapy with vincristine, doxorubicin, cyclophosphamide, and etoposide.
   COG renal tumor studies have aimed to further refine the treatment of Wilms tumor. AREN0532 demonstrated excellent outcomes with a 4-year event-free survival of 90% and overall survival of 100% for patients younger than 2 years of age with small, stage I FH Wilms tumor after nephrectomy and observation alone. The majority of those whose disease relapsed had loss of heterozygosity (LOH) of 1p and 16q or 1q gain. Increased therapy with doxorubicin for those patients improved 4-year event-free survival for 75% to 84%. AREN0533 demonstrated that whole-lung radiation could be eliminated for children with stage IV FH WT and lung metastases only

whose lung nodules responded completely to 6 weeks of vincristine, dactinomycin, and doxorubicin with maintenance of excellent event-free survival. AREN0321 intensified therapy for patients with anaplastic Wilms tumor but with increased toxicity. AREN0534 improved survival in patients with bilateral Wilms tumor while preserving renal tissue using a prenephrectomy chemotherapy regimen of vincristine, dactinomycin, and doxorubicin, surgical resection within 12 weeks of diagnosis, and response- and histology-based postoperative therapy. This approach improved 4-year event-free survival from 56% to 82% for patients with bilateral Wilms tumor.

Current chemotherapy regimens for stages I and II with favorable histology usually involve two chemotherapy agents: vincristine and dactinomycin. Stage III and IV FH Wilms tumors and anaplastic Wilms tumor, clear cell sarcoma of the kidney, and malignant rhabdoid tumor are treated with three or more chemotherapy agents depending on stage and histology. These agents include vincristine, dactinomycin, doxorubicin, cyclophosphamide, carboplatin, etoposide, or ifosfamide. The choice of chemotherapy used depends on the stage and status of current research treatment protocols.

17. What is the prognosis of patients with renal tumors?

Five-year survival for patients with Wilms tumor is over 90%. Stage I, II, and III FH tumors have a 4-year survival rate of 95% to 100%. Stage IV and V FH tumors have a 4-year survival rate of 85% to 100%. Survival rates for tumors with a focal and diffuse anaplastic histology range from 70% to 100% and 30% to 85%, respectively. Patients with renal clear cell sarcoma of the kidney have an overall survival of 85%. Patients with rhabdoid tumor of the kidney had the worst outcome, with a 4-year relapse free survival of 25%.

BIBLIOGRAPHY

1. Aldrink JH, Heaton TE, Dasgupta R, et al. Update on Wilms tumor. *J Ped Surg.* 2019;54:390–397.
2. Bahrami A, Joodi M, Maftooh M, et al. The genetic factors contributing to the development of Wilms tumor and their clinical utility in its diagnosis and prognosis. *J Cell Physiol.* 2018;233:2882–2888.
3. Kotagal M, Geller J. Aggressive pediatric renal tumors. *Sem in Ped Surg.* 2019;28:1055–8586.
4. Liu EK, Suson KD. Syndromic Wilms tumor: a review of predisposing conditions, surveillance, and treatment. *Transl Androl Urol.* 2020;9 (5):2370–2381.
5. Mansfield SA, Lamb MG, Stanek JR, et al. Renal tumors in children and young adults older than 5 years of age. *J Pediatr Hematol Oncol.* 2020;42(4):287–291.
6. Neville HL, Ritchey ML, Wilms tumor. Overview of National Wilms Tumor Study Group results. *Urol Clin North Am.* 2000;27:435–442.
7. Wang J, Li M, Tang D, Gu W, Mao J, Shu Q. Current treatment for Wilms Tumor: COG and SIOP standards. *World Jnl Ped Surgery.* 2019;2:1–4.

CHAPTER 38

HODGKIN LYMPHOMA IN CHILDREN AND ADOLESCENTS

Justine M. Kahn, MD, MS and Kara M. Kelly, MD

1. **Describe the incidence and epidemiology of Hodgkin lymphoma in children and adolescents.**
   There are approximately 1200 new cases of Hodgkin lymphoma (HL) diagnosed in the United States annually among children and adolescents. Among adolescents, HL is associated with a higher socioeconomic background. In contrast, the incidence of HL among young children tends to increase with increasing family size and lower socioeconomic status. The mixed cellularity histologic subtype is more common in these younger patients. In low-income countries, an early peak occurs before adolescence, where it is also associated with Epstein-Barr virus (EBV) infection, mixed cellularity histology, and male sex.

2. **What is the epidemiologic relationship between HL and Epstein-Barr virus?**
   An infectious etiology for Hodgkin has long been suggested by its epidemiologic characteristics, and much of the data point specifically to EBV. High EBV antibody titers have been detected in young patients with HL, suggesting that enhanced activation of EBV may precede the development of HL. EBV is more often associated with HL occurring in patients with primary or secondary immunodeficiencies, such as human immunodeficiency virus (HIV) infection and after solid organ transplant.

3. **Name the subtypes of HL.**
   The World Health Organization (WHO) histologic classification recognizes two major subtypes of HL: *classical HL (cHL)* and *nodular lymphocyte predominant HL (nLPHL)*. The primary distinctions between these two are on the basis of histology and immunohistochemical staining pattern.
   A. cHL has four histologic subtypes:
   - Nodular sclerosis (most common): The primary *histologic subtype* of cHL is nodular sclerosis (up to 70% of cases). This is the most common cHL histology and often involves neck and mediastinum.
   - Mixed cellularity: The majority of the remaining cases exhibit the mixed cellularity histology. This is the second most common cHL, patients are younger than 10 years old, and EBV frequently involved. Often there is advanced disease at presentation.
   - Lymphocyte-depleted.
   - Lymphocyte-rich (least common).
   B. nLPHL accounts for 10% to 20% of pediatric HL, usually presents with early-stage disease (IA, IIA), and has a male predominance, indolent course, and good prognosis but can have late and occasionally multiple relapses and transformation to T-cell/histiocyte rich large B-cell lymphoma.

4. **Describe the clinical presentation of HL.**
   - Painless lymphadenopathy
   - Persistent cough, shortness of breath, or chest pain related to the presence of a mediastinal mass (in approximately two-thirds)
   - Constitutional symptoms

5. **Define "B" symptoms.**
   B symptoms describe the extent of systemic or constitutional symptoms that accompany a diagnosis of HL. Presenting with any or all of the following defines having B-symptoms.
   - Unintentional weight loss of at least 10% in 6 months
   - Drenching night sweats
   - Unexplained fevers of at least 38°C for 3 consecutive days

6. **What is included in the diagnostic workup for suspected HL?**
   Workup should begin with a thorough history to determine the presence or absence of B-symptoms, as well as family history, other medical conditions, and infectious history. Physical examination should focus on palpation of lymph nodes, auscultation of lungs, and palpation of the abdomen assessing for hepatosplenomegaly. The diagnosis of HL requires histologic confirmation with an excisional lymph node biopsy. Fine-needle aspiration of a lymph node should be avoided because a negative biopsy will not rule out a diagnosis of HL because of the rarity of the Hodgkin-Reed-Sternberg (HRS) cells within the lymph node. Diagnostic imaging includes a chest radiograph, both posteroanterior (PA) and lateral, and a positron emission tomography/computed tomography (PET/CT) scan is used to determine the metabolic activity of involved nodes and extralymphatic organs, including the bone and bone marrow.

All involved sites should be assigned a Deauville score. Contrast-enhanced CT scan of the neck, chest, abdomen, and pelvis should be included. Bilateral bone marrow biopsy has largely been replaced by PET scan.

7. **How is bulky disease defined?**
   - In current Children's Oncology Group (COG) protocols, mediastinal lymphadenopathy is defined as bulky if it exceeds 33% of the maximum intrathoracic cavity on a PA chest radiograph.
   - Nonmediastinal nodal aggregate: 6 cm in transverse dimension on axial CT or longest dimension on coronal or sagittal reformatted CT

8. **What are "E" lesions? How do they differ from extranodal lesions?**
   E lesions are the extension of HL involvement into extralymphatic structures. These must be distinguished from isolated extranodal lesions.
   - *E lesions* are defined by *extension* from involved nodes into adjacent structures, such as the lung, pleura, or chest wall.
   - *Extranodal lesions* are lesions in the liver, isolated lesions within the lung parenchyma, or bone marrow involvement. All are considered stage IV disease.

9. **Describe the staging of HL.**
   The Ann Arbor staging system is used to stage HL, which spreads predictably along contiguous lymph nodes until it is very advanced. Stages are subclassified into "A" or "B" based on the absence or presence of systemic systems. Presence or absence of bulky disease is also incorporated into final risk stratification.
   - Stage I: Single node region (I) or single extranodal organ or site (IE).
   - Stage II: Two or more node regions on the same side of the diaphragm (II) or one node region and localized extranodal site on the same side of the diaphragm (IIE).
   - Stage III: Node regions are involved on both sides of the diaphragm (III) and may include a localized extranodal site (IIIE), the spleen (IIIS), or both (IIISE).
   - Stage IV: Diffuse/disseminated involvement of at least one extranodal site.
   - *Substage classifications are based on defined clinical features and are used in risk stratification.*
   - Substage A indicates asymptomatic disease.
   - Substage B indicates the presence of B symptoms
   - Bulk disease is not part of the Ann Arbor classification but has been used to by some groups in risk stratification.

10. **Describe the pathologic classification of Hodgkin Reed-Sternberg cells.**
    Hodgkin Reed-Sternberg (HRS) cells are classically associated with HL and generally make up only 1% of the neoplastic mass. They are neoplastic, large multinucleated cells with two mirror-image nuclei (owl eyes). HRS cells are derived from germinal center B cells but have lost their B-cell identity. They secrete active cytokines to recruit inflammatory cells, which is why the majority of the infiltrate (or microenvironment) in an involved lymph node is made up of nonneoplastic T cells, B cells, eosinophils, neutrophils, macrophages, and plasma cells. The inflammatory background is key to the clinical behavior of HRS cells because there is bidirectional signaling between the cells and their microenvironment. Immunohistochemistry stains for HRS cells are positive for CD30 and CD15, which is relevant for targeted therapies.

11. **Describe the principles of therapy for Hodgkin lymphoma.**
    Enrollment in an ongoing clinical trial is recommended for all patients, when possible.
    Treatment of pediatric HL has continued to evolve in attempts to strike the optimal balance between maintaining high rates of overall survival (OS) and reducing the long-term morbidity and mortality associated with chemotherapy or radiation therapy (RT), with strategies that are often quite different than those used for adults with HL. There are three main principles to therapy:
    A. Multimodal: Multiagent chemotherapy and radiation are standard.
    B. Risk-directed: Disease severity determines the intensity of therapy.
       a. Stage/prognostic factors at diagnosis
    C. Response-adapted: Objective response to therapy via PET or CT (during or after planned treatment completion) dictates therapy augmentation or de-escalation.

12. **Describe the principles of radiotherapy.**
    RT is increasingly a less common component of HL treatment. Long-term toxicity is a major consideration when using RT; thus recent trials in pediatrics have used functional imaging with [^{18}F]fluorodeoxyglucose (FDG) PET during treatment (interim PET) to assess early chemotherapy response and adjust subsequent therapy based on response to initial treatment cycles. This has allowed for omission of consolidation RT in many patients with both early and advanced stage disease.
    - Involved field radiation (IFRT) is radiation to the area where the lymphoma is located, including adjacent lymph nodes and surrounding normal tissue.
    - Involved site radiation therapy (ISRT) involves targeting only the lymph nodes that originally contained lymphoma and smaller nearby areas the cancer extended into. This is largely replacing IFRT.

13. **Using contemporary therapies, what are the expected event-free survival and overall survival rates for pediatric and adolescent HL?**
About 10% to 15% of patients with early stage and 15% to 30% with advanced-stage HL fail to respond or relapse after primary conventional treatment. Fortunately, salvage regimens and second-line treatments for HL are extraordinarily effective, and thus OS rates at 5 years approach 98% for the majority of pediatric and adolescent patients.

14. **Describe the Deauville Score for patients with a PET scan.**
PET scans are used to identify areas of metabolic uptake of lymphoma in patients with HL. FDG uptake correlates with anaerobic glycolysis. For patients with active disease, avidity is evaluated by comparison with uptake in liver and the mediastinal blood pool to assign a score on the *5-point Deauville scale (DS):*
A. No uptake
B. Uptake lesser or equal to mediastinal blood pool
C. Uptake greater than mediastinal blood pool but lesser or equal to liver
D. Moderately increased uptake, greater than liver
E. Markedly increased uptake, greater than liver and/or new lesions

15. **Describe the utility of post-treatment surveillance after therapy completion.**
Early detection of asymptomatic recurrent disease by imaging studies does not affect OS outcomes in HL. For that reason, surveillance imaging after a complete radiographic response is *not routinely* recommended outside the context of a clinical trial, especially beyond 12 to 18 months from completion of treatment. Physical exam is the optimal approach to assessing for disease recurrence, and if recurrence is suspected, a biopsy is required to confirm the relapse.

16. **What is the difference between relapsed HL and refractory HL?**
Refractory: A small minority (~5%) of pediatric patients with HL will have primary refractory disease, defined as the absence of a complete response after initial therapy.
Relapsed: Among patients who do achieve a complete response, as many as 25% will experience a subsequent relapse, with risk of relapse related to initial disease characteristics and early response to therapy. The majority of relapses occur within the first year.

17. **How is relapsed HL managed?**
When relapse or progression is suspected, histologic confirmation with tissue biopsy is recommended before initiating treatment of relapsed/refractory disease. Optimal salvage treatment has not been defined in children and adolescents, and it is for this reason that enrollment on a clinical trial is always the best first choice for treatment of recurrent disease. In general, the treatment options include standard-dose chemotherapy and/or immunotherapy (reinduction therapy), high-dose chemotherapy with autologous stem cell rescue (ASCR), or novel approaches. Some patients with low-risk features at time of relapse (low stage at diagnosis, limited number of cycles of initial chemotherapy treatment, relapse beyond 1 year) may be successfully treated with standard-dose chemotherapy and/or immunotherapy with radiation therapy only.

18. **What are the emerging treatments for HL, such as immune therapies and targeted agents?**
Recent approaches in the treatment of HL combine novel immunotherapies such as brentuximab vedotin (BV) and antiprogrammed cell death protein 1 (PD-1) antibodies (nivolumab and pembrolizumab), which were originally used primarily in the relapsed setting but which have been moved to upfront therapy in recent clinical trials.
Brentuximab vedotin is an antibody–drug conjugate that selectively targets cells expressing the CD30 antigen, which is uniformly expressed in classical HL.
HRS cells produce molecules that inhibit T-cell–mediated immune responses. Specifically, PD-L1 expressed on HRS cells engages PD-1 expressed on T cells, induces immune checkpoint inhibition, and causes T-cell exhaustion. Thus anti-PD-1 antibodies have shown important efficacy in treating HL, particularly in the relapsed setting, and now are under investigation in the upfront setting for adolescents and young adults with advanced stage disease.

19. **Describe common late effects associated with HL therapy.**
Lifelong monitoring for surveillance for late organ toxicities is highly recommended, preferably at a center with expertise in cancer survivorship or with a primary care provider familiar with survivorship guidelines.

	Exposure	*Late sequelae*
Second malignant neoplasms	Radiotherapy	• Breast cancers: Risk is highest 15–20 years after radiation, is highest for girls who received radiation at age 10 years or older, and declines with increasing age. • Thyroid and nonmelanoma skin cancers are the most commonly reported second cancers; in older cohorts, gastrointestinal and lung cancers are beginning to appear with increasing frequency. • Therapy-related leukemias: Myelodysplasia and acute myeloid leukemia [t-MDS/AML]

	Alkylating agents; topoisomerase II inhibitors, radiation	
Endocrine	Radiotherapy	Thyroid dysfunction
Cardiovascular	Radiotherapy	Cardiac fibrosis, coronary artery disease, carotid artery stenosis
	Anthracyclines	Diastolic dysfunction; cardiomyopathy
Pulmonary	Radiotherapy	Pulmonary fibrosis, pneumonitis, compromised diffusion capacity
	Bleomycin	

BIBLIOGRAPHY

1. Castellino SM, Parsons SK, Pei Q, et al. A Randomized Phase III Trial of Brentuximab Vedotin (Bv) for de Novo High-Risk Classical Hodgkin Lymphoma (cHL) in Children and Adolescents - Study Design and Incorporation of Secondary Endpoints in Children's Oncology Group (COG) AHOD1331. 2018. https://childrensoncologygroup.org/ahod1331.
2. Ehrhardt MJ, Flerlage JE, Armenian SH, Castellino SM, Hodgson DC, Hudson MM. Integration of pediatric Hodgkin lymphoma treatment and late effects guidelines: seeing the forest beyond the trees. *J Natl Compr Canc Netw.* 2021;19(6):755–764.
3. Flerlage JE, Hiniker SM, Armenian S, et al. Pediatric Hodgkin lymphoma, version 3.2021. *J Natl Compr Canc Netw.* 2021;19(6):733–754.
4. Giulino-Roth L, Keller FG, Hodgson DC, et al. Current approaches in the management of low risk Hodgkin lymphoma in children and adolescents. *Br J Haematol.* 2015;169:647–660.
5. Kelly KM. Hodgkin lymphoma in children and adolescents: improving the therapeutic index. *Hematology (Am Soc Hematol Educ Program).* 2015;2015:514–521.
6. Lo AC, Dieckmann K, Pelz T, et al. Pediatric classical Hodgkin lymphoma. *Pediatr Blood Cancer.* 2021;68(Suppl. 2):e28562.
7. Mauz-Körholz C, Metzger ML, Kelly KM, et al. Pediatric Hodgkin lymphoma. *Journal of Clinical Oncology.* 2015;33(27):2975–2985.
8. NCCN Clinical Practice Guidelines in Oncology. *Pediatric Hodgkin Lymphoma.* 2021. https://www.nccn.org/guidelines/guidelines-detail?category=1&id=1498.

CHAPTER 39

NON-HODGKIN LYMPHOMA IN CHILDREN AND ADOLESCENTS

Nitya Gulati, MBBS and Nader Kim El-Mallawany, MD

1. **Describe the epidemiology of non-Hodgkin lymphoma in children and adolescents.**

   Non-Hodgkin lymphoma (NHL) is a heterogeneous category that includes a wide diversity of malignancies derived from lymphocytic cell origin. Although the World Health Organization (WHO) classification of lymphoid neoplasms includes more than 50 distinct diagnostic entities, many of them are extremely rare in the pediatric population.[1] Five lymphomas account for more than 90% of all pediatric NHL diagnoses (Table 39.1). Burkitt lymphoma (BL) is the most common, followed by T-cell lymphoblastic lymphoma (T-LBL), diffuse large B-cell lymphoma (DLBCL), anaplastic large cell lymphoma (ALCL), and primary mediastinal B-cell lymphoma (PMBL).[2,3] There are unique geographic distinctions in the epidemiology of childhood NHL; endemic BL is the most common overall childhood cancer in equatorial regions of sub-Saharan Africa where *Plasmodium falciparum* infection is holoendemic, whereas East Asia and Central and South America have a higher incidence of the rare Epstein-Barr virus (EBV)-associated T and natural killer (NK)-cell lymphomas and lymphoproliferative disorders.[4]

   NHL is the fourth most common cancer of childhood and fifth most common in adolescence, occurring more often in males in both groups.[3] Risk of developing NHL is well-established in patients with underlying immune deficiency, including inherited cell-mediated and humoral immunodeficiency syndromes, disorders of cell repair, and acquired immunodeficiency in the form of human immunodeficiency virus (HIV) infection or post-transplant immune suppression.[5] Pathogenesis in the setting of immune deficiency is often attributed to viral infection with EBV and human herpesvirus-8 (HHV-8).[6] Nonetheless, cases of pediatric NHL in the setting of underlying immune deficiency or dysregulation represent a small proportion of overall diagnoses, and the vast majority of lymphomas occur de novo.

2. **Provide an overview of the classification of NHL in the pediatric population.**

   The WHO classification categorizes NHL based on the cell compartment of origin as B versus T/NK cell (Table 39.2).[1] The majority of pediatric NHL arise from mature lymphocytes. Mature B-cell NHL is most common, including BL, DLBCL, and PMBL.[2] Several histologic variants of DLBCL have recently been defined and are typically grouped with BL/DLBCL. ALCL is the most common mature T-cell NHL of childhood, whereas other mature B/T/NK-cell NHLs are categorized as rare. Lymphoblastic lymphoma arises in precursor lymphocytes and represents approximately 25% of NHLs in children. Contrary to patterns in lymphoblastic leukemia, T-LBL accounts for the majority (~75%) of lymphoblastic lymphomas compared with B-cell LBL.[2]

3. **What are some considerations specific to the adolescent/young adult population?**

   The high incidence of NHL in adolescents and young adults (AYA) emphasizes its epidemiological importance. Some important issues pertaining specifically to the AYA population include:

   - Although BL is common in pediatric oncology and treated with intensive multiagent chemotherapy, such regimens are poorly tolerated by the rare older adult with BL. Nevertheless, considering the superior survival advantage associated with pediatric mature B-NHL regimens and its tolerability in younger adults, there is rationale for incorporating pediatric-based therapeutic strategies for young adults with BL.[7]
   - Some of the rare NHLs that infrequently occur in children (e.g., nonanaplastic mature T/NK-cell NHL) do not have an established pediatric-specific treatment paradigm; therefore extrapolation from adult oncology guidelines may be necessary to offer evidence-based strategies for the rare pediatric patients.[8]
   - The biology of DLBCL occurring in the pediatric population appears distinct from that described in adults.[9,10] On the other hand, there seems to be substantial overlap between the biology of childhood versus adult BL.[11] It remains to be proven whether NHL occurring in younger patients represents a distinct biological phenomenon or if extrapolation from the molecular mechanisms established in adult disease may apply and enlighten the development of targeted therapies for children.[12]
   - Strong consideration must be taken for pediatric and AYA patients regarding the potential late effects of chemotherapy, immunotherapy, and radiation therapy. This includes a comprehensive review of fertility preservation.[13]

4. **Which staging system is used for pediatric NHL?**

   The St. Jude NHL staging classification was developed by Sharon Murphy over 35 years ago and is the most widely accepted tool to define disease extent in pediatric NHL (Table 39.3).[14] Nevertheless, there has been significant advancement in the evaluation, treatment, and prognosis of pediatric NHL since the St. Jude staging system was first proposed. A revised international pediatric NHL staging system (IPNHLSS) attempts to incorporate technological

Table 39.1 Overview of the Clinical Characteristics for the Most Common Non-Hodgkin Lymphomas (NHLs) of Childhood and Adolescence

DISEASE	CELL OF ORIGIN	MOLECULAR HALLMARKS	% OF NHL	TYPICAL CLINICAL PRESENTATION	POTENTIAL ACUTE COMPLICATIONS	TYPICAL UPFRONT THERAPY[B]	EFS
Burkitt[a]	Mature B	*CMYC* rearrangements (disease-defining)	35–40	abdominal mass(es)	TLS, spinal cord compression	FAB/LMB regimen – rituximab risk-stratified into low (Group A), intermediate (Group B), and high-risk (Group C) strata	>90%
T-lymphoblastic	Precursor T	variable	20–25	mediastinal mass	acute airway obstruction, SVC syndrome, TLS	Similar to T-ALL with escalating methotrexate, nelarabine role yet undetermined for lymphoma	80%–85%
DLBCL[a]	Mature B	variable	10–15	abdominal mass(es), peripheral LAD	TLS	Same as for Burkitt lymphoma	>90%
ALCL	Mature T	*ALK* rearrangements (disease-defining)	~10	diffuse nodal involvement, often extranodal too	TLS, malignancy-associated HLH	ALCL99 regimen + brentuximab	~75%
PMBL	Mature B	9p24 alterations (in approximately half)	~5	mediastinal mass	acute airway obstruction, SVC syndrome	da-EPOCH + rituximab	70%–75%

Please note that more than 50 distinct diagnostic entities fall under the umbrella classification of NHL (i.e., lymphomas that are not Hodgkin). Not included in this table are the rare NHLs, which account for approximately 5% to 10% of childhood NHL. These rare lymphomas are listed in the 2016 World Health Organization Classification of Lymphoid Neoplasms, and include numerous malignancies of mature B, T, and NK-cell origin and post-transplant lymphoproliferative disorders.

[a]Please note that gray-zone aggressive mature B-cell NHL histologies that are intermediate between Burkitt and DLBCL would be treated the same, including high grade B-cell lymphoma, not otherwise specified, Burkitt-like lymphoma with 11q aberration, high-grade B-cell lymphoma with *MYC* and *BCL2* and/or *BCL6* rearrangements. Other variants of DLBCL include large B-cell lymphoma with *IRF4* rearrangement and mediastinal gray-zone lymphoma (also known as B-cell lymphoma, unclassifiable, with features intermediate between DLBCL and classical Hodgkin lymphoma).

[b]ALCL therapy only has one dose of intrathecal chemotherapy. PMBL and Group A (i.e., low-risk) Burkitt/DLBCL regimens have none. All others have numerous doses of intrathecal chemotherapy throughout the treatment course.

ALCL, Anaplastic large cell lymphoma; *da-EPOCH,* dose-adjusted EPOCH; *DLBCL,* diffuse large B-cell lymphoma; *EFS,* event-free survival (estimated); *HLH,* hemophagocytic lymphohistiocytosis; *LAD,* lymphadenopathy; *PMBL,* primary mediastinal B-cell lymphoma; *SVC,* superior vena cava; *T-ALL,* T-cell acute lymphoblastic leukemia; *TLS,* tumor lysis syndrome.

Table 39.2 Contextual Categorization of Non-Hodgkin Lymphomas (NHLs) and Lymphoproliferative Disorders in Children and Adolescents Based on Cell of Origin and Incidence in the Pediatric Population

CATEGORY	B-CELL COMPARTMENT	T/NK-CELL COMPARTMENT
COMMON	Burkitt Lymphoma	T-cell Lymphoblastic Lymphoma
	Diffuse Large B-cell Lymphoma (DLBCL)	ALK+ Anaplastic Large Cell Lymphoma (ALCL)
	Primary Mediastinal B-cell Lymphoma	
LESS COMMON & RARE	B-cell Lymphoblastic Lymphoma	Peripheral T-cell Lymphoma, NOS
	High-grade B-cell Lymphoma, NOS	ALK-negative ALCL
	Burkitt-Like Lymphoma with 11q Aberration	Extranodal NK/T-cell Lymphoma
	High-grade "Double-Hit" B-cell Lymphoma[a]	Subcutaneous Panniculitis-like T-cell Lymphoma
	Large B-cell Lymphoma with *IRF4* Rearrangement	Hepatosplenic (Gamma-Delta) T-cell Lymphoma
	T-cell/histiocyte-rich Large B-cell Lymphoma	Primary Cutaneous Gamma-Delta T-cell Lymphoma
	Mediastinal Gray-Zone Lymphoma[b]	Mycosis Fungoides
	Pediatric-type Follicular Lymphoma	Lymphomatoid Papulosis
	Pediatric Nodal Marginal Zone Lymphoma	Primary Cutaneous ALCL
VERY RARE[c]	Extranodal Marginal Zone Lymphoma	Angioimmunoblastic T-cell Lymphoma
	EBV+ DLBCL, NOS	Systemic EBV+ T-cell Lymphoma of Childhood
	Lymphomatoid Granulomatosis	T/NK-cell Chronic Active EBV
	Primary CNS Lymphoma	Aggressive NK-cell Leukemia
	Plasmablastic Lymphoma	T-cell Large Granular Lymphocytic Leukemia
	Primary Effusion Lymphoma	Primary Cutaneous CD4+ Small/Medium T-cell LPD
	Multicentric Castleman Disease	Enteropathy-associated T-cell Lymphoma
		Adult T-cell Leukemia/Lymphoma

[a]Also known as high-grade B-cell lymphoma, with MYC and BCL2 and/or BCL6 rearrangements.
[b]Also known as B-cell lymphoma, unclassifiable, with features intermediate between DLBCL and classical Hodgkin lymphoma.
[c]Please note that numerous additional lymphoma diagnoses exist on the 2016 version of the World Health Organization Classification of Lymphoid Neoplasms; however, they are not all included in this table because of the extremely rare nature of their occurrence in children.
CNS, Central nervous system; *EBV*, Epstein-Barr virus; *LPD*, lymphoproliferative disorder; *NK*, natural killer; *NOS*, not otherwise specified.

advances in molecular diagnostic methods, the detection of minimal disseminated disease, and advanced imaging technologies.[15] Some pragmatic distinctions of the pediatric NHL staging system include the following: Stage IV is limited to central nervous system (CNS) or bone marrow involvement, whereas clinical presentation with nonresected abdominal disease or mediastinal mass is automatically stage III, even if disease involvement is restricted to one side of the diaphragm.

5. **Describe the diagnostic workup and evaluation for children with suspected NHL.**
Besides a thorough history and physical examination to delineate the extent of disease and evaluate for end-organ damage because of potential oncological emergencies as described later, the initial diagnostic workup is detailed in Box 39.1. The oncological emergencies to consider are tumor lysis syndrome, acute upper airway obstruction, superior vena cava syndrome, spinal cord compression or cranial nerve defects, and malignancy-associated hemophagocytic lymphohistiocytosis.

6. **What are general treatment considerations for pediatric NHL?**
Typically multiagent chemotherapy achieves high cure rates without the need for surgical resection or radiation therapy in pediatric NHL cases. Intrathecal chemotherapy is incorporated in most treatment regimens, even for CNS-negative patients, with the following exceptions: no intrathecal chemotherapy is required for PMBL or Group A BL/DLBCL, and only a single dose of intrathecal chemotherapy is included in the ALCL regimen. CNS involvement is typically

Table 39.3 St. Jude Staging for Pediatric Non-Hodgkin Lymphoma

STAGE	DESCRIPTION
I	A single tumor (extranodal) or single anatomic area (nodal), excluding the mediastinum or abdomen
II	A single extranodal tumor with regional node involvement
	Two or more nodal areas on the same side of the diaphragm
	Two single extranodal tumors on the same side of the diaphragm, with or without regional node involvement
	A primary gastrointestinal tract tumor grossly and completely excised, with or without associated mesenteric nodes only
III	Two single extranodal tumors on opposite sides of diaphragm
	Two or more nodal areas on opposite sides of diaphragm
	All of the primary intrathoracic tumors (mediastinal, pleural, thymic)
	All extensive primary intraabdominal disease
	All paraspinal or epidural tumors, regardless of the other tumor site(s)
IV	Any of the above with initial central nervous system and/or bone marrow involvement ($<$25% malignant cells)

Box 39.1 Work-Up for a Child With Suspected Non-Hodgkin Lymphoma (NHL)

Laboratory Studies

Complete blood count (CBC) may be normal in NHL. Presence of anemia, thrombocytopenia, or leukopenia/neutropenia may be because of extensive bone marrow infiltration, splenic involvement, or bleeding because of gastrointestinal tract involvement.

Serum chemistries (hyperkalemia, hyperphosphatemia with/without hypocalcemia, with/without abnormal renal function because of tumor lysis syndrome [TLS])

Uric acid (hyperuricemia because of TLS)

Lactate dehydrogenase (LDH; often elevated because of high tumor burden, rapidly proliferative NHL such as Burkitt lymphoma [BL], diffuse large B-cell lymphoma [DLBCL], or lymphoblastic lymphoma [LBL], or extensive liver/spleen involvement. Normal LDH does not rule out NHL.)

Liver function studies (baseline evaluation)

Coagulation studies (baseline evaluation)

Serum ferritin (if suspicion for malignancy-associated hemophagocytic lymphohistiocytosis is present)

Baseline Imaging Studies

Chest x-ray (during initial evaluation to evaluate for mediastinal mass causing airway compression)

Computed tomography (CT) neck, chest, abdomen, and pelvis with intravenous (IV) contrast (historic gold standard for staging and disease evaluation)

Positron emission tomography (PET)/CT (increasingly used at the time of diagnosis and to assess treatment responses; however, extent of its utility remains to be defined)

Ultrasound or magnetic resonance imaging (MRI): if needed or if unable to perform the previous studies. MRI particularly useful to evaluate for intradural extension in patients with concern of central nervous system (CNS) involvement.

Diagnostic Biopsy

Excisional or incisional biopsy is preferred to get adequate tissue for histopathology, immunohistochemistry (IHC), flow cytometry, fluorescence in-situ hybridization (FISH), molecular diagnostics

    Core needle biopsies acceptable alternative if tissue biopsy is unsafe/unfeasible

    Fine-needle aspiration (FNA; least preferred because of high chance for false negative)

Bilateral bone marrow biopsies and aspiration for histopathology, cytogenetics/FISH, and flow cytometry

Diagnostic lumbar puncture (suggested for all NHL, although CNS involvement is very in primary mediastinal B-cell lymphoma)

---

successfully treated by incorporating high-dose methotrexate with or without high-dose cytarabine, except for CNS-positive patients with T-LBL, who also receive cranial radiation therapy. Radiation therapy is not included in frontline treatment regimens, except for patients with PMBL with biopsy-proven residual disease at the end of therapy. Finally, targeted therapies are increasingly incorporated into frontline regimens (e.g., rituximab for mature B-NHL and brentuximab for ALCL).[16,17] Current and future clinical trials are investigating the incorporation of additional targeted agents and the potential for dose reductions in cytotoxic chemotherapy for lower-risk patients. Hematopoietic stem cell transplantation (HSCT) is typically reserved for patients with relapsed or refractory disease.

7. Describe (A) the pathology/molecular characteristics and (B) clinical features and treatment outcomes of pediatric mature B-cell NHL.

   A. BL and DLBCL are often referred to as the pediatric mature B-NHL.[18,19] Although distinct hematopathological characteristics are appreciated in typical cases, the two lymphomas share considerable histologic and clinical overlap. Ultimately, translocation of the *C-MYC* oncogene (on chromosome 8) with either a heavy or light chain immunoglobulin gene partner is the defining biological characteristic of BL—most commonly t(8;14) but also t(8;22) and t(2;8). *C-MYC* rearrangements in pediatric DLBCL are rare. There are also some less common gray-zone high-grade mature B-NHL that fall along the spectrum of disease between BL and DLBCL, as well as additional gray-zone variants of DLBCL (see Tables 39.1 and 39.2).[1] Ultimately, they are typically treated uniformly in pediatric patients.

   B. BL and DLBCL most commonly present with intra-abdominal primary disease sites, including involvement of the gastrointestinal (GI) tract presenting with intussusception. Peripheral lymphadenopathy and involvement of the head and neck region are more common in DLBCL, whereas bone marrow and CNS involvement are more common in BL. Building on the backbone of the FAB/LMB96 protocol,[20] contemporary FAB/LMB-based therapy achieves cure for greater than 90% of all patients.[16] This treatment regimen is a risk-stratified approach that categorizes patients into low-risk (Group A, completely resected localized disease), Intermediate-risk (Group B), and high-risk strata (Group C, CNS-positive, and/or leukemia presentation), with regimens that vary in intensity.[21–23] More recently, the higher risk subset of patients from Group B (stage III/IV with elevated lactate dehydrogenase [LDH]), as well as patients from Group C, were included in an international randomized clinical trial combining the anti-CD20 monoclonal antibody rituximab with the FAB/LMB96 chemotherapy backbone.[16] This study demonstrated superior 3-year event-free survival (EFS) for those patients randomized to receive rituximab (93.9% vs. 82.3%). Thus rituximab has since been incorporated in frontline therapy.[16]

   The other contemporary therapy with equivalent survival outcomes to the FAB/LMB protocol is the BFM mature B-NHL regimen.[24,25] Both regimens use comparable risk-stratification platforms and combination chemotherapy with emphasis on alkylating agents and high-dose methotrexate, plus the addition of high-dose cytarabine for high-risk patients.[18,19,26] Ultimately, the combination of rituximab with either the LMB or BFM chemotherapy backbone achieves cure for the vast majority of children, including the highest risk patients. Nevertheless, those patients with relapsed or refractory disease are extremely difficult to salvage, despite treatment advances in HSCT, and represent a formidable clinical challenge.[27–30]

8. Provide an (A) overview of T- versus B-cell lineage LBL and (B) describe recent advances in the treatment approach for T-LBL.

   A. T-cell lineage represents approximately 75% of all pediatric lymphoblastic lymphomas.[2,31] Although the vast majority of patients with T-LBL present with a primary mediastinal mass and advanced-stage III/IV disease, B-LBL is most often characterized by localized stage I/II presentation involving lymph nodes of the head and neck, skin/subcutaneous tissue, or bone.[32,33] Approximately one-fifth of patients with LBL will present with bone marrow disease, whereas CNS involvement is relatively uncommon overall—especially compared with T-cell ALL.[34,35] Extent of bone marrow infiltration distinguishes LBL (0%–25% involvement) from its leukemic counterpart, acute lymphoblastic leukemia (ALL, defined as greater than 25% involvement).

   B. Curative outcomes for children with T-LBL have steadily improved over the past quarter-century, with approximately 80% to 85% of children achieving long-term EFS.[35,36] Recent studies have demonstrated the critical role of incorporating asparaginase intensively into the multiagent chemotherapy regimens used for ALL and the seemingly counterintuitive survival advantage of intermediate-dose escalating methotrexate over high-dose infusions.[32,37] Prospective risk-stratification platforms are yet to be established because clinical features, such as the presence of minimal disseminated disease in the diagnostic bone marrow (i.e., at least 1% involvement), initial stage, radiographic response to induction therapy, and early T-cell precursor immunophenotype, have been inconsistently associated with prognostic impact.[32,36–39] Additionally, the future role of promising therapeutics such as nelarabine, bortezomib, and daratumumab for T-LBL remains undefined.[37] Extrapolating from the poor prognostic significance of end-of-consolidation minimal residual disease in T-cell ALL, some experts voice concern over the potential adverse prognostic significance of having biopsy-proven residual disease at end-of-consolidation for children with T-LBL as well.[36] Long-term cure is rarely achieved for children with refractory or relapsed T-LBL and is only possible in patients who respond to salvage therapy followed by allogeneic HSCT.[30,40]

9. Describe (A) the pathobiology of ALCL and (B) provide an overview of the salient clinical features and treatment strategy for ALK+ ALCL.

   A. ALCL is a CD30+ mature T-cell lymphoma and is subdivided into ALK+, ALK-negative, and primary cutaneous disease.[1] Tumor cells express CD30 in a membrane-bound fashion and often show an aberrant T-cell phenotype with frequent T-cell antigen deletion. Some cases without demonstration of any T-cell phenotype are called "null-cell phenotype" (both entities are clinicopathologically and genetically identical and thus considered the same entity).[41–43] ALK+ ALCL expresses ALK proteins and is characterized by rearrangement of the *ALK* gene on chromosome 2q23 with several translocation partners, the most common being nucleophosmin *(NPM)* on chromosome 5q35 (t (2; 5)). Other common partners include genes such as *TPM3, ATIC, TFG, CLTC, MSN,* or *TPM4*. In adults, the prognosis of *ALK*-rearranged cases is superior to those without ALK alterations and is independent of the *ALK* fusion partner. Nevertheless, the prognostic impact in pediatric ALCL is difficult to ascertain because of the rarity of ALK-negative disease in children.[43] ALK-negative ALCL is morphologically indistinguishable from ALK+ ALCL; recurrent genetic alterations established in ALK-negative disease include rearrangements of DUSP22 and TP63.[44]

B. ALK+ ALCL is most common in the first three decades (median age of approximately 12 years) with a slight male predominance (male to female ratio 1.5:1). Patients frequently present with B symptoms and advanced stage III/IV disease. The vast majority (>90%) of cases have nodal involvement, often diffusely present above and below the diaphragm. In addition, extranodal involvement, such as skin, bone, lung, and liver, is not uncommon.[45] Bone marrow involvement is variable (<10% on basic morphologic analysis but 15%–30% if stained for CD30 and ALK and ~50% by polymerase chain reaction detection). CNS involvement occurs in less than 5% of cases.[46] Approximately 10% of children with ALCL can present with hemophagocytic lymphohistiocytosis (HLH) or HLH-like symptoms.[47]

Pediatric ALCL is a chemo-sensitive disease with high response rates to various chemotherapy regimens resulting in EFS and overall survival (OS) ranging from 65% to 75% and 70% to 90%, respectively.[17] Although no single regimen has emerged as definitively superior, the ALCL99 chemotherapy regimen is often considered frontline therapy because of its tolerability and short overall duration (4–5 months). The Children's Oncology Group (COG) recently reported outcomes based on frontline treatment with the anti-CD30 monoclonal antibody brentuximab vedotin plus ALCL99 backbone chemotherapy. The 2-year EFS was 79.1% with an OS of 97%, and only one patient experienced an event during therapy. Although there was no control arm to evaluate the impact of brentuximab in a randomized fashion, the authors commented that therapy was well-tolerated, and there were no on-therapy relapses.[17]

Overall, despite the wide range of chemotherapy regimens tested to date, none have improved the failure rate of approximately 25% that still occurs. Most patients relapse soon after completion of chemotherapy (median time to relapse 1.7 months).[48] Fortunately, most patients are still treatment-responsive at relapse, with astounding complete response rates of approximately 80% reported in phase I/II clinical trials using monotherapy with the ALK-inhibitor crizotinib.[49] Recent data from Europe have demonstrated superior long-term outcomes after consolidation of reinduction therapy with allogeneic HSCT for those patients that experience early relapse (defined as occurring ≤12 months after diagnosis). Alternatively, weekly vinblastine monotherapy has shown high response rates and long-lasting remission in patients with late relapse and CD3-negative disease.[48]

10. (A) How is the biology of PMBL different from DLBCL, and (B) what are some distinctions in the therapeutic approach?

A. PMBL arises from medullary thymic B-cells and characteristically presents with a bulky anterior mediastinal mass. Although PMBL was historically classified as a subtype of DLBCL, its clinical, histological, and biological features lie along a spectrum between DLBCL and nodular sclerosis classical Hodgkin lymphoma (HL), with which it shares approximately one-third of its genes and has common driver mutations.[50] JAK-STAT signaling activation has been identified as critical to the pathogenesis of PMBL.[51] More than half of PMBL cases have genomic gains of chromosome 9p24, which includes multiple genes, including JAK2 and the programmed death ligands.[52]

B. Around the turn of the century, children with PMBL were treated the same as patients with DLBCL and experienced inferior outcomes compared with their counterparts on both LMB and BFM regimens (EFS ranging between 67%–70% PMBL vs. ~85% for other mature B-NHL).[53,54] Although treatment regimens for adults with PMBL historically used consolidation radiation therapy after B-NHL chemotherapy regimens, outcomes from those early pediatric studies were based on radiotherapy-free treatment. Prospective and retrospective adult studies evaluating the use of the dose-adjusted EPOCH (infusional vincristine/doxorubicin/etoposide plus prednisone and cyclophosphamide) with rituximab (da-EPOCH-R) regimen offered compelling evidence that EFS in the 80% to 90% range could be achieved with minimal exposure to radiation therapy for adult patients.[55–57] Subsequently, a prospective international phase II clinical trial was performed to determine the efficacy of da-EPOCH-R (without radiation) in children and adolescents with PMBL. The results were not yet published at the time of writing; however, interim reports at international conferences reported the EFS to be approximately 70%. With EFS outcome being less than hoped for, the current COG PMBL study (ANHL1931) will continue with the same da-EPOCH-R backbone, randomized to include nivolumab in a multicenter, multiconsortium AYA trial. Patients with biopsy-proven residual disease at the end of therapy will receive consolidation radiation therapy in that study.

11. Describe the categorization, clinical features, and treatment approach for post-transplant lymphoproliferative disorders.

Post-transplant lymphoproliferative disorders (PTLD) represent a heterogeneous group of diverse diagnostic entities that occur in patients receiving immune suppression after solid organ or allogeneic HSCT. Conceptually, prototypical PTLD encompasses the spectrum of lymphoproliferation driven by EBV infection ranging from early lesion/nondestructive PTLD to polymorphic/destructive PTLD to monomorphic/destructive PTLD with DLBCL histology.[6] Post-transplant monomorphic lymphomas (such as BL and HL) are also broadly categorized as PTLD, despite distinctions in disease pathogenesis, frequency of EBV involvement, clinical features, treatment considerations, and survival outcomes (Table 39.4).[58,59] Such disparate differences—especially in treatment strategies and survival—suggest that these diagnostic entities should be considered separately rather than lumped together.

Table 39.4 Categorizing Post-Transplant Epstein-Barr Virus (EBV) Infection and Associated Post-Transplant Lymphoproliferative Disorders (PTLDs)

CATEGORY	LYMPHOCYTIC INFILTRATE	HISTOLOGY	TYPICAL THERAPY	EBV ASSOCIATION	THINK OF AS …
EBV Viremia	None	Normal	RI and clinical observation	Always	Post-transplant EBV infection (primary vs reactivation)
Early Lesion	Nondestructive	Plasmacytic hyperplasia Infectious mononucleosis-like florid follicular hyperplasia	Most likely to respond to RI	Almost always EBV+	EBV-driven reactive lymphoid hyperplasia
Polymorphic	Destructive	Polymorphous infiltrate with various stages of B-cell maturation, often clonal	May respond to RI, but often requires rituximab	Usually EBV+ (> 90%)	Lymphoid neoplasia
Monomorphic	Destructive	DLBCL	Up to 50% respond to rituximab alone Alternatively, low-dose CPR	Often EBV+	Lymphoid neoplasia vs De Novo Lymphoma
Monomorphic	Destructive	Burkitt lymphoma T/NK-cell lymphoma Plasma cell neoplasm	Require disease-specific multiagent chemotherapy	Often EBV-negative	De Novo Lymphoma occurring posttransplant
Hodgkin Lymphoma	Destructive	Classical Hodgkin lymphoma	Requires disease-specific multiagent chemotherapy	Usually EBV+ (> 90%)	De Novo Lymphoma occurring posttransplant

CPR, Cyclophosphamide (low-dose), prednisone, and rituximab chemotherapy regimen; *DLBCL*, diffuse large B-cell lymphoma; *NK*, natural killer; *RI*, reduction of immune suppression.

The clinical features of PTLD vary considerably. Patients can present with systemic symptoms (fevers, night sweats, weight loss), involvement of lymphoid organs (lymphadenopathy, hepatosplenomegaly, tonsillar/adenoidal hypertrophy) or extranodal tissue (GI symptoms such as malabsorption, nausea/vomiting, or bloody stool), or with dysfunction of the allograft. Fulminant PTLD is rare but severe and characterized by rapid progression of multiorgan failure with cytopenias. The onset of EBV-associated PTLD is typically preceded by a substantial increase in viral load and the proliferation of EBV-infected B cells. Frequent monitoring of the EBV viral load in peripheral blood is a valuable screening test for EBV-associated PTLD.[58,59]

Treatment of PTLD depends entirely on the underlying histology. Initial considerations include the reduction of immune suppression if feasible without risking the allograft. For patients with the prototypical spectrum of PTLD, including early lesion/nondestructive, polymorphic, and monomorphic DLBCL, reduction in immune suppression may be all that is required to restore EBV-specific immunity and achieve durable remission. Nevertheless, patients with polymorphic PTLD and monomorphic DLBCL often require systemic therapy, typically either rituximab or rituximab plus low-dose chemotherapy (cyclophosphamide plus prednisone).[59,60] For patients with non-DLBCL monomorphic PTLD or DLBCL that does not respond to rituximab plus low-dose chemotherapy, multiagent histology-specific chemotherapy is required for definitive treatment.[61] Recent development of adoptive cellular immunotherapies that target EBV-specific antigens offer promise for novel, less toxic therapeutic approaches for a subset of patients with immunogenic, EBV[+] disease.[58]

12. Provide context for the occurrence of rare NHL.

Although the most common childhood/adolescent histologies have been described, some rare NHL require consideration (see Table 39.2). The most common rare B-cell NHLs include indolent lymphomas such as follicular lymphoma and marginal zone lymphoma, both of which have pediatric-specific disease entities with significant clinical and biological distinctions from disease typically seen in adults.[62] Other rare B-cell NHLs described in the pediatric population include EBV-associated neoplasms that may or may not be linked with underlying immunodeficiency syndromes such as EBV[+] DLBCL, NOS; lymphomatoid granulomatosis; primary CNS lymphoma; plasmablastic lymphoma; and primary effusion lymphoma.

In the T/NK-cell compartment, a long list of rare lymphomas demonstrates extreme clinical heterogeneity with distinct patterns of organ involvement, disease presentation, and survival outcomes.[63,64] For example, survival for peripheral T-cell lymphoma (PTCL), NOS—the most common of the rare T/NK-NHL in children—is reported as approximately 50% after treatment with multiagent chemotherapy. In sharp contrast, long-term survival for patients with hepatosplenic gamma-delta T-cell lymphoma is rare in the absence of aggressive chemotherapy regimens followed by allogeneic HSCT.[62] Alternatively, some of the rare T/NK-cell NHL with primarily cutaneous disease presentations are characterized by favorable survival outcomes without intensive chemotherapy. Finally, a category of EBV-associated lymphoid neoplasms exists in the T/NK-cell compartment, representing some of the most lethal and challenging diagnostic entities in pediatric NHL.[65]

REFERENCES

1. Swerdlow SH, Campo E, Pileri SA, et al. The 2016 revision of the World Health Organization classification of lymphoid neoplasms. *Blood.* 2016;127(20):2375–2390.
2. Minard-Colin V, Brugieres L, Reiter A, et al. Non-Hodgkin lymphoma in children and adolescents: progress through effective collaboration, current knowledge, and challenges ahead. *J Clin Oncol.* 2015;33(27):2963–2974.
3. Ward E, DeSantis C, Robbins A, Kohler B, Jemal A. Childhood and adolescent cancer statistics, 2014. *CA Cancer J Clin.* 2014;64 (2):83–103.
4. Ozuah NW, El-Mallawany NK. Childhood and adolescence non-Hodgkin lymphomas in low- and middle-income countries. In: Abla O, Attarbaschi A (eds). *Non-Hodgkin's Lymphoma in Childhood and Adolescence.* Springer International Publishing, 2019:337–351.
5. Thacker N, Abla O. Epidemiology of Non-Hodgkin Lymphomas in Childhood and Adolescence. In: Abla O, Attarbaschi A (eds). *Non-Hodgkin's Lymphoma in Childhood and Adolescence.* Springer International Publishing, 2019:15–22.
6. Natkunam Y, Gratzinger D, Chadburn A, et al. Immunodeficiency-associated lymphoproliferative disorders: time for reappraisal? *Blood.* 2018;132(18):1871–1878.
7. Hoelzer D, Walewski J, Dohner H, et al. Improved outcome of adult Burkitt lymphoma/leukemia with rituximab and chemotherapy: report of a large prospective multicenter trial. *Blood.* 2014;124(26):3870–3879.
8. Hochberg J, El-Mallawany NK, Abla O. Adolescent and young adult non-Hodgkin lymphoma. *Br J Haematol.* 2016;173(4):637–650.
9. Deffenbacher KE, Iqbal J, Sanger W, et al. Molecular distinctions between pediatric and adult mature B-cell non-Hodgkin lymphomas identified through genomic profiling. *Blood.* 2012;119(16):3757–3766.
10. Oschlies I, Klapper W, Zimmermann M, et al. Diffuse large B-cell lymphoma in pediatric patients belongs predominantly to the germinal center type B-cell lymphomas: a clinicopathologic analysis of cases included in the German BFM (Berlin-Frankfurt-Munster) Multicenter Trial. *Blood.* 2006;107(10):4047–4052.
11. Klapper W, Szczepanowski M, Burkhardt B, et al. Molecular profiling of pediatric mature B-cell lymphoma treated in population-based prospective clinical trials. *Blood.* 2008;112(4):1374–1381.
12. Miles RR, Shah RK, Frazer JK. Molecular genetics of childhood, adolescent and young adult non-Hodgkin lymphoma. *Br J Haematol.* 2016;173(4):582–596.
13. Ehrhardt MJ, Hochberg J, Bjornard KL, Brinkman TM. Long-term survivors of childhood, adolescent and young adult non-Hodgkin lymphoma. *Br J Haematol.* 2019;185(6):1099–1110.
14. Murphy SB. Classification, staging and end results of treatment of childhood non-Hodgkin's lymphomas: dissimilarities from lymphomas in adults. *Semin Oncol.* 1980;7(3):332–339.

15. Rosolen A, Perkins SL, Pinkerton CR, et al. Revised International Pediatric Non-Hodgkin Lymphoma Staging System. *J Clin Oncol.* 2015;33(18):2112–2118.
16. Minard-Colin V, Auperin A, Pillon M, et al. Rituximab for high-risk, mature B-cell non-Hodgkin's lymphoma in children. *N Engl J Med.* 2020;382(23):2207–2219.
17. Lowe EJ, Reilly AF, Lim MS, et al. Brentuximab vedotin in combination with chemotherapy for pediatric patients with ALK+ ALCL: results of COG trial ANHL12P1. *Blood.* 2021;137(26):3595–3603.
18. El-Mallawany NK, Cairo MS. Advances in the diagnosis and treatment of childhood and adolescent B-cell non-Hodgkin lymphoma. *Clin Adv Hematol Oncol.* 2015;13(2):113–123.
19. Egan G, Goldman S, Alexander S. Mature B-NHL in children, adolescents and young adults: current therapeutic approach and emerging treatment strategies. *Br J Haematol.* 2019;185(6):1071–1085.
20. Cairo MS, Sposto R, Gerrard M, et al. Advanced stage, increased lactate dehydrogenase, and primary site, but not adolescent age (>/= 15 years), are associated with an increased risk of treatment failure in children and adolescents with mature B-cell non-Hodgkin's lymphoma: results of the FAB LMB 96 study. *J Clin Oncol.* 2012;30(4):387–393.
21. Gerrard M, Cairo MS, Weston C, et al. Excellent survival following two courses of COPAD chemotherapy in children and adolescents with resected localized B-cell non-Hodgkin's lymphoma: results of the FAB/LMB 96 international study. *Br J Haematol.* 2008; 141(6):840–847.
22. Patte C, Auperin A, Gerrard M, et al. Results of the randomized international FAB/LMB96 trial for intermediate risk B-cell non-Hodgkin lymphoma in children and adolescents: it is possible to reduce treatment for the early responding patients. *Blood.* 2007;109(7): 2773–2780.
23. Cairo MS, Gerrard M, Sposto R, et al. Results of a randomized international study of high-risk central nervous system B non-Hodgkin lymphoma and B acute lymphoblastic leukemia in children and adolescents. *Blood.* 2007;109(7):2736-43.
24. Woessmann W, Seidemann K, Mann G, et al. The impact of the methotrexate administration schedule and dose in the treatment of children and adolescents with B-cell neoplasms. a report of the BFM Group Study NHL-BFM95. *Blood.* 2005;105(3):948–958.
25. Meinhardt A, Burkhardt B, Zimmermann M, et al. Phase II window study on rituximab in newly diagnosed pediatric mature B-cell non-Hodgkin's lymphoma and Burkitt leukemia. *J Clin Oncol.* 2010;28(19):3115–3121.
26. Ozuah NW, Lubega J, Allen CE, El-Mallawany NK. Five decades of low intensity and low survival: adapting intensified regimens to cure pediatric Burkitt lymphoma in Africa. *Blood Adv.* 2020;4(16):4007–4019.
27. Rigaud C, Auperin A, Jourdain A, et al. Outcome of relapse in children and adolescents with B-cell non-Hodgkin lymphoma and mature acute leukemia: a report from the French LMB study. *Pediatr Blood Cancer.* 2019;66(9):e27873.
28. Cairo M, Auperin A, Perkins SL, et al. Overall survival of children and adolescents with mature B cell non-Hodgkin lymphoma who had refractory or relapsed disease during or after treatment with FAB/LMB 96: a report from the FAB/LMB 96 study group. *Br J Haematol.* 2018;182(6):859–869.
29. Woessmann W, Zimmermann M, Meinhardt A, et al. Progressive or relapsed Burkitt lymphoma or leukemia in children and adolescents after BFM-type first-line therapy. *Blood.* 2020;135(14):1124–1132.
30. Burkhardt B, Taj M, Garnier N, et al. Treatment and outcome analysis of 639 relapsed non-Hodgkin lymphomas in children and adolescents and resulting treatment recommendations. *Cancers (Basel).* 2021;13(9).
31. Burkhardt B, Oschlies I, Klapper W, et al. Non-Hodgkin's lymphoma in adolescents: experiences in 378 adolescent NHL patients treated according to pediatric NHL-BFM protocols. *Leukemia.* 2011;25(1):153–160.
32. Termuhlen AM, Smith LM, Perkins SL, et al. Disseminated lymphoblastic lymphoma in children and adolescents: results of the COG A5971 trial: a report from the Children's Oncology Group. *Br J Haematol.* 2013;162(6):792–801.
33. Termuhlen AM, Smith LM, Perkins SL, et al. Outcome of newly diagnosed children and adolescents with localized lymphoblastic lymphoma treated on Children's Oncology Group trial A5971: a report from the Children's Oncology Group. *Pediatr Blood Cancer.* 2012;59(7):1229–1233.
34. Burkhardt B. Paediatric lymphoblastic T-cell leukaemia and lymphoma: one or two diseases? *Br J Haematol.* 2010;149(5):653–668.
35. Burkhardt B, Hermiston ML. Lymphoblastic lymphoma in children and adolescents: review of current challenges and future opportunities. *Br J Haematol.* 2019;185(6):1158–1170.
36. Teachey DT, O'Connor D. How I treat newly diagnosed T-cell acute lymphoblastic leukemia and T-cell lymphoblastic lymphoma in children. *Blood.* 2020;135(3):159–166.
37. Hayashi RJ, Winter SS, Dunsmore KP, et al. Successful outcomes of newly diagnosed T lymphoblastic lymphoma: results from Children's Oncology Group AALL0434. *J Clin Oncol.* 2020;38(26):3062–3070.
38. Coustan-Smith E, Sandlund JT, Perkins SL, et al. Minimal disseminated disease in childhood T-cell lymphoblastic lymphoma: a report from the Children's Oncology Group. *J Clin Oncol.* 2009;27(21):3533–3539.
39. Conter V, Valsecchi MG, Buldini B, et al. Early T-cell precursor acute lymphoblastic leukaemia in children treated in AIEOP centres with AIEOP-BFM protocols: a retrospective analysis. *Lancet Haematol.* 2016;3(2):e80–e86.
40. Burkhardt B, Reiter A, Landmann E, et al. Poor outcome for children and adolescents with progressive disease or relapse of lymphoblastic lymphoma: a report from the Berlin-Frankfurt-Muenster Group. *J Clin Oncol.* 2009;27(20):3363–3369.
41. Lamant L, McCarthy K, d'Amore E, et al. Prognostic impact of morphologic and phenotypic features of childhood ALK-positive anaplastic large-cell lymphoma: results of the ALCL99 study. *J Clin Oncol.* 2011;29(35):4669–4676.
42. Mussolin L, Le Deley MC, Carraro E, et al. Prognostic factors in childhood anaplastic large cell lymphoma: long term results of the International ALCL99 Trial. *Cancers (Basel).* 2020;12(10).
43. Lowe EJ, Gross TG. Anaplastic large cell lymphoma in children and adolescents. *Pediatr Hematol Oncol.* 2013;30(6):509–519.
44. Parrilla Castellar ER, Jaffe ES, Said JW, et al. ALK-negative anaplastic large cell lymphoma is a genetically heterogeneous disease with widely disparate clinical outcomes. *Blood.* 2014;124(9):1473–1480.
45. Le Deley MC, Reiter A, Williams D, et al. Prognostic factors in childhood anaplastic large cell lymphoma: results of a large European intergroup study. *Blood.* 2008;111(3):1560–1566.
46. Williams D, Mori T, Reiter A, et al. Central nervous system involvement in anaplastic large cell lymphoma in childhood: results from a multicentre European and Japanese study. *Pediatr Blood Cancer.* 2013;60(10):E118–E121.
47. Pasqualini C, Minard-Colin V, Saada V, et al. Clinical analysis and prognostic significance of haemophagocytic lymphohistiocytosis-associated anaplastic large cell lymphoma in children. *Br J Haematol.* 2014;165(1):117–125.

48. Knörr F, Brugières L, Pillon M, et al. Stem cell transplantation and vinblastine monotherapy for relapsed pediatric anaplastic large cell lymphoma: results of the international, prospective ALCL-Relapse Trial. *J Clin Oncol.* 2020;38(34):3999–4009.
49. Mossé YP, Voss SD, Lim MS, et al. Targeting ALK With crizotinib in pediatric anaplastic large cell lymphoma and inflammatory myofibroblastic tumor: a Children's Oncology Group Study. *J Clin Oncol.* 2017;35(28):3215–3221.
50. Rosenwald A, Wright G, Leroy K, et al. Molecular diagnosis of primary mediastinal B cell lymphoma identifies a clinically favorable subgroup of diffuse large B cell lymphoma related to Hodgkin lymphoma. *J Exper Med.* 2003;198(6):851–862.
51. Viganò E, Gunawardana J, Mottok A, et al. Somatic IL4R mutations in primary mediastinal large B-cell lymphoma lead to constitutive JAK-STAT signaling activation. *Blood.* 2018;131(18):2036–2046.
52. Twa DD, Chan FC, Ben-Neriah S, et al. Genomic rearrangements involving programmed death ligands are recurrent in primary mediastinal large B-cell lymphoma. *Blood.* 2014;123(13):2062–2065.
53. Gerrard M, Waxman IM, Sposto R, et al. Outcome and pathologic classification of children and adolescents with mediastinal large B-cell lymphoma treated with FAB/LMB96 mature B-NHL therapy. *Blood.* 2013;121(2):278–285.
54. Seidemann K, Tiemann M, Lauterbach I, et al. Primary mediastinal large B-cell lymphoma with sclerosis in pediatric and adolescent patients: treatment and results from three therapeutic studies of the Berlin-Frankfurt-Münster Group. *J Clin Oncol.* 2003;21(9):1782–1789.
55. Dunleavy K, Pittaluga S, Maeda LS, et al. Dose-adjusted EPOCH-rituximab therapy in primary mediastinal B-cell lymphoma. *N Engl J Med.* 2013;368(15):1408–1416.
56. Giulino-Roth L, O'Donohue T, Chen Z, et al. Outcomes of adults and children with primary mediastinal B-cell lymphoma treated with dose-adjusted EPOCH-R. *Br J Haematol.* 2017;179(5):739–747.
57. Giulino-Roth L. How I treat primary mediastinal B-cell lymphoma. *Blood.* 2018;132(8):782–790.
58. Wistinghausen B, Gross TG, Bollard C. Post-transplant lymphoproliferative disease in pediatric solid organ transplant recipients. *Pediatr Hematol Oncol.* 2013;30(6):520–531.
59. Mynarek M, Schober T, Behrends U, Maecker-Kolhoff B. Posttransplant lymphoproliferative disease after pediatric solid organ transplantation. *Clin Dev Immunol.* 2013;2013, 814973.
60. Gross TG, Orjuela MA, Perkins SL, et al. Low-dose chemotherapy and rituximab for posttransplant lymphoproliferative disease (PTLD): a Children's Oncology Group Report. *Am J Transplant.* 2012;12(11):3069–3075.
61. Maecker B, Jack T, Zimmermann M, et al. CNS or bone marrow involvement as risk factors for poor survival in post-transplantation lymphoproliferative disorders in children after solid organ transplantation. *J Clin Oncol.* 2007;25(31):4902–4908.
62. Attarbaschi A, Abla O, Arias Padilla L, et al. Rare non-Hodgkin lymphoma of childhood and adolescence: a consensus diagnostic and therapeutic approach to pediatric-type follicular lymphoma, marginal zone lymphoma, and nonanaplastic peripheral T-cell lymphoma. *Pediatr Blood Cancer.* 2020;67(8):e28416.
63. Xavier AC, Suzuki R. Treatment and prognosis of mature (non-anaplastic) T- and NK-cell lymphomas in childhood, adolescents, and young adults. *Br J Haematol.* 2019;185(6):1086–1098.
64. Flower A, Xavier AC, Cairo MS. Mature (non-anaplastic, non-cutaneous) T-/NK-cell lymphomas in children, adolescents and young adults: state of the science. *Br J Haematol.* 2019;185(3):418–435.
65. El-Mallawany NK, Curry CV, Allen CE. Haemophagocytic lymphohistiocytosis and Epstein-Barr virus: a complex relationship with diverse origins, expression and outcomes. *Br J Haematol.* 2021.

CHAPTER 40

NEURO-ONCOLOGY

Luca Szalontay, MD and Stergios Zacharoulis, MD

1. How common are childhood central nervous system tumors?

Approximately 3500 cases of pediatric central nervous system (CNS) tumors are diagnosed each year in the United States with an incidence of 6.1 per 100,000.[1] They are the most common solid tumors in the pediatric age group and are the leading cause of cancer-related death in this population.

2. How are brain tumors classified?

Brain tumors are classified on the basis of cell origin, histology, and molecular alterations. The international classification of human tumors published by the World Health Organization (WHO) was initiated in 1957, and its goal has been to clearly define the classification and grading of tumors, which is accepted and used worldwide. In 2016 the WHO published an update to classification of CNS tumors that, for the first time, combined molecular alterations together with histologic findings in the diagnoses. With the rapid advances in understanding how molecular findings impact diagnosis, grading of brain tumors, management, and prognosis, an updated WHO CNS tumor classification was released in 2021.[2]

3. Which CNS tumors are associated with a cancer predisposition syndrome?

About 5% of childhood CNS tumors are linked to specific inherited genetic disorders. Table 40.1 summarizes the most important cancer predisposition syndromes associated with CNS tumors.

4. What are the symptoms of the brain tumors?

Supratentorial tumors include tumors of the cerebral hemispheres, basal ganglia, thalamus, and hypothalamus. These tumors can show signs of increased intracranial pressure, such as early morning headache or headache that goes away after vomiting. In addition, these tumors may be accompanied by focal deficits, such as memory loss, weakness, visual changes, hearing loss, speech problems, and deterioration of school performance. They can often present with *seizure* when the tumor involves the temporal lobe. A constellation of symptoms, called *diencephalic syndrome,* occurs in the presence of a hypothalamic-optic chiasmatic tumor, including failure to thrive and severe emaciation despite normal caloric intake, hyperactivity, euphoria, anemia without pallor, hypoglycemia, and hypotension.

Infratentorial tumors include tumors of the cerebellum and brainstem. When infratentorial tumors block cerebrospinal fluid (CSF) outflow, headache and vomiting may be the presenting signs; they can also become apparent with localizing signs such as cranial nerve palsies or ataxia (loss of balance and trouble walking).

In infants, symptoms can be nonspecific but may include irritability, loss of appetite, and developmental delay or regression.

Figure 40.1 summarizes the symptoms associated with different brain areas.[3]

5. What are the symptoms of a spinal cord tumor?

Spinal tenderness on percussion correlates with the site of the tumor in up to 80% of patients. *Muscle weakness* or *numbness* in the arms or legs is also a common symptom. Sensory level changes and *decreased reflexes* can also suggest spinal cord involvement. The collection of nerves at the end of the spinal cord is known the cauda equina; compression of these nerve roots can cause loss of bowel or bladder function and saddle anesthesia. Spinal cord compression most commonly occurs in the thoracic area (70%) compared with the lumbar (20%) and cervical (10%) regions.

6. How have recent advances in neuroimaging helped in the management of CNS tumors?

Magnetic resonance imaging (MRI) is the standard imaging modality in the evaluation of CNS tumors. Not only does it generate high-resolution maps of tissue anatomy, but also functional imaging techniques like MR spectroscopy, perfusion imaging, and diffusion-weighted MRI can interrogate tumor biology, guide biopsy and resection, and help monitoring disease response. Correlation between tumor location/enhancement and medulloblastoma subgroups has been recently demonstrated that MRI can serve as a surrogate for genomic testing.[4]

7. What are the symptoms of posterior fossa syndrome?

Posterior fossa syndrome, also known as cerebellar mutism, refers to a group of symptoms noted most commonly after surgery for posterior fossa tumors in the pediatric population. These signs and symptoms include mutism or speech disturbances, dysphagia, decreased motor movement, cranial nerve palsies, and emotional lability. They develop in 1 to 4 days after surgery and may take weeks to months to resolve.[5]

Table 40.1 Cancer Predisposition Syndromes Associated With Central Nervous System Tumors

CANCER PREDISPOSITION SYNDROME	MUTATED GENE	CLINICAL FEATURES	ROLE OF MUTATED GENE	TUMOR ASSOCIATION
Neurofibromatosis 1	NF1	Café-au-lait macules, neurofibromas, freckling in axillary and inguinal region, Lisch nodules, learning disabilities, bone deformities	Negative regulator of the *Ras* proto-oncogene	Optic pathway glioma, glioblastoma, brainstem glioma, peripheral malignant nerve sheet tumor
Neurofibromatosis 2	NF2	Vestibular schwannoma, neurofibromas, meningioma, cataract	Merlin (schwannomin) is a cell membrane-related protein that acts as a tumor suppressor	Bilateral vestibular schwannoma, meningioma, glioma
Tuberous sclerosis complex	TSC1, TSC2	Seizures, skin angiofibroma, focal hypopigmentation, cardiac rhabdomyoma, renal angiomyolipoma, retinal astrocytic hamartomas, developmental delay	Hamartin *(TSC1)* and tuberin *(TSC2)* are heterodimerizing tumor suppressor proteins	Subependymal giant cell astrocytoma
Von Hippel-Lindau syndrome	pVHL	Renal angiomas, clear cell renal cell carcinoma, pheochromocytoma, endolymphatic sac tumor, serous cystadenomas	pVHL protein is a tumor suppressor that forms a complex and targets certain proteins for proteasomal degradation	Hemangioblastoma of brain and spine
Turcot syndrome	APC	Multiple adenomatous colon polyps, increased risk of colorectal cancer and central nervous system tumors	Negative regulator that controls β-catenin concentrations	Medulloblastoma
	hMLH1, hPMS2		DNA mismatch repair	Glioblastoma
Gorlin syndrome	PTCH1	Developmental abnormalities, bone cysts, increased risk of basal cell carcinoma and medulloblastoma	Receptor for sonic hedgehog	Medulloblastoma
	SUFU		Negative regulator in the hedgehog/smoothened signaling pathway	
Li Fraumeni syndrome	TP53	Multiple cancer types and primary sites (breast, sarcomas, brain tumors, adrenocortical carcinoma) at an early onset	Tumor suppressor protein, regulates genes involved in cell cycle arrest, apoptosis, senescence, DNA repair and changes in metabolism	Choroid plexus carcinoma, glioblastoma, medulloblastoma

Continued on following page

Table 40.1 Cancer Predisposition Syndromes Associated With Central Nervous System Tumors (*Continued*)

CANCER PREDISPOSITION SYNDROME	MUTATED GENE	CLINICAL FEATURES	ROLE OF MUTATED GENE	TUMOR ASSOCIATION
Fanconi anemia	BRCA2/ FANCD1	Developmental abnormalities, bone marrow failure, predisposition to medulloblastoma	Double-strand DNA break repair, vital in homologous recombination	Medulloblastoma
	PALB2		Partner and localizer of BRCA2	
Rubenstein Taybi syndrome	CREBBP	Microcephaly, growth deficiency, dysmorphic features, intellectual disability, increased risk of brain tumors	CREB-binding protein–coactivator of transcription factors	Medulloblastoma
Ataxia Telangiectasia	ATM	Cerebellar atrophy, telangiectasias, immunodeficiency, radiosensitivity, malignancies	Protein kinase involved in the repair of DNA double-strand breaks	Meningioma, glioblastoma, pilocytic astrocytoma

8. Which chemotherapy is able to cross the blood-brain barrier, and which agents can be administered intrathecally?

The blood-brain barrier is a network of blood vessels and cells that maintains relatively constant levels of nutrients, water, and hormones in the brain and protects against circulating toxins and pathogens. For a chemotherapy to work in tumors localized to the CNS, it must have the ability to cross the blood-brain barrier. This greatly limits the number of chemotherapies that can be used in the treatment of brain tumors. The most commonly used agents are temozolomide, vincristine, carmustine (BCNU), lomustine (CCNU), cisplatin, carboplatin, etoposide, irinotecan, methotrexate, procarbazine, thiotepa, and cyclophosphamide.

Thiotepa, etoposide, cytarabine, methotrexate, and a novel formulation of nitrosourea (BCNU) are agents used for intrathecal administration of CNS malignancies. It can deliver high drug concentration to the CSF while minimizing systemic toxicities through an Ommaya-reservoir or when performing a lumbar puncture.

9. A 14-year-old girl presents with unsteady gait, dizziness, headache, and vomiting. MRI shows a lateral cerebellar hemispheric tumor with cystic and solid components. What is the likely diagnosis, and which signal transduction pathway is the most often involved in these tumors?

The child most likely has juvenile pilocytic astrocytoma. They are usually resectable with an excellent survival after surgery alone. Emerging evidence indicates that the Ras-RAF-ERK signaling pathway is hyperactive in gliomas, not only because of its upstream regulators but also because of somatic mutations, copy number changes, and active fusion proteins, as shown in Figure 40.2.[6] *BRAF-KIAA* fusions are common in cerebellar and optic pathway pilocytic tumors and lead to constitutive activation of the BRAF protein, whereas *BRAF* mutations are more common in gangliogliomas, pleomorphic xanthoastrocytomas, and cerebral pilocytic astrocytoma.[7] One of the most studied entities is the BRAF V600E mutation, which constitutively activates the pathway maintaining tumor proliferation. Anti-Ras/RAF therapy is being actively exploited for patients with these tumors. Vemurafenib or dabrafenib interrupts the BRAF/MEK step and works in patients whose cancer harbors the V600E mutation. Trametinib, selumetinib, or binimetinib blocks the pathway at the level of the downstream effector MEK. They are often used in combination to prevent resistance. There is an ongoing clinical trial comparing traditional chemotherapy (carboplatin and vincristine) with targeted therapy as a first-line management.

10. A 7-year-old boy presents with progressive vomiting, morning headaches, and unsteadiness of 6 weeks' duration. MRI reveals a contrast-enhancing tumor filling the fourth ventricle, resulting in obstructive hydrocephalus. What is the most likely diagnosis, and what are the characteristics of the different subgroups?

Medulloblastoma is the most common malignant brain tumor of childhood, accounting for about 20% of all childhood brain tumors. Standard treatment includes surgery, craniospinal irradiation, and adjuvant chemotherapy. Analysis of

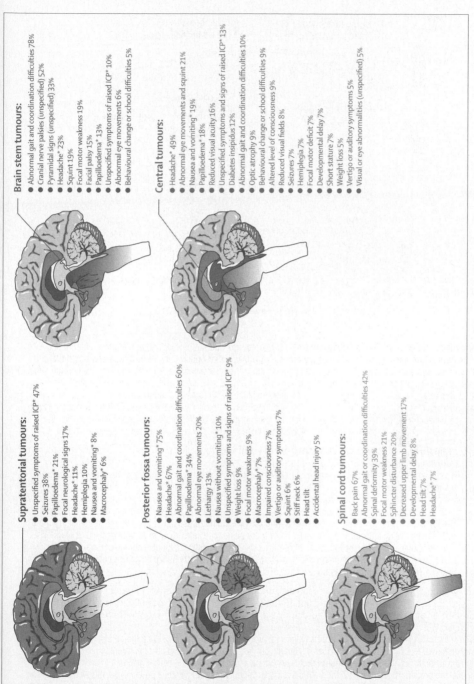

Supratentorial tumours:
- Unspecified symptoms of raised ICP* 47%
- Seizures 38%
- Papilloedema* 21%
- Focal neurological signs 17%
- Headache* 11%
- Hemiplegia 10%
- Nausea and vomiting* 8%
- Macrocephaly* 6%

Posterior fossa tumours:
- Nausea and vomiting* 75%
- Headache* 67%
- Abnormal gait and coordination difficulties 60%
- Papilloedema* 34%
- Abnormal eye movements 20%
- Lethargy 13%
- Nausea without vomiting* 10%
- Unspecified symptoms and signs of raised ICP* 9%
- Weight loss 9%
- Focal motor weakness 9%
- Macrocephaly* 7%
- Impaired consciousness 7%
- Vertigo or auditory symptoms 7%
- Squint 6%
- Stiff neck 6%
- Head tilt
- Accidental head injury 5%

Spinal cord tumours:
- Back pain 67%
- Abnormal gait or coordination difficulties 42%
- Spinal deformity 39%
- Focal motor weakness 21%
- Sphincter disturbance 20%
- Decreased upper limb movement 17%
- Developmental delay 8%
- Head tilt 7%
- Headache* 7%

Brain stem tumours:
- Abnormal gait and coordination difficulties 78%
- Cranial nerve palsies (unspecified) 52%
- Pyramidal signs (unspecified) 33%
- Headache* 23%
- Squint 19%
- Focal motor weakness 19%
- Facial palsy 15%
- Papilloedema* 13%
- Unspecified symptoms of raised ICP* 10%
- Abnormal eye movements 6%
- Behavioural change or school difficulties 5%

Central tumours:
- Headache* 49%
- Abnormal eye movements and squint 21%
- Nausea and vomiting* 19%
- Papilloedema* 18%
- Reduced visual acuity 16%
- Unspecified symptoms and signs of raised ICP* 13%
- Diabetes insipidus 12%
- Abnormal gait and coordination difficulties 10%
- Optic atrophy 9%
- Behavioural change or school difficulties 9%
- Altered level of consciousness 9%
- Reduced visual fields 8%
- Seizures 7%
- Hemiplegia 7%
- Focal motor deficit 7%
- Developmental delay 7%
- Short stature 7%
- Weight loss 5%
- Vertigo or auditory symptoms 5%
- Visual or eye abnormalities (unspecified) 5%

Figure 40.1 Clinical presentation of childhood central nervous system (CNS) tumors. *ICP,* Intracranial pressure. *Symptoms or signs caused by increased intracranial pressure (ICP). (From Wilne S, Collier J, Kennedy C, Koller K, Grundy R, Walker D. Presentation of childhood CNS tumours: a systematic review and meta-analysis. *Lancet Oncol.* 2007;8:685–695.)

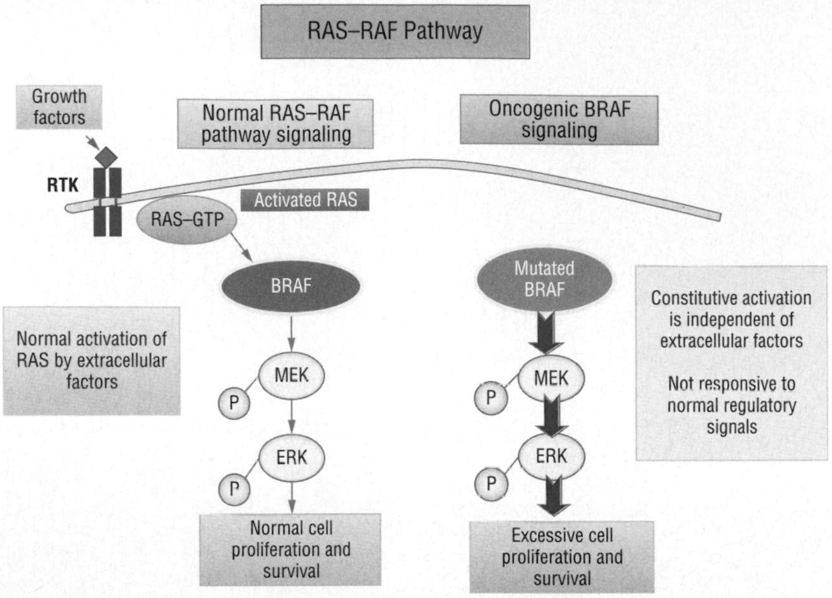

Figure 40.2 RAS-RAF-ERK pathway. (From Munoz-Couselo E, Soberino Garcia J, Perez-Garcia JM, et al. Recent advances in the treatment of melanoma with BRAF and MEK inhibitors. *Ann Trans Med.* 2015;3:207.)

molecular features divided medulloblastoma into four subgroups and not only helped in understanding the behavior of the tumor but also offered insight into the prognosis, providing an opportunity for individualized treatment. Group 1 tumors showing activation of the Wnt pathway have the best prognosis. Tumors with activation of the sonic hedgehog (SHH) pathway (Group 2) have an intermediate prognosis with the exception of the ones harboring TP53 mutations, which have poor prognosis. Medulloblastomas with high-level amplification MYC proto-oncogene with aberrant MYC expression (Group 3) have the worst prognosis. Group 4 medulloblastoma is a heterogenous group with amplification of MYCN and CDK6 and cytogenetic abnormalities including isochromosome 17q. It has an intermediate prognosis with 30% to 40% metastasis. These subgroups are summarized in Figure 40.3.[8]

11. **A 4-year-old boy presents with headache and vomiting, and MRI shows a tumor filling the fourth ventricle and also extending into the upper cervical spinal cord, with evidence of obstructive hydrocephalus. What is the most likely diagnosis, and what are the important prognostic factors in the tumor?**
    Ependymoma is a glial neoplasm derived from ependymal cells, which form the inner lining of the ventricles. Posterior fossa ependymomas may extend inferiorly through the foramen magnum in about 30% of the cases. There are several prognostic factors that can help predict the outcome. Complete resection of ependymoma results in more than 60% survival. Cranial location compared with primary spinal cord ependymomas, younger age at diagnosis, anaplastic histology, subtotal resection, and certain molecular characteristics, including chromosome 1q gain, 6q loss, and RELA fusion, all indicate worse prognosis. Risk stratification based on these variables can guide management of ependymoma patients, optimizing the combination of treatment modalities.

12. **A 6-year-old girl developed progressive cranial neuropathy, motor weakness, and disturbance of speech and swallowing in the past 2 weeks. MRI shows an expansile lesion occupying the center of the pons. What is the diagnosis and the most likely genetic finding on molecular analysis?**
    Diffuse intrinsic pontine glioma (DIPG) carries the worst prognosis of any childhood brain tumor, being nearly uniformly fatal within 18 to 24 months. Surgery does not impact survival, and the only standard treatment improving symptoms is involved field radiation therapy. The molecular hallmark of DIPG and other midline gliomas is an alteration in the histone protein (H3K27M mutation). DNA is usually wrapped around the histone proteins, but this alteration opens up the DNA, making it more vulnerable to mutations. Histone-deacetylase inhibitors have been promising candidates in DIPG clinical trials. The major difficulty in treating DIPG is overcoming the blood-brain barrier; however, new approaches are rapidly emerging, including convection-enhanced delivery of drugs, focused ultrasound to temporarily disrupt the blood-brain barrier, and liposomes or nanoparticles to be used as drug carriers.

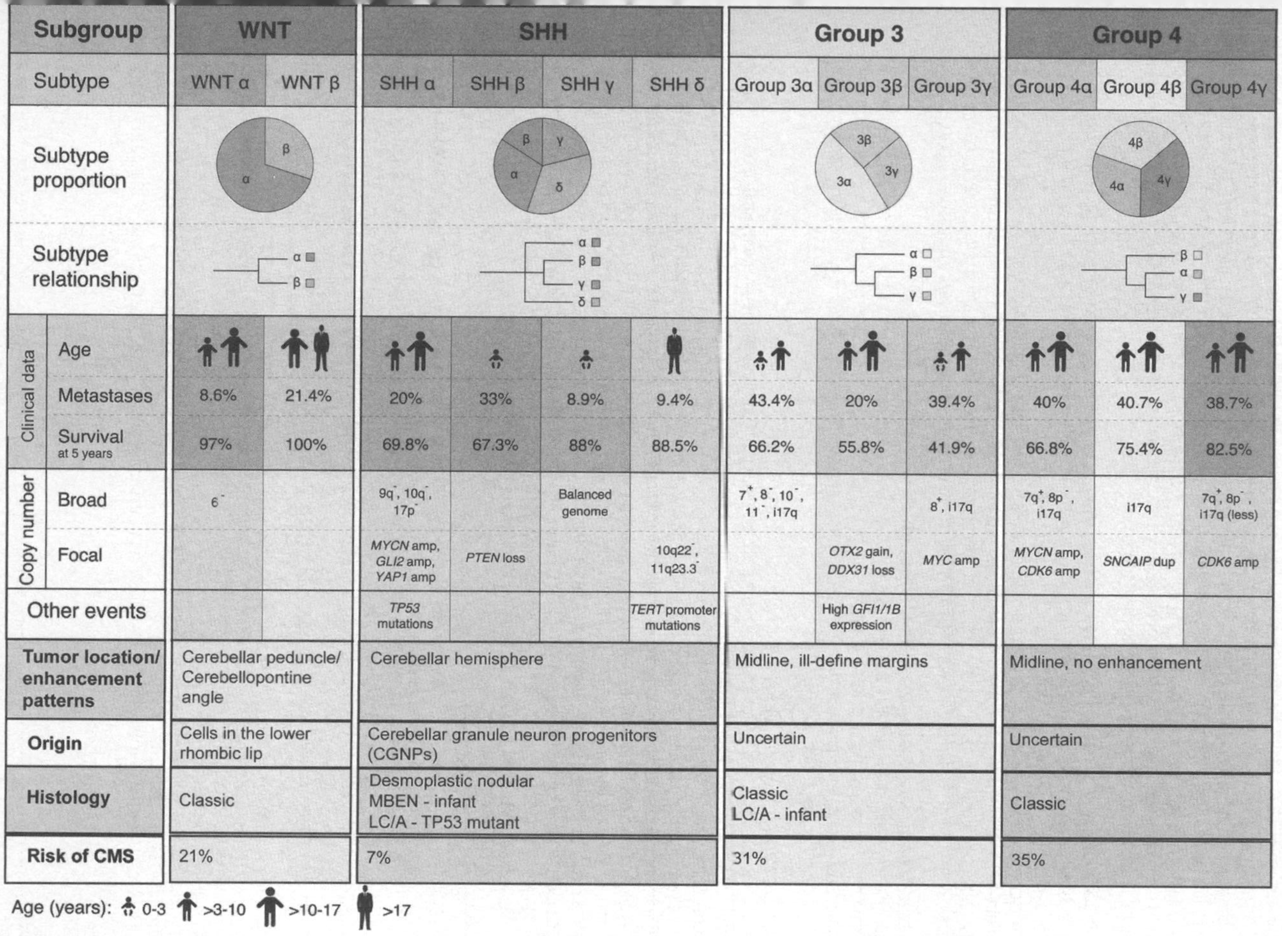

Subgroup	WNT		SHH				Group 3			Group 4		
Subtype	WNT α	WNT β	SHH α	SHH β	SHH γ	SHH δ	Group 3α	Group 3β	Group 3γ	Group 4α	Group 4β	Group 4γ
Subtype proportion												
Subtype relationship												
Clinical data: Age												
Clinical data: Metastases	8.6%	21.4%	20%	33%	8.9%	9.4%	43.4%	20%	39.4%	40%	40.7%	38.7%
Clinical data: Survival at 5 years	97%	100%	69.8%	67.3%	88%	88.5%	66.2%	55.8%	41.9%	66.8%	75.4%	82.5%
Copy number: Broad	6^-		$9q^-$, $10q^-$, $17p^-$		Balanced genome		7^+, 8^-, 10^-, 11^-, i17q		8^+, i17q	$7q^+$, $8p^-$, i17q	i17q	$7q^+$, $8p^-$, i17q (less)
Copy number: Focal			*MYCN* amp, *GLI2* amp, *YAP1* amp	*PTEN* loss		$10q22^-$, $11q23.3^-$		*OTX2* gain, *DDX31* loss	*MYC* amp	*MYCN* amp, *CDK6* amp	*SNCAIP* dup	*CDK6* amp
Other events			*TP53* mutations			*TERT* promoter mutations		High *GFI1/1B* expression				
Tumor location/ enhancement patterns	Cerebellar peduncle/ Cerebellopontine angle		Cerebellar hemisphere				Midline, ill-define margins			Midline, no enhancement		
Origin	Cells in the lower rhombic lip		Cerebellar granule neuron progenitors (CGNPs)				Uncertain			Uncertain		
Histology	Classic		Desmoplastic nodular MBEN - infant LC/A - TP53 mutant				Classic LC/A - infant			Classic		
Risk of CMS	21%		7%				31%			35%		

Age (years): 0-3 >3-10 >10-17 >17

Figure 40.3 Medulloblastoma subgroups. *CMS*, Cerebellar mutism syndrome; *LC/A*, large cell/anaplastic; *MBEN*, medulloblastoma with extensive nodularity; *SHH*, Sonic hedgehog; *WNT*, wingless. (From Cavalli FMG, Remke M, Rampasek L, et al. Intertumoral heterogeneity within medulloblastoma subgroups. *Cancer Cell.* 2017;31:737–754.)

13. **A 16-year-old boy presents with a 4-week history of headache, vomiting, and diplopia. He has elevated serum and CSF alpha-fetoprotein (AFP). What is the most likely diagnosis?**

    CNS germ cell tumors originate from pluripotent germ cells and can be divided into pure germinomas and nongerminomatous germ cell tumors (NGGCTs).[9] They often present in the adolescent years with a classic triad of symptoms of diabetes insipidus, panhypopituitarism, and visual disturbances, and the most common locations are the pineal and suprasellar regions. Germinomas are often nonsecretory and most effectively treated with chemotherapy and radiation, whereas patients with NGGCTs can have elevated tumor markers (AFP or β-human chorionic gonadotropin [HCG]) and require surgical resection, chemotherapy, and radiation for treatment with the exception of mature teratomas, which are often curable with surgery alone. Growing teratoma syndrome is a rare entity that presents with an enlarging tumor mass during appropriate chemotherapy and normalized serum markers. The most likely etiology of this phenomenon is that in NGGCTs, chemotherapy only destroys the immature malignant cells, leaving the mature benign teratomatous elements to grow.

14. **An 8-year-old boy presents with headache, vomiting, and excessive thirst with polyuria. MRI of the brain reveals a cystic-solid tumor in the suprasellar region. What is the most likely diagnosis, and how would you treat this patient?**

    Craniopharyngiomas represent 6% to 9% of all pediatric brain tumors and originate from embryonic tissue located in the Rathke's pouch, which forms the anterior pituitary gland. Treatment is maximum surgical resection, but total removal can be difficult because of invasion of adjacent structures. Focal radiotherapy is often used in progressive disease. Although overall survival is excellent, many patients have long-term sequalae of the disease and its treatment.

15. **What is radiation necrosis, and how is it treated?**

    Although uncommon, brain necrosis is a serious complication after radiation therapy. Most cases present within a year of treatment. It poses a considerable diagnosis challenge because it is difficult to differentiate from tumor recurrence. MR spectroscopy or perfusion-weighted MRI can provide additional information. Treatment includes surgery, corticosteroids, or bevacizumab.[10]

16. **What are the long-term effects of brain tumor treatment?**

    Late adverse effects of cancer treatment are a significant source of morbidity in the growing population of pediatric CNS tumor survivors. Radiation therapy, especially craniospinal irradiation, is particularly damaging to the developing brain resulting in significant neurocognitive impairment. Proton therapy is thought to lessen the risk of neuropsychological complications and secondary malignancies compared with photon therapy, but these benefits have yet to be confirmed. Radiation to the hypothalamic-pituitary axis can result in significant hormone deficiencies, which generally occurs 5 years after treatment and is strongly correlated to the total radiation dose. Ototoxicity can be caused by both radiation and extensive use of cisplatin. Secondary malignancies including glioblastoma, meningiomas, and soft tissue sarcomas years after cranial radiation and myelodysplastic syndromes or acute myeloid leukemia after alkylator chemotherapy are rare but serious adverse effects of prior treatment. Patients with cancer predisposition syndromes have a higher risk of developing secondary neoplasms. Brain tumor diagnosis also has a significant economic and social impact on the survivors' lives.

REFERENCES

1. Ostrom QT, Patil N, Cioffi G, Waite K, Kruchko C, Barnholtz-Sloan JS. CBTRUS Statistical Report: primary brain and other central nervous system tumors diagnosed in the United States in 2013-2017. *Neuro Oncol.* 2020;22(Suppl 2):iv1–96.
2. Louis DN, Perry A, Wesseling P, et al. The 2021 World Health Organization Classification of tumours of the central nervous system: a summary. *Neuro Oncol.* 2021;23:1231–1251.
3. Wilne S, Collier J, Kennedy C, Koller K, Grundy R, Walker D. Presentation of childhood CNS tumours: a systematic review and meta-analysis. *Lancet Oncol.* 2007;8:685–695.
4. Perreault S, Ramaswamy V, Schrol AS, et al. MRI surrogates for molecular subgroups. *Am J Neuroradiol.* 2014;35:1263–1269.
5. Schreiber JE, Palmer SL, Conklin HM, et al. Posterior fossa syndrome and long-term neuropsychological outcomes among children treated for medulloblastoma on a multi-institutional, prospective study. *Neuro Oncol.* 2017;19:1673–1682.
6. Munoz-Couselo E, Garcia JS, Perez-Garcia JM, et al. Recent advances in the treatment of melanoma with BRAF and MEK inhibitors. *Ann Trans Med.* 2015;3:207.
7. Ryall S, Tabori U, Hawkins C. Pediatric low-grade glioma in the era of molecular diagnostics. *Acta Neuropathol Commun.* 2020;8:30.
8. Cavalli FMG, Remke M, Rampasek L, et al. Intertumoral heterogeneity within medulloblastoma subgroups. *Cancer Cell.* 2017;31:737–754.
9. Fetcko K, & Dey M. Primary central nervous system germ cell tumors: a review and update. *Med Res Arch.* 2018;6:1719.
10. Omay SB, Komli-Kofi A, Baehring JM. Nonneoplastic mass lesions of the central nervous system. In: Newton HB (ed). *Handbook of Neuro-Oncology Neuroimaging.* 2nd ed. Elsevier Ltd., 2016:653–665.

POST-TRANSPLANT LYMPHOPROLIFERATIVE DISORDER (PTLD)

Manuela Orjuela, MD, ScM, Lianna J. Marks, MD, and Bradley Gampel, MD

1. **What infectious agent plays a central role in the development of most post-transplant lymphoproliferative disorder and why?**

   Epstein-Barr virus (EBV), a ubiquitous human herpesvirus transmitted primarily via saliva, is causally involved in most lymphoproliferative disease. Initial infection with EBV occurs during childhood but persists as a latent infection throughout life. EBV colonizes antibody-producing B cells and thus evades recognition and destruction by cytotoxic T cells. EBV infection is largely controlled by memory EBV-specific cytotoxic T lymphocytes (EBV-CTL) and remains an asymptomatic infection in B cells. EBV carries a set of latent genes that induce cellular proliferation when expressed in resting B cells. This cell proliferation when unregulated or accompanied by additional genetic events can lead to malignant transformation. EBV infection in patients with compromised T-cell immunity after transplantation because of immunosuppression leads to the development of post-transplant lymphoproliferative disorder (PTLD). Other DNA viruses such as human immunodeficiency virus (HIV; HTLVIII), human herpesvirus 8 (HHV8, also known as Kaposi sarcoma–associated virus), cytomegalovirus (CMV), and hepatitis C virus (HCV) have also been associated with the development of lymphoproliferative diseases.

2. **How does PTLD present clinically?**

   PTLD involves a diverse spectrum of symptoms, including isolated adenopathy, hepatitis, lymphoid interstitial pneumonitis, meningo-encephalitis, an infectious mononucleosis-like syndrome, or a septic shock–like presentation. Although PTLD can arise after any organ transplant, the cells of origin in patients who have undergone a bone marrow transplant are usually donor cells, whereas in patients who have undergone solid organ transplants (SOT), PTLD arises in cells that are of host origin. Nevertheless, clinical manifestations do not appear to differ by cell of origin.

   PTLD appears to arise as a defective response to a viral infection, most commonly EBV. This defective response is in part because of immune dysregulation, stemming from an absence of EBV-CTL. This inability to clear EBV-infected B cells leads to B-cell proliferation with the potential for malignant transformation.

3. **What histologic and genetic changes are described in PTLD?**

   The updated 2016 World Health Organization classification of histologic presentation of PTLD ranges from benign florid follicular hyperplasia or lesions with polymorphic cellular infiltration to lesions with monomorphic, lymphoblastic cell populations or classical Hodgkin lymphoma (HL) PTLD. These lesions can be polyclonal, oligoclonal, or monoclonal, even within different lesions in the same patient. Although PTLD may appear histologically identical to non-Hodgkin lymphoma (NHL) or even HL, it is genetically distinct. The EBV gene expression in PTLD is like that seen in EBV-positive large cell lymphoma, not Burkitt lymphoma or HL. Cytogenetic abnormalities commonly found in Burkitt or Hodgkins disease (HD), such as those involving *MYC, NRAS, HRAS* and *KRAS, TP53, BCL2*, and *BCL6*, are rare in PTLD.

4. **Describe the period after transplant associated with the highest incidence of occurrence of PTLD.**

   Incidence of PTLD occurs primarily during the first 6 months after transplantation, coinciding with the period of greatest immunosuppression. More than 90% of early (<6 months after transplant) cases of PTLD are EBV positive, when EBV-CTL immunity is lowest. PTLD at this stage is more often polymorphic and often responds to decreased immunosuppression without additional therapy. A second peak in incidence of PTLD occurs 2 years after transplant. These cases of PTLD are referred to as "late-onset" and have a much higher prevalence of EBV negativity, generally require more aggressive therapy, and generally have a poorer prognosis compared with early-onset PTLD. These late PTLD may be a different disease and appear more akin to lymphoproliferative disorders observed in other immunodeficient states (e.g., acquired immunodeficiency syndrome [AIDS] and primary immunodeficiencies), which are not always of B-cell origin or associated with EBV.

5. **How frequent is PTLD, and what factors increase the likelihood of developing the disorder after SOT?**

   Data from the Organ Procurement and Transplantation Network show there are over 100 cases of newly diagnosed PTLD per year in children and adolescents in the United States. Frequency of PTLD in SOT recipients varies by organ transplanted: 1% to 5% in renal, heart, and liver transplants; 10% to 30% in lung, small bowel, and multiple organ grafts; and with frequency of rejection episodes requiring intensified immunosuppression (especially the use of T-cell antibody therapy), EBV seronegativity at time of transplant, and younger age of recipients (especially <5 years of age, at which time children are more likely to be EBV seronegative in industrialized countries).

6. Describe the most common treatment approach for PTLD.

Treatment of PTLD requires controlling the EBV-induced B-cell proliferation and facilitating the development of an appropriate EBV-CTL response. The initial step for treating PTLD is reduction of immunosuppression to enhance alloreactive T-cell immunity and thus the development of EBV-specific CTLs. However, this increases the risk of organ rejection and graft loss. Decreased immunosuppression can be sufficient for controlling PTLD, especially when localized or polyclonal. Antiviral agents (acyclovir or ganciclovir) may be useful in prophylaxis or delaying primary EBV infection or reactivation, but results are mixed. Surgery can be used to cure disease only when it is localized.

For patients with CD20+ PTLD that does not respond to reduction in immunosuppression or patients who are at high risk of developing rejection and are not candidates for reduction in immunosuppression, rituximab monotherapy is the next line of treatment (see question 7 for exceptions). Rituximab, an anti-CD20 monoclonal antibody, targets CD20, a transmembrane protein present on almost all B cells, and decreases B-cell proliferation. CD20 positivity predicts improved outcomes in children with PTLD, independent of therapy with rituximab. In adult trials, risk-stratified sequential treatment of patients beginning with rituximab for four cycles, followed by additional rituximab in those with a complete response or the addition of chemotherapy with R-CHOP (rituximab, cyclophosphamide, doxorubicin, vincristine and prednisone) in patients with a partial response or progressive disease has led to good outcomes and decreased treatment-related mortality.

Because PTLD arises from an underlying immunodeficient environment, treatment regimens developed for AIDS-associated lymphomas, such as DA-EPOCH-R (dose-adjusted etoposide, prednisone, vincristine, cyclophosphamide, doxorubicin, and rituximab), have also been trialed in advanced PTLD with comparable efficacy and tolerability compared with R-CHOP. A COG trial of rituximab with low-dose chemotherapy including cyclophosphamide and prednisone demonstrated safety and efficacy and has become a frequently used treatment for this age group.

7. How does treatment differ for specific histological subtypes of PTLD such as Hodgkin lymphoma, Burkitt lymphoma, primary central nervous system lymphoma, and T-cell lymphoma?

These PTLD subtypes typically do not respond to reduction of immunosuppression or rituximab monotherapy and should be treated with regimens that are based on the standard of care chemoimmunotherapy for the specific histology. Nevertheless, patients with PTLD frequently have compromised renal or other organ function because of their immunosuppressive regimens or pretransplant comorbidities and may require dose modifications in their chemotherapy to minimize treatment-related toxicities. Patients with HL PTLD treated with somewhat modified standard Hodgkin chemotherapy protocols have favorable outcomes although dose modifications were common due to patient comorbidities, and overall survival and event-free survival appear less than for nonimmunocompromised patients treated on the same protocol. Burkitt lymphoma PTLD is considered aggressive and appears to require Burkitt lymphoma immunochemotherapy, although again often requiring dose modification, especially during administration of high-dose methotrexate. PTLD that involves the CNS has a generally poor prognosis. Treatment approaches are informed from adult CNS lymphoma protocols and include chemotherapy with high-dose methotrexate, cytarabine, higher dose intravenous and intrathecal rituximab, consolidation with radiotherapy, and /or EBV-CTLs. T-cell lymphoma PTLD, including peripheral T-cell lymphoma, hepatosplenic T-cell lymphoma, and anaplastic large cell lymphoma are extremely rare, are often not associated with EBV, tend to be late-onset PTLD, and typically also have a poor prognosis.

8. What is the role of adoptive T-cell therapy in PTLD?

Adoptive T-cell therapy (i.e., donor leukocyte infusion) has been used in an attempt to boost CTL activity. In BMT, donor leukocytes from the marrow donor can be used; however, in solid organ transplant, the donors are often no longer available. In addition, the lymphocyte proliferation occurs in host, not donor cells, so the immunologic recognition, specificity, and efficacy of donor leukocytes are uncertain. One alternative for SOT has been to give patients EBV-CTLs, which are generated ex vivo, and have demonstrated responses in EBV+ PTLD. These EBV-CTLs can be autologous CTLs, generated from the patient's own cells, or third-party CTLs, generated from healthy EBV seropositive donors matched at one HLA allele. The benefit of third-party CTLs is that they can be rapidly available for patients, whereas autologous cells can take several weeks to generate. Both types of EBV-CTLs are generally well tolerated and can generate good responses but are still in phase II or III clinical trials and are not yet widely available.

BIBLIOGRAPHY

1. Crawford DH. Biology and disease associations of Epstein-Barr virus. *Philos Trans R Soc Lond B Biol Sci.* 2001;356(1408):461–473.
2. DeStefano CB, Malkovska V, Rafei H, et al. DA-EPOCH-R for post-transplant lymphoproliferative disorders. *Eur J Haematol.* 2017;99 (3):283–285.
3. Dierickx D, Habermann TM. Post-transplantation lymphoproliferative disorders in adults. *N Engl J Med.* 2018;378(6):549–562.
4. Gross TG, Orjuela MA, Perkins SL, et al. Low-dose chemotherapy and rituximab for posttransplant lymphoproliferative disease (PTLD): a Children's Oncology Group Report. *Am J Transplant.* 2012;12(11):3069–3075.
5. Kampers J, Orjuela-Grimm M, Schober T, et al. Classical Hodgkin lymphoma-type PTLD after solid organ transplantation in children: a report on 17 patients treated according to subsequent GPOH-HD treatment schedules. *Leuk Lymphoma.* 2017;58(3):633–638.

6. Orjuela MA, Alobeid B, Liu X, et al. CD20 expression predicts survival in paediatric post-transplant lymphoproliferative disease (PTLD) following solid organ transplantation. *Br J Haematol*. 2011;152(6):733–742.

7. Schultze-Florey RE, Tischer S, Kuhlmann L, et al. Dissecting Epstein-Barr virus-specific T-cell responses after allogeneic EBV-specific T-cell transfer for central nervous system posttransplant lymphoproliferative disease. *Front Immunol*. 2018;9:1475.

8. Wistinghausen B, Gross TG, Bollard C. Post-transplant lymphoproliferative disease in pediatric solid organ transplant recipients. *Pediatr Hematol Oncol*. 2013;30(6):520–531.

CHAPTER 42

RETINOBLASTOMA

Manuela Orjuela, MD, ScM and Bradley Gampel, MD

1. Describe the underlying genetic defect in retinoblastoma.

Retinoblastoma, a primitive neuroectodermal cell tumor, develops as a result of an absence of pRb, the retinoblastoma protein, which functions as a regulator of the cell cycle by modifying transcription factors, which allow progression into the S phase. Lack of functional pRb primarily occurs as a result of mutations in *RB1*, the retinoblastoma gene. These mutations can occur in germline or somatic cells. As predicted by Knudson's two-hit hypothesis, both *RB1* alleles must be affected for a tumor to develop.

2. What are the presenting signs for retinoblastoma?

Most (>50%) children with retinoblastoma present with leukocoria. Children with more advanced tumors can present with a dilated pupil in their affected eye. In these patients, the leukocoria is more easily visible. Leukocoria is usually first noted by a close relative. It is best visualized when the pupil is dilated and light strikes the eye obliquely, such as in indoor flash photographs. Families will often notice in recent photographs that the affected eye has a white pupil and the other one has a red pupil. Less frequently, children can present with esotropia, exotropia, or amblyopia. These symptoms are because of visual loss in the affected eye. Rarely, children can present with heterochromia, or rubeosis iridis. Children with retinoblastoma rarely complain of pain unless they have developed secondary glaucoma (increased intraocular pressure). Discomfort from increased intraocular pressure can cause anorexia. Children with increased intraocular pressure usually have poor vision in the affected eye at diagnosis and usually require prompt enucleation (see later). The pain and anorexia resolve immediately after enucleation.

3. Describe the staging classification for retinoblastoma.

There are multiple staging classification systems for retinoblastoma, including the TNM (tumor, node, metastasis) staging system, which combines the International Classification for Intraocular Retinoblastoma (IIRC) and the International Retinoblastoma Staging System (IRSS), and the Reese-Ellsworth classification system. The TNM system is used by The American Joint Committee on Cancer. The Children's Oncology Group (COG) uses a combination of the IIRC and ICSS. The IIRC is used by ophthalmologists to stage intraocular disease and is guided by likelihood of eye preservation. The IRSS is primarily used to stage extraocular disease. The most widely used system is the TNM. These staging systems are still being operationalized.

4. How do you evaluate a child who presents with possible retinoblastoma?

The diagnosis of retinoblastoma is made clinically because tissue diagnosis is unnecessary if a child is evaluated by an ophthalmologist with expertise in handling the disease. Initial evaluation includes an examination under anesthesia, an ultrasonogram looking for characteristic calcifications, and magnetic resonance imaging (MRI) to evaluate optic nerve involvement, extraocular extension, and central nervous system (CNS) involvement. If there is concern that the disease may have spread to the optic nerve or extraocular tissues (such as orbital soft tissue or preauricular lymph nodes), a lumbar puncture and bilateral bone marrow aspirates and biopsies are also indicated.

5. What proportion of retinoblastoma is unilateral? At what age does unilateral disease usually present?

Sixty-five percent of retinoblastoma is unilateral, with a mean age at diagnosis of 24 months. Most children affected by retinoblastoma are diagnosed before the age of 6 years.

6. Discuss how bilateral retinoblastoma is genetically different from unilateral retinoblastoma.

Children with bilateral retinoblastoma usually have *RB1* mutations in their germline. Therefore all cells (including retinal cells) have one defective RB1 allele. Ninety percent of children with bilateral retinoblastoma have new germline mutations occurring preferentially on the paternally inherited allele. Only 15% of children with unilateral disease have germline mutations. Most children with unilateral disease have *RB1* mutations present only in their retinal cells.

7. How does this biologic difference manifest itself clinically?

Children with bilateral disease present earlier than unilateral disease, with a mean age at diagnosis of 11 months, although disease can be detected prenatally. Bilateral disease can involve multifocal and asynchronous tumors. Each eye must be staged separately. Tumors can develop as late as 28 months of age and can continue developing until age 7. A small proportion of children with bilateral retinoblastoma develop pineal tumors (trilateral retinoblastoma).

8. **What proportion of retinoblastoma is familial?**
   Only 10% of newly diagnosed cases of retinoblastoma occur in children with a prior family history of retinoblastoma. Nevertheless, each child of a patient with a germline *RB1* mutation has a 45% risk of developing bilateral disease.

9. **How is intraocular disease treated?**
   The goal of treating intraocular disease is to eliminate the tumor and save vision. If there is no salvageable vision at diagnosis, ophthalmologists usually recommend enucleation. If there is still salvageable vision, the management can be complex with numerous options. Small tumors can be treated with chemotherapy, laser photocoagulation, thermotherapy, or cryotherapy. There are four routes of delivery of chemotherapy: the intravenous, intra-arterial, periocular, and intravitreal techniques.

   The type of treatment used is not only dependent on the staging but also the patient's age. Intra-arterial chemotherapy is typically done for patients 6 months and older. A patient under 6 months old may get bridging systemic chemotherapy until they are large enough to allow technically safe administration of chemotherapy in the ophthalmic artery. Intra-arterial chemotherapy has been shown to be safe and effective in the treatment of advanced intraocular retinoblastoma (e.g., stage D in the IIRC). Chemotherapy agents used most frequently include melphalan, followed by carboplatin and topotecan. In intravitreal chemotherapy, chemotherapy (melphalan or topotecan) is instilled in the vitreous to target vitreal seeds, which are challenging to treat given their lack of direct blood supply. With both intra-arterial and intravitreal therapy, patients need to be monitored for cytopenias similar to systemic chemotherapy and other local inflammatory toxicities at the sites of chemotherapy delivery. For bilateral disease, systemic chemotherapy (with carboplatin, vincristine, and with or without etoposide) may be attempted as first-line therapy to salvage patient vision depending on intraocular tumor group.

10. **Describe the options for therapy for extraocular disease.**
    Orbital disease (stage III) requires enucleation followed by chemotherapy. Chemotherapy agents include carboplatin, etoposide, vincristine, cyclophosphamide, and cisplatin. Sometimes this can be followed by radiation therapy. If localized soft tissue spread is noted at diagnosis, chemoreduction may be attempted before enucleation to avoid orbital exenteration. Metastatic disease (stage IV) requires intensive chemotherapy and, frequently, consolidation with autologous bone marrow transplantation. The goal of vision salvage is secondary to prevent spread of the disease to the CNS. Survival rates for metastatic disease without CNS involvement have greatly improved to over 70%. Unfortunately for patients who do have CNS involvement, survival rates remain below 10%. In contrast, survival rates for ocular and orbital disease are above 85%, whereas those for retinal disease are above 95%.

11. **Children with bilateral retinoblastoma are at risk for developing secondary malignancies as they get older. Which tumors do they develop? When are they at risk for developing these tumors?**
    Patients who have germline mutations of *RB1* and survive their retinoblastoma are at increased risk of developing sarcoma (bone or soft tissue), melanoma, or brain tumors. This increased risk results from the acquisition of a second (somatic cell) mutation in the remaining normal RB1 allele, thereby leading to an absence of pRb-dependent regulation in that particular cell. This risk is particularly increased in areas exposed to radiation. The risk of osteogenic sarcoma is highest between the ages of 10 and 20 years. The risk for developing brain tumors is highest between the ages of 25 and 35 years. Carriers of *RB1* mutations also have an increased risk for developing early-onset (before age 55 years) smoking-induced lung cancers. The overall lifetime risk for secondary malignancies is approximately 30%.

12. **Discuss how the age at which children receive radiation therapy affects their chance for development of secondary malignancies.**
    Risk for secondary malignancies is highest in children with germline mutations who receive radiation therapy before their first birthday. These children are at greatly increased risk for developing sarcomas in the soft tissues of their heads (between the ages of 5 and 25 years) and in the bones of their skulls (the highest risk occurring between ages 12 and 25 years). They also have a lower but still increased risk for developing brain tumors. Children with germline mutations who receive radiation after their first birthday are still at increased risk for developing all of these tumors, but their risk is significantly less than that of those who receive radiation as infants.

BIBLIOGRAPHY

1. Abramson DH, Frank CM, Susman M, et al. Presenting signs of retinoblastoma. *J Pediatr.* 1998;132(3, pt. 1):505–508.
2. Chantada GL, Sampor C, Bosaleh A, Solernou V, Fandiño A, de Dávila MT. Comparison of staging systems for extraocular retinoblastoma: analysis of 533 patients. *JAMA Ophthalmol.* 2013;131(9):1127–1134.
3. Chantada G, Doz F, Antoneli CB, et al. A proposal for an international retinoblastoma staging system. *Pediatr Blood Cancer.* 2006;47(6):801–805.
4. Eng C, Li FP, Abramson DH, et al. Mortality from second tumors among long-term survivors of retinoblastoma. *J Natl Cancer Inst.* 1993;85:1121–1128.
5. Linn Murphree A. Intraocular retinoblastoma: the case for a new group classification. *Ophthalmol Clin North Am.* 2005;18(1):41-53, viii.
6. Wong FL, Boice JD, Jr Abramson DH, et al. Cancer incidence after retinoblastoma. Radiation dose and sarcoma risk. *JAMA.* 1997;278(15):1262–1267.
7. Zheng L, Lee WH. The retinoblastoma gene: a prototypic and multifunctional tumor suppressor. *Exp Cell Res.* 2001;264(1):2–18.

CHAPTER 43

LANGERHANS CELL HISTIOCYTOSIS (LCH)

Kristin Lieb, MD and Justine M. Kahn, MD

1. What are the former names of Langerhans cell histiocytosis?

What is known today as Langerhans cell histiocytosis (LCH) was first described in the early 1900s. By 1953, the diagnoses of eosinophilic granuloma, Hand-Schüller-Christian disease, Letterer-Siwe disease, and Hashimoto-Pritzker disease were grouped together as a disease spectrum known as Histiocytosis X. The "X" stood for "unknown," representing the lack of understanding of the underlying pathology.[6] In 1973 Nezelof and colleagues coined the term LCH with the identification of Birbeck granules, thought to be pathognomonic of Langerhans cells, which until recently, was considered the pathogenic cell.[2]

2. What is the cause of LCH?

The underlying etiology has long been debated. dysfunctional or exaggerated inflammatory response versus neoplastic disorder. It has since been determined that LCH is secondary to a clonal expansion or neoplasm of myeloid precursor cells that differentiate into dendritic cells.

3. Discuss the clinical presentations of LCH.

Patients may present with a wide spectrum of disease involving one organ system (single-system) or more than one (multisystem).[2,4]

Single-system: The most common presentations include bone or skin lesions.
- Lytic bone lesions typically involve the skull, followed by the spine, limbs, or pelvis.
- Skin involvement is noted in approximately one-third of children with LCH, classically an erythematous papule that may ulcerate or depigment.
- Lymph node involvement occurs in less than 10% of children.

Multisystem: Other organ systems that can be involved include the liver, spleen, bone marrow, lungs, and central nervous system (CNS). The aggressive presentation of multisystem disease is usually seen in children younger than 2 years. The presentation is often similar to an acute leukemia, with evidence of bone marrow suppression, hepatosplenomegaly, and constitutional symptoms.
- Lungs: Involvement may be manifested by respiratory distress with tachypnea, retractions, and persistent cough. Chronic respiratory failure may ensue as a result of widespread cyst and bullae formation. Rupture of a bullous lesion may lead to pneumothorax.
- Bone, skin, and lymph node involvement usually coexist with a presentation similar to single-system disease.
- Gingival disease is marked by early loss of deciduous teeth and gum hypertrophy.
- Auditory canal involvement is manifested by persistent ear drainage nonresponsive to antibiotics.

4. Describe the epidemiology of LCH.

LCH occurs in approximately 5 out of 1,000,000 children, with an average age of diagnosis of 3 years.[5] Males and females are affected near equally, and Hispanic children are more commonly affected than other ethnicities.

5. What is the classification system for LCH?

After confirmatory diagnosis, a patient is first described as having single-system or multisystem organ disease.[3] Second, the patient is classified as with or without risk organ (RO) involvement, which includes the liver, spleen, and/or bone marrow. See Figure 43.1.

6. What is the most frequent endocrinopathy in LCH?

The most frequent endocrinopathy in LCH is diabetes insipidus (DI), which may occur before, concurrently, or subsequent to the development of the disease in other sites, especially with bone lesions of the skull.

7. How is LCH diagnosed?

After clinical suspicion, diagnosis is confirmed with a biopsy, most commonly of skin if involved because it is the least invasive.
- Immunohistochemistry staining shows CD1a+ and CD207+ (langerin). Historically, electron microscopy was used showing Birbeck granules; however, that method has fallen out of favor.[4]
- Molecular studies are also performed. Activating mutations within the MAP kinase pathway responsible for regulation of cell growth often are present; the most frequent mutation identified is the *BRAFV600E* mutation.[1]

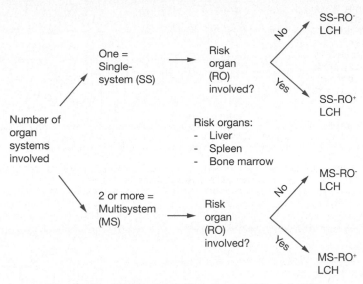

Figure 43.1 Classification system for Langerhans cell histiocytosis (LCH).

8. **Discuss the treatment approach for single-system LCH.**
   Because single-system LCH rarely has been incorporated in clinical trials, a standard of care has not been established. Treatment approaches are typically based on the organ system involved and if the disease is a solitary or multifocal lesion.
   - For solitary bone lesions, surgical curettage with or without local corticosteroid injection is often effective to obtain a complete response.
   - Multifocal bone lesions or unifocal lesions arising from CNS-risk craniofacial areas (orbital, temporal, sphenoid, ethmoid, or mastoid bones, paranasal sinuses, or the anterior or middle cranial fossa) require treatment approaches similar to multisystem LCH.
   - In contrast, solitary skin lesions often regress spontaneously and typically require observation only. If the lesion does not regress, progresses, or becomes symptomatic, patients can be treated topically, with low-dose systemic chemotherapy and/or corticosteroids.[4]

9. **Describe the treatment approach for multisystem LCH.**
   Upfront therapy involves a backbone of steroids (prednisone) and vinblastine for at least 12 months and is most successful in patients with RO⁻ disease.[6] Patients with RO⁺ disease are more likely to have refractory or recurrent disease; studies are ongoing to determine optimal treatment regimens and duration. Given the understanding of the myeloid lineage derivation of LCH, alternative chemotherapy regimens have been tested with higher success rates, including cytarabine, cladribine, and clofarabine.[2]
   For high-risk patients who cannot tolerate intense chemotherapy regimens or respond poorly despite treatment, reduced intensity conditioning followed by hematopoietic stem cell transplantation (HSCT) can be considered.[2]

10. **What are the other targeted therapy options?**
    Potential targeted therapy includes inhibitors of the MAPK pathway, such as the MEK1 inhibitor trametinib, and inhibitors of BRAF, such as vemurafenib.[1]

11. **What are the prognostic factors of LCH?**
    Prognosis relates to disease severity. Single-system disease, affecting the bones, skin, or lymph nodes, has a favorable prognosis, whereas multisystem disease, particularly RO⁺, has an unfavorable prognosis. Additionally, patients who respond poorly to the initial course of therapy or who have disease recurrence, observed more frequently in multisystem-RO⁺ patients, tend to have more morbidity and mortality.[6]
    Studies have not clearly identified an association between genetic mutations and disease prognosis. Although not directly prognostic, patients with *BRAFV600E* mutations are more likely to have multisystem than single-system disease.[2]

12. **What are the potential late sequelae from LCH?**
    Inactive lesions may have late sequelae that significantly affect the quality of life of LCH survivors.[4,5] The risk of complications is particularly high for patients with multisystem disease and multiple reactivations. Complications include:

- Orthopedic problems
- Short stature
- Poor dentition
- Deafness
- Diabetes insipidus
- Pulmonary fibrosis
- Hepatic cirrhosis
- Neurodegeneration

BIBLIOGRAPHY

1. Abla O, Rollins B, Ladisch S. Langerhans cell histiocytosis: progress and controversies. *Br J Haematol.* 2019;187:559–562.
2. Allen CE, Merad M, McClain KL. Langerhans-cell histiocytosis. *N Engl J Med.* 2018;379(9):856–868.
3. Hutter C, Minkov M. Insights into the pathogenesis of Langerhans cell histiocytosis: the development of targeted therapies. *Immunotargets Ther.* 2016;5:81–91.
4. Krooks J, Minkov M, Weatherall AG. Langerhans cell histiocytosis in children. *J Am Acad Dermatol.* 2018;78(6):1047–1056.
5. Rodriguez-Galindo C, Allen CE. Langerhans cell histiocytosis. *Blood.* 2020;135(16):1319–1331.
6. Thacker NH, Abla O. Pediatric Langerhans cell histiocytosis: state of science and future directions. *Clin Adv Hematol Oncol.* 2019;17(2):122–131.

CHAPTER 44

HEMOPHAGOCYTIC LYMPHOHISTIOCYTOSIS

Jess Hochberg, MD and Prakash Satwani, MD

1. **What is the definition of hemophagocytic lymphohistiocytosis?**

   Hemophagocytic lymphohistiocytosis (HLH) is a rare but potentially fatal clinical syndrome of severe pathologic immune activation, characterized by signs and symptoms of excessive inflammation. It commonly appears in infancy but can be found in any age group. There are both genetic (primary) and acquired (secondary) forms. Immunologic basis for HLH is presumed because of its inflammatory nature and findings of specific cytotoxic and immune abnormalities in patients. HLH remains a syndromic disorder with a unique pattern of clinical findings and diagnostic criteria.

2. **What are the clinical signs of HLH?**
   - Fever
   - Hepatosplenomegaly
   - Lymphadenopathy
   - Jaundice
   - Rash
   - Easy bruisability and pallor
   - Central nervous system (CNS) involvement (seizures, ataxia, hemiplegia, mental status changes, and irritability)
   - Abdominal pain, vomiting, and diarrhea
   - Feeding problems with failure to thrive (especially in infants)

3. **How is HLH diagnosed?**

   The prompt diagnosis of HLH can be difficult because individual signs or symptoms may overlap with a number of clinical entities. A methodical approach is necessary to initiate effective treatment in a timely manner. Most of the diagnostic patterns of HLH are caused by pathologic inflammation. The Histiocyte Society used a standard definition of HLH in the HLH-94 clinical trial, which was later revised for the HLH-2004 trial and serves as the current diagnostic criteria for HLH (Box 44.1). Confirmatory genetic testing is useful to predict the risk of future recurrence, determine criteria for hematopoietic cell transplant (HCT), and identify predisposition syndromes that may affect additional family members but should not delay diagnosis and initiation of treatment.

   A high index of suspicion is required for diagnosing HLH; children with unexplained fever of more than 5 days duration should have a serum ferritin checked. Ferritin is an acute phase reactant. Ferritin levels of greater than 3000 ng/mL should raise suspicion for HLH and levels greater than 10,000 ng/mL are strongly associated with HLH. It is advisable that serum ferritin is analyzed on a few occasions because in the early phase of HLH ferritin may not be very elevated.

4. **What are pathologic features of HLH?**

   The pathologic hallmark of this disease is an aggressive proliferation and accumulation of lymphocytes and mature macrophages, often displaying hemophagocytosis (Figure 44.1), seen anywhere within the spleen, lymph nodes, bone marrow, liver, and cerebral spinal fluid in affected patients. The uncontrolled growth is nonmalignant and does not appear clonal. In the liver, histology consistent with chronic persistent hepatitis is commonly found.

5. **What leads to the development of HLH?**

   The development of HLH is centered around triggering of the immune system, with the majority of cases triggered by viral infection. Nevertheless, any infectious agent can result in HLH in a susceptible host. The primary defense mechanism against viruses is provided by natural killer (NK) cells. Patients with familial HLH have defective NK cell function in which NK cells are unable to eliminate viruses, which results in the activation of T-cells. Because T cells do not have prior memory of eliminating viruses, ineffective activation and proliferation of T cells occurs, and these T cells secrete various cytokines, leading to the activation of macrophages. Activated macrophages further secrete various cytokines, leading to various symptoms related to HLH and ultimately organ injury (Figure 44.2).

   Primary HLH is linked to chromosomes 9 and 10 and in approximately 50% to 75% of patients, the disease is hereditary, with an autosomal recessive trait pattern. Various mutations, deletions, or insertions that cause frameshift or missense mutation in perforin genes *(PRF1* and *PRF2)*, MUNC 13-4, and syntaxin 11 and others have been reported (Table 44.1). These lead to impaired perforin production and function, granule exocytosis, intracellular trafficking, and cytolytic activity involving the interactions between NK cells and its target. In patients with

Box 44.1 Diagnostic Criteria for HLH

Diagnosis of HLH requires one of either 1 or 2
1. Molecular diagnosis consistent with HLH
2. Five out of eight of these diagnostic criteria:
   - Fever
   - Splenomegaly
   - Cytopenias (must affect $\geq$ 2 of 3 lineages in the peripheral blood)
   - -Hg <9; Platelets <100; Neutrophils <1000
   - Hypertriglyceridemia (fasting $\geq$265 mg/dL) and/or hypofibrinogenemia ($\leq$1.5 g/L)
   - Hemophagocytosis in bone marrow, spleen, or lymph nodes
   - Low or absent NK-cell activity
   - Ferritin $\geq$500 mg/L
   - Soluble CD25 (sIL-2 receptor) $\geq$2400 U/mL

HLH, Hemophagocytic lymphohistiocytosis; *NK,* natural killer; *sIL,* soluble interleukin.

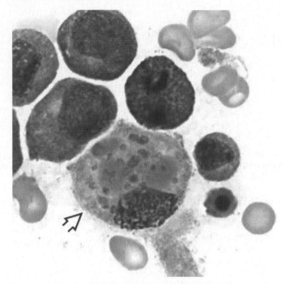

Figure 44.1 Hemophagocytosis in bone marrow aspirate. (From Wang HL. Hemophagocytic syndromes. In Lamps LW, Kakar S (eds). *Diagnostic Pathology, Diagnostic Pathology: Hepatobiliary and Pancreas.* 2nd ed. Elsevier, 2017:284–285.)

acquired HLH, the impairment of NK cells and cytotoxic T cells is less understood but may be related to viral and/or cytokine effects on specific immune functions.

6. **Are there atypical clinical findings seen in HLH?**
   Although the most typical findings of HLH are fever, hepatosplenomegaly, and cytopenias, other common findings include hypertriglyceridemia, coagulopathy with hypofibrinogenemia because of liver dysfunction, elevated serum transaminases, pulmonary dysfunction, and neurological symptoms because of CNS disease. Additional nonspecific findings may also include lymphadenopathy, skin rash, jaundice, and edema. Patients with HLH almost always have evidence of liver inflammation, which may range from very mild transaminitis to fulminant liver failure. Any unexplained liver failure with cytopenias and elevated inflammatory indices should suggest HLH and prompt further workup.

7. **How are primary and acquired HLH different?**
   Primary HLH is typically inherited in an autosomal recessive or X-linked manner, although it can be sporadic. Genetics subgroups can be divided further into familial HLH and immune deficiencies such as Chédiak-Higashi syndrome, Griscelli syndrome, and X-linked proliferative syndrome (XLP1 and XLP2). In primary HLH, the onset of disease is typically in infancy in up to 80% of cases, although late-onset cases in adolescence and adulthood have been published.

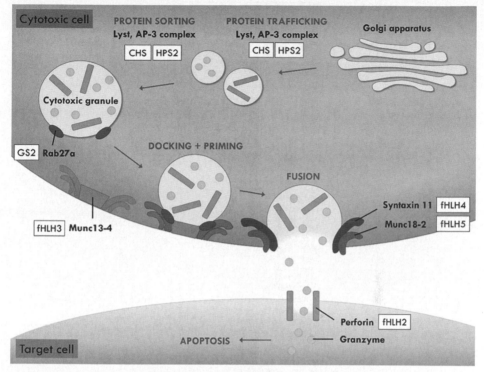

Figure 44.2 Immune defects in hemophagocytic lymphohistiocytosis (HLH). (From Brisse E, Wouters CH, Matthys P. Hemophagocytic lymphohistiocytosis (HLH): a heterogeneous spectrum of cytokine-driven immune disorders. *Cytokine Growth Factor Rev.* 2015;26:263–280.)

Acquired (secondary) HLH can occur in all age groups and is not known to have an underlying genetic cause. It was first described after viral infections (particularly Epstein-Barr virus [EBV], cytomegalovirus [CMV], and herpes simplex virus [HSV]); however, any infection could serve as a trigger for HLH. An important distinction between the two entities involves risk of recurrence. Although mortality may be significant for either primary or secondary HLH, the risk of recurrence in cases of secondary HLH is less and patients may have complete resolution without need for further treatment.

8. How are HLH and macrophage activation syndrome different?
Once thought to be different entities, macrophage activation syndrome (MAS) has long been recognized by the rheumatology community and is now considered more likely a special subtype of HLH. MAS occurs in children and adults with autoimmune diseases, commonly systemic onset juvenile rheumatoid arthritis or lupus erythematosus and manifests as fever, hepatosplenomegaly, hepatitis, lymphadenopathy, and disseminated intravascular coagulation with less frequently cytopenias. MAS has close immunologic and genetic resemblance to HLH with patients showing depressed NK function, depressed expression of perforin, and elevated sCD25. As with HLH, MAS can be triggered by viruses, but many of the drugs used in treatment of autoimmune disease have also been implicated.

9. What illness or disease entities are associated with secondary HLH?
In addition to autoimmune disorders, many other conditions can lead to the clinical picture of HLH, including malignancies (leukemia, lymphoma, solid tumors), infections (viral, bacterial, or fungal), and inherited immune syndromes. Many patients with underlying immune defects are found to have a bacterial, viral, or fungal infection that may serve as a trigger for the HLH in the context of a dysfunctional immune system. EBV is the most frequent infection associated with HLH. EBV-associated HLH varies widely from inflammation that resolves spontaneously to unrelenting disease requiring HSCT. EBV infection may trigger HLH in patients with underlying familial disease and patients with XLP. Initial presentation of EBV-induced, self-resolving HLH can later develop into aggressive recurrent HLH even without identification of underlying immune defect.

10. What is the treatment for HLH?
The primary purpose of HLH treatment is to suppress the immune response and life-threatening inflammatory process that underlies the disorder. The HLH-94 protocol included an 8-week induction therapy with

Table 44.1 Genetic Mutations in Primary HLH

	FHL1	FHL2	FHL3	FHL4	FHL5	GRISCELLI SYNDROME	CHEDIAK-HIGASHI SYNDROME	XLP1	XLP2
Gene	unknown	*PRF1*	*UNC13D*	*STX11*	*STXBP2*	*RAB27A*	*LYST*	*SH2D1A*	*XIAP*
Locus	9q21.3–22	10q21–22	17q25	6q24	19p13	15q21	1q42.1–42.2	Xq24–26	Xq25
Protein, Function		Perforin, pore forming	Munc13-4, priming factor	Syntaxin 11, membrane fusion	Munc18-2, syntaxin binding	Rab27a, tethering	Lyst, lysosomal fusion protein	SAP, lymphocyte activation	XIAP, inhibitor apoptosis

HLH, Hemophagocytic lymphohistiocytosis

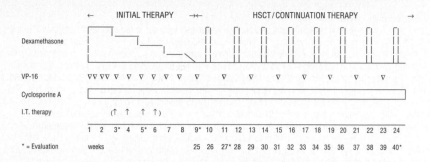

Figure 44.3 Hemophagocytic lymphohistiocytosis (HLH)-2004 treatment schema. (Adapted from Henter JI, Horne A, Arico M, et al. HLH-2004: diagnostic and therapeutic guidelines for hemophagocytic lymphohistiocytosis. *Pediatr Blood Cancer.* 2007;48:124–131.)

dexamethasone, etoposide, and intrathecal methotrexate, followed by continuation therapy until allogeneic hematopoietic cell transplantation (alloHCT). The follow-up study, HLH-2004, modified the original treatment regimen by incorporating cyclosporine dosing to the beginning of induction therapy to allow for more complete suppression of the inflammatory response and by adding hydrocortisone to intrathecal therapy (Figure 44.3). HLH-2004 designates all patients with either primary or acquired HLH undergo 8 weeks of induction therapy. Those patients with documented genetic mutations or familial HLH or those with persistent disease proceed with continuation therapy consisting of dexamethasone pulses, etoposide, and cyclosporine until time of alloHCT. Patients with acquired HLH who have resolution of disease are monitored. If at any time there is recurrence of symptoms or biologic markers, continuation therapy is initiated, and alloHCT is recommended. This is now considered standard therapy.

Addition of cyclosporine in HLH-2004 study was not associated with improvement in induction treatment outcomes and could potentially lead to adverse events. Current recommendation is to follow the HLH-94 protocol for management of HLH.

11. **How is CNS disease treated?**
Almost 70% of patients with primary HLH have nonspecific abnormalities detectable with a computed tomography (CT) scan or magnetic resonance imaging (MRI) of the brain. The most common abnormalities include periventricular white matter involvement, with enlarged ventricular system, gray matter disorders, and brainstem and corpus callosum disease. Involvement of meninges is uncommon. CNS inflammation may recur as treatment doses are tapered. All patients should receive a careful neurologic examination; lumbar puncture and brain MRI should be performed in patients who are clinically stable. Changes in mental status at any time during therapy should be investigated. The majority of CNS symptoms respond to systemic treatment with dexamethasone because it has good CNS penetration. Intrathecal methotrexate therapy is recommended for patients with CNS involvement not improving during systemic HLH-94 therapy. Timing of intrathecal methotrexate should be dictated by the patients' clinical condition. During the early phase of illness, patients may have severe bleeding diathesis. Patients may also have high blood methotrexate levels after intrathecal methotrexate because of slow clearance as a result of liver and renal dysfunction, which could add to further toxicity.

Risk of posterior reversible encephalopathy syndrome appears to be significant during induction therapy and may be related to hypertension in the setting of cyclosporine and dexamethasone use. CNS involvement suggests an underlying genetic etiology with substantial risks for long-term morbidity that would be an indication for alloHCT. Nevertheless, severe neurological impairment may exclude patients from alloHCT.

12. **What is the survival rate for HLH?**
Without therapy, primary HLH is uniformly fatal and survival of patients with active familial HLH is less than 6 months. The HLH-94 trial led to reported survival of 55%, with a median follow-up of 3 years. Approximately 50% of patients treated on the HLH-94 study experienced a complete resolution of HLH, whereas 30% experienced a partial resolution and approximately 20% died before alloHCT. Even with response, recurrences are almost guaranteed and alloHCT is necessary for any chance of cure. Most deaths on clinical trials occurred during the first few weeks of treatment, likely reflecting the irreversible organ damage caused by uncontrolled inflammation or infections. The overall survival (OS) reported in the HLH-2004 study was similar to the HLH-94 study, which is disappointing and reflects the challenges and need for a better treatment algorithm that incorporates novel-targeted therapies.

   Outcomes for secondary HLH vary from 20% to 65% in various studies and depend on disease association, underlying trigger for HLH, comorbidities, and response to induction treatment. Patients with malignancy-associated HLH or those with refractory disease fare much worse. Patients with refractory or recurrent disease who are able to attain a response and proceed with alloHCT overall have a much better prognosis.

13. **What new agents have been developed for HLH?**
The main goal of conventional therapies in primary HLH is to suppress the inflammatory response to allow patients to proceed to alloHCT, which is the only known cure for this disease. Despite the use of aggressive chemoimmunotherapy regimens, there has been no significant decrease in mortality over the past two decades. In addition, most treatment regimens have substantial toxic effects, leading to unacceptable rates of morbidity and mortality. The discovery that elevated interferon (IFN)-γ levels in patients with hemophagocytic lymphohistiocytosis correlate with active disease led to targeting this pathway. Emapalumab is a fully human IgG1 anti–interferon-γ monoclonal antibody that binds IFN-γ and neutralizes its biologic activity. A landmark clinical trial combining emapalumab and dexamethasone in both previously treated (refractory or recurrent) and untreated primary HLH patients showed response rates of 65%, with 74% of patients alive at last follow-up. This promising data led to the recent U.S. Food and Drug Administration (FDA) approval of emapalumab for patients with relapsed, refractory, or progressive primary HLH. Serum biomarker CXCL-9 levels should be monitored among patients undergoing treatment with emapalumab.

   Patients refractory to upfront therapy for HLH have a worse prognosis. In refractory cases, successful treatment with alemtuzumab, ruxolitinib, and IL-1 blocker has been reported as single case reports or small case series.

14. **What are the indications for allogeneic hematopoietic cell transplantation?**
   - Children with primary HLH in complete remission
   - Asymptomatic children with biallelic HLH associated mutations if the sibling(s) presented in infancy
   - Recurrent episodes of HLH among patients without HLH associated mutations
   - Adults with recurrent/refractory disease with HLH associated mutations

15. **When is the appropriate time for allogeneic hematopoietic cell transplantation?**
The optimal timing for alloHCT depends on donor availability and the clinical condition of the patient. HLA typing should be performed on the patient as soon as possible. Once the diagnosis of primary HLH is established (takes around 3–4 weeks from the presentation), HLA typing on available siblings should be performed. All the siblings in the family should also be screened for HLH mutation identified in the index case. An HLA matched sibling without HLH mutation is the obvious first choice for donation of hematopoietic cells. Nevertheless, an HLA-matched sibling heterozygous for HLH mutation is also acceptable if the first scenario is not met.

   In case the HLA-matched sibling is not available, 10/10 HL-matched unrelated donor is the next option followed by haploidentical family donors.

   From a patient perspective, it is preferable that the patient has achieved complete remission of HLH before the alloHCT. Complete remission is defined as no fever, no splenomegaly, ferritin less than 2000 ng/mL, absolute neutrophil count up to 1.0×10^9/L, platelet count up to 1.0×10^9/L, fibrinogen less than 150 mg/dL. Patients with refractory disease not in complete remission after failing several salvage regimens should also be considered for alloHCT as these patients have a small chance of survival after alloHCT compared with no alloHCT.

16. **Are their unique challenges associated with alloHCT for HLH patients?**
Yes, it is preferred that HLH patients have recovered from liver injury and have normal liver functions before alloHCT. Preparative chemotherapy administration before alloHCT can result in significant liver injury resulting in the development of sinusoidal obstruction syndrome (SOS), which could be fatal. Another complication responsible for poor outcome after alloHCT is acute lung injury resulting in respiratory failure.

17. **What kind of conditioning regimen before alloHCT is optimal for HLH patients?**
Optimal pretransplant conditioning regimens for HLH are a matter of debate. Reduced intensity conditioning regimens are associated with less risk of SOS but higher risk of graft rejection and mixed chimerism. Myeloablative conditioning increases the risk of SOS and pulmonary injury. Nevertheless, the probability of donor cell engraftment is much higher.

18. What are the outcomes after alloHCT?

Among alloHCT recipients in the HLH-2004 study, the 5-year OS after alloHCT was 66%. Nevertheless, patients who received alloHCT in complete remission had much higher OS compared with patients not in complete remission (81% vs. 59%, $P = .035$). The 5-year OS was 71% vs. 52%, $P = .40$ among patients with confirmed familial HLH versus unconfirmed HLH. In a prospective study (RICHI), patients with familial HLH received a uniform conditioning regimen (alemtuzumab/fludarabine/melphalan). The 1-year and 18-month rates of OS were 82% and 68%, respectively.

Based on these two prospective studies, one can conclude that alloHCT outcomes are suboptimal, which, in part, could be related to the selection of optimal conditioning regimen. Recently in a retrospective study, outcomes were compared based on the conditioning regimens. The 5-year OS did not differ, however, by conditioning regimens, OS was 68% (fludarabine/melphalan), 75% (fludarabine/melphalan/thiotepa), 86% (fludarabine/busulfan), and 64% (busulfan/cyclophosphamide), respectively. Fludarabine/melphalan regimen had a significantly higher risk of graft failure, and busulfan/cyclophosphamide and fludarabine/busulfan regimens were associated with higher incidence of SOS. This retrospective study concludes that fludarabine/melphalan/thiotepa may be a preferred conditioning regimen for HLH disorders.

BIBLIOGRAPHY

1. Allen CE, Marsh R, Dawson P, et al. Reduced-intensity conditioning for hematopoietic cell transplant for HLH and primary immune deficiencies. *Blood.* 2018;132(13):1438–1451.
2. Bergsten E, Horne A, Arico M, et al. Confirmed efficacy of etoposide and dexamethasone in HLH treatment: long-term results of the cooperative HLH-2004 study. *Blood.* 2017;130:2728–2738.
3. Bergsten E, Horne A, Myrberg I, et al. Stem cell transplantation for children with hemophagocytic lymphohistiocytosis: results from the HLH-2004 study. *Blood Adv.* 2020;4(15):3754–3766.
4. Brisse E, Wouters CH, Matthys P. Hemophagocytic lymphohistiocytosis (HLH): a heterogeneous spectrum of cytokine-driven immune disorders. *Cytokine Growth Factor Rev.* 2015;26(3):263–280.
5. Gholam C, Grigoriadou S, Gilmour KC, et al. Familial haemophagocytic lymphohistiocytosis: advances in the genetic basis, diagnosis and management. *Clin Exp Immunol.* 2011;163:271–283.
6. Henter JI, Samuelsson-Horne A, Arico M, et al. Treatment of hemophagocytic lymphohistiocytosis with HLH-94 immunochemotherapy and bone marrow transplantation. *Blood.* 2002;100:2367–2373.
7. Horne A, Janka G, Maarten Egeler R, et al. Haematopoietic stem cell transplantation in haemophagocytic lymphohistiocytosis. *Br J Haematol.* 2005;129:622–630.
8. Jordan MB, Allen CE, Weitzman S, et al. How I treat hemophagocytic lymphohistiocytosis. *Blood.* 2011;118:4041–4052.
9. Locatelli F, Jordan MB, Allen C, et al. Emapalumab in children with primary hemophagocytic lymphohistiocytosis. *N Engl J Med.* 2020;382:1811–1822.
10. Marsh RA, Hebert K, Kim S, Dvorak CC, et al. Comparison of hematopoietic cell transplant conditioning regimens for hemophagocytic lymphohistiocytosis disorders. *J Allergy Clin Immunol.* 2021;S0091-6749(21):01205–01207.
11. Ravelli A. Macrophage activation syndrome. *Curr Opin Rheumatol.* 2002;14:548–552.
12. Zinter MS, Hermiston ML. Calming the storm in HLH. *Blood.* 2019;134:103–104.

IV
STEM CELL AND CELLULAR THERAPIES

CHAPTER 45

PRINCIPLES AND PRACTICE OF PEDIATRIC HEMATOPOIETIC CELL TRANSPLANTATION

Megan Askew, MD and Prakash Satwani, MD

1. Describe the types of transplant and their indications.

Type of Transplant	Details of Transplant	Indications	Disadvantages
Autologous hematopoietic stem cell transplantation (autoHCT)	• Use patient's own hematopoietic cells. • Give granulocyte colony-stimulating factor (G-CSF) and/or Plerixafor to mobilize cells to collect. • Collect after initial cycle(s) of chemotherapy. • Goal collection: 5 million/kg of CD34$^+$ cells (higher if multiple transplants planned) • Goal: High doses of chemotherapy will eliminate chemotherapy-resistant malignant cells, autoHCT to regenerate bone marrow	Malignant conditions • Relapsed Hodgkin and non-Hodgkin lymphoma • High risk or relapsed neuroblastoma • High-risk brain tumors (i.e., children <3 years as replacement for radiation)	• No graft versus malignancy effect
Allogeneic hematopoietic stem cell transplantation (alloHCT)[a]	• Use donor hematopoietic cells. • Goal: To provide one of the following: graft versus malignancy effect, replacement of missing genes in hematopoietic/immune system, replete failed bone marrow, replace missing enzyme	Malignant conditions • ALL (refractory, relapsed) • AML (High risk for relapse NUP-98 and KMT2A mutations, monosomy 7, induction failure, relapsed, secondary) • MDS • JMML • CML (refractory to multiple tyrosine kinase inhibitors and blast crisis) • Lymphoma (relapses after autoHCT) Nonmalignant conditions • Hemoglobinopathies (SCD, Thalassemia) • Bone marrow failure (SAA, PNH, FA, DKC) • Inborn errors of immune system (SCID, WAS, CGD, LAD, Chediak Higashi, HLH) • Inborn errors of metabolism (Mucopolysaccharidosis, Krabbe disease, X-linked adrenoleukodystrophy, metachromatic leukodystrophy)	• Risk of graft versus host disease

[a]Syngeneic alloHCT is when donor is an identical twin. Indication for syngeneic alloHCT is limited to severe acquired aplastic anemia.

ALL, Acute lymphoblastic leukemia; *AML*, acute myeloid leukemia; *CGD*, chronic granulomatous disease; *CML*, chronic myeloid leukemia; *DKC*, dyskeratosis congenita; *FA*, Fanconi anemia; *HLH*, hemophagocytic lymphohistiocytosis; *JMML*, juvenile myelomonocytic leukemia; *LAD*, leukocyte adhesion defect; *MDS*, myelodysplastic syndrome; *SAA*, severe aplastic anemia; *SCD*, sickle cell disease; *SCID*, severe combined immunodeficiency; *WAS*, Wiskott-Aldrich syndrome.

2. **What is human leukocyte antigen typing, and how is it used for allogeneic hematopoietic stem cell transplantation?**
Human leukocyte antigen (HLA) typing has had a tremendous impact on allogeneic hematopoietic stem cell transplantation (alloHCT) outcomes. HLA genes are part of the major histocompatibility complex, responsible for alloreactivity because of minor and major HLA mismatch between patient and donor. HLA genes are located on chromosome 6, and HLA antigens are divided into two groups. Class I consists of HLA-A, HLA-B, and HLA-C and Class II includes HLA-DP, HLA-DQ, and HLA-DRBI.

HLA typing can be performed on blood samples or buccal swabs. The current standard is to perform matching by analyzing DNA at the allelic level, which is more precise than antigen typing. Over the decades, the level of matching for unrelated donors has evolved from matching at 8 alleles (HLA-A, HLA-B, HLA-C, and HLA-DRBI) to 10 alleles (HLA-A, HLA-B, HLA-C, HLA-DQ, and HLA-DRBI). When several 10 out of 10 (10/10) HLA-matched donors are available, typing can be extended to 12 alleles (to include HLA-DPB1). A better match is associated with better outcomes because of lower risk of graft versus host disease (GVHD) and graft rejection.

For sibling and haploidentical donors, HLA typing should be performed at 10 HLA alleles. In the past, siblings were typed at 6 alleles (HLA-A, HLA-B, and HLA-DRBI). Occasionally, however, 6 out of 6 HLA-matched siblings may not be a 10/10 match.

For unrelated umbilical cord blood (CB) transplants, HLA typing has also evolved. In the past, antigen typing was performed for HLA-A, HLA-B, and allelic typing for HLA-DRB1; however, CB is now typed at the allelic level for all 6 loci.

3. **What are the different types of donors considered for alloHCT?**
AlloHCT donors can be broadly divided into two groups: HLA-matched sibling donors (MSD) and alternate donors. Alternate donors can be further subdivided into mismatched family donors (50%–90% HLA matched) or unrelated donors, which include adult unrelated donors and unrelated umbilical CB (HLA matched [100% matching] or mismatched [70%–90% match]).

The use of an MSD is the gold standard and is associated with best overall outcomes because of lower risk of acute GVHD. Conversely, a MSD is associated with higher incidence of leukemia relapse, likely because of lower alloreactivity provided by donor immune system. When an HLA-matched sibling is unavailable, a 10/10 HLA-matched unrelated donor (MUD) is preferred. If 10/10 MUD is also unavailable, depending on a center's experience, haploidentical or unrelated umbilical cord can be chosen as donor for alloHCT.

4. **What types of hematopoietic cell sources can be used for alloHCT?**
Hematopoietic cells can be obtained from the bone marrow (BM), peripheral blood (PBSC), or umbilical CB. BM harvests from related and unrelated donors are performed under general anesthesia. The most common side effect is procedural pain, which typically resolves in 1 to 2 weeks. Some centers use granulocyte colony-stimulating factor (G-CSF) mobilization to increase the number of CD34$^+$ cells in the BM, especially when the donor's weight is lower than the recipient's weight.

For PBSC donation, G-CSF is administered to the donors for 4 to 5 days. Most donors require temporary placement of a double lumen catheter (i.e., in the internal jugular vein) for an apheresis procedure. The procedure takes approximately 4 to 6 hours to complete and may require a second day of apheresis.

In pediatrics, BM is the preferred stem cell source for alloHCT because it is associated with a lower incidence of chronic graft versus host disease (cGVHD). This is particularly true for patients with nonmalignant diseases when GVHD is not beneficial for cure. For patients with pre-alloHCT comorbidities, especially infectious concerns, PBSC is used because neutrophil recovery is much faster.

5. **How are donor and cell sources selected for alloHCT?**
When multiple MSDs and MUDs are available, the purpose of optimal donor selection is to minimize the risk of severe aGVHD and donor safety. The following factors are considered in donor selection:
   A. **Age:** For HLA-matched siblings, younger donors have higher CD34$^+$ cells/μL; however, BM harvest in children under 2 years old can be difficult. Beyond 2 years of age, younger donor is preferred, unless there is a large weight discrepancy between the patient and donor. The maximum volume of BM that can be harvested from a donor is 20 mL/kg. If a patient's weight is greater than 10 kg compared with the donor's weight, CD34$^+$ cell collection may be inadequate. For unrelated donors, the upper age limit is 62 years old. Younger donors are still preferred.
   B. **Sex:** Female lymphocytes can identify the Y antigen in males; hence, male recipients of female hematopoietic cells are at high risk for GVHD. If everything is equal, in the case of male recipients, male donors are preferred.
   C. **Parity:** Transplacental migration of fetal lymphocytes and other proteins can result in maternal HLA allosensitization. Allosensitization from donors with past pregnancies can result in a higher risk of GVHD; hence, nulliparous female are preferred donors.
   D. **Cytomegalovirus (CMV) status**: Preference is given to donors who have similar CMV serological profiles to the recipient. CMV reactivation post-alloHCT is associated with inferior outcomes. The risk of CMV reactivation is lowest when both recipient and donor are CMV serology negative, intermediate when both are positive, and highest when either recipient or donor is positive.

E. **ABO blood type:** Major mismatch of blood group between recipient and patient can result in a higher incidence of graft failure and pure red cell aplasia. Residual host B-cells and plasma cells can produce anti-A, anti-B, or both antibodies, which can attach to early erythroid precursors, resulting in elimination of those cells.

F. **Cell source:** Occasionally, donors are deemed unfit for either BM or PBSC donation. Depending on the clinical situation, this may impact donor choice.

6. **What is T-cell depletion? How and why is it performed?**

T-cell depletion is performed to optimize the stem cell source before the infusion. In most cases, the goal is to decrease the risk of GVHD by reducing the number of T-cells ex vivo or in vivo. Depletion of T-cells, however, is associated with a higher risk of leukemia relapse, graft failure, and viral infections.

In ex vivo T-cell depletion, the PBSC product undergoes cell separation by magnetic beads and columns. Different methods include CD34 enrichment and alpha-beta T-cell depletion. In CD34-selected graft manipulation, a highly purified population of CD34 stem cells is obtained, and a small, predetermined number of T-cells are added back to the product before infusion. Alternatively, in alpha-beta T-cell depletion, the alpha-beta T cells presumed responsible for GVHD are removed, whereas gamma-delta T cells remain in product to provide graft versus malignancy and antiviral effects.

In vivo graft manipulation uses various medications to deplete infused donor T-cells. Commonly used medications are the monoclonal antibodies, antithymocyte globulin (ATG) and alemtuzumab. ATG is produced from the injection of fetal thymus tissue in horses or rabbits, resulting in the development of antibodies that can bind to T-cells. Alemtuzumab is an anti-CD52 monoclonal antibody; CD52 is expressed on most immune cells. ATG or alemtuzumab is infused during conditioning and binds to host T-cells to reduce the risk of graft rejection. Because both of these antibodies have a long half-life, they also bind to the infused donor T cells after transplant, resulting in decreased incidence of GVHD.

7. **Why are conditioning regimens used before transplant? What are the types of conditioning regimens used?**

The majority of patients receive chemotherapy, and some receive total body irradiation (TBI) therapy before infusion of hematopoietic cells. The purpose of the conditioning regimen is to partially or completely eliminate the BM and immune system. In patients with malignant diseases, it is also used to minimize disease burden so that the donor immune system has a better chance to eliminate minimal residual disease.

Conditioning Regimen	Explanation	Advantages	Disadvantages	Indications	Examples
Myeloablative conditioning (MAC) regimens	• Highest doses of chemotherapy and/or TBI	• Provide maximum ablation of bone marrow • Improved chances of engraftment • Improved antileukemia activity	• Increased risk of organ injury	• ALL • AML • JMML • Transfusion dependent thalassemia	• Busulfan (12.8–16 mg/kg) + cyclophosphamide (100–200 mg/kg) • TBI (12 Gray) + cyclophosphamide (100–120 mg/kg) ± thiotepa (10 mg/kg)
Reduced Intensity Conditioning (RIC) Regimens	• Lower doses of chemotherapy • Intense immunotherapy to decrease risk of graft rejection	• Minimize organ damage	• Increased risk of graft rejection in patients with nonmalignant disease, despite immunotherapy • Increased risk of viral infections	• SCD • HLH • Patients with pretransplant comorbidities precluding them from receiving MAC regimen	• Fludarabine (150–180 mg/m^2) + melphalan (140 mg/m^2) + alemtuzumab • Fludarabine (150–180 mg/m^2) + cyclophosphamide (60 mg/kg) + ATG • Fludarabine (150–180 mg/m^2) + busulfan (6.4–8 mg/kg) + ATG

| Reduced toxicity conditioning (RTC) regimens | • Doses of chemotherapy between RIC and MAC regimen dosing • Use one alkylator (vs. two in MAC regimens) and replace other alkylator with Fludarabine | • Reduce organ injury • Lower risk of graft rejection compared with RIC regimens | • Higher risk of graft rejection compared with MAC regimens | • SCD • AML | • Busulfan (12.8–16 mg/kg) + Fludarabine (150–180 mg/m^2) • Alemtuzumab or ATG |

ALL, Acute lymphoblastic leukemia; *AML*, acute myeloid leukemia; *HLH*, hemophagocytic lymphohistiocytosis; *JMML*, juvenile myelomonocytic leukemia; *SCD*, sickle cell disease; *TBI*, total body irradiation.

8. **Why do some patients receive total body irradiation?**
   Radiation therapy has strong antileukemia activity. Total body irradiation (TBI) is the preferred conditioning regimen for patients with acute lymphoblastic leukemia (ALL) and is associated with a better leukemia-free survival (LFS). It can, however, cause neurological deficits in children, especially among patients who are younger than 3 years old, so some physicians may choose to instead use a chemotherapy-based conditioning regimen for those patients. TBI is associated with a significant number of long-term side effects.

9. **Describe the steps involved in proceeding with alloHCT.**
   A. **Donor Procurement**: Once a patient has met the indication for alloHCT and the family has received counseling about risks and benefits, the donor search is started. First, the patient and biological siblings undergo HLA typing with results taking approximately 1 week. If there is no 10/10 HLA-matched sibling, the patient's HLA typing is entered into the National Marrow Donor Program Match (Be the Match) and a list of potential unrelated donors (adults and CB) is generated. If available, suitable donors undergo history and physical examination. It takes approximately 6 to 8 weeks to procure product from an adult unrelated donor. When a 10/10 HLA-matched unrelated donor is not available, depending on their experience, some centers prefer to perform transplant using haploidentical donors from within the family, whereas others prefer CB transplant. In some patients, particularly those with leukemia, the window to perform an alloHCT could be very narrow, and thus an unrelated donor may not be an optimal source.
   B. **Disease Control:** LFS is affected by pre-alloHCT minimal residual disease (MRD) status. Patients who are MRD negative have superior LFS. Reasonable attempts should be made to bring MRD levels to negative. Nevertheless, it is crucial to balance the risk of organ injury and infections from additional chemotherapy versus lower risk post-alloHCT. The desired MRD negative level is less than 1 leukemia cell per 10,000 normal cells in the BM. In recent times, more and more patients with primary immune dysregulation are undergoing alloHCT; in those patients, it is paramount to have inflammation under excellent control. Excess inflammation can result in stormy course in the peritransplant period. Patients with ongoing inflammation at the time of transplant should continue to receive disease-specific anti-inflammation therapy.
   C. **Organ Function and Infection:** All patients have to undergo liver, renal, cardiac, and pulmonary function tests. Patients with pretransplant organ dysfunction are at high risk of post-transplant complications. Occasionally, the intensity of the conditioning regimen or chemotherapeutic agents used have to be adjusted because of organ dysfunction. Patients with active infections also have a higher risk of complications. Every attempt should be made to control infections before alloHCT. In patients with severe combined immunodeficiency or severe aplastic anemia, however, some physicians may choose to proceed to transplant despite active infection because reconstitution of the immune system might be the only strategy to cure these patients.

10. **Define engraftment and immune reconstitution after alloHCT.**
    Engraftment is one of the most crucial events to occur after HCT. Lack of cellular reconstitution predisposes patients to various infections and disease recurrence. Neutrophil engraftment is defined by absolute neutrophil count (ANC) greater than 500/μL × 3 days with the first day of ANC greater than 500/μL being considered the day of neutrophil engraftment. The rule of thumb for neutrophil engraftment is 2, 3, and 4 weeks for PBSC, BM, and CB, respectively.
    Platelet engraftment is defined as platelet count greater than 20,000/μL for 7 days without platelet transfusion. This typically occurs approximately 2 weeks after neutrophil engraftment.
    T-cell reconstitution is crucial for antiviral immunity. T-cell count also depends on the cell source (PBSC > BM > CB) and immunotherapy used pretransplant. Patients receiving alemtuzumab tend to have delayed T-cell reconstitution compared with patients receiving ATG. Ex vivo T-cell depletion can also result in delayed T-cell recovery.
    B-cell recovery after alloHCT is also important because B cells produce the immunoglobulins required for the prevention of bacterial infections. Patients with GVHD, unrelated donor alloHCT recipients, and those treated with

rituximab may need intravenous gamma globulin (IVIG) infusion for a few months post-alloHCT with the goal to maintain immunoglobulin G (IgG) levels greater than 400 mg/dL.

11. Explain the use of chimerism analysis after alloHCT.

Chimerism analysis is used to assess the proportion of donor cells in the PBSC or BM of the transplant recipient. It is a DNA analysis using donor- and patient-specific STR (single tandem repeat) or VNTR (variable nucleotide tandem repeat). Chimerism can be performed on the whole sample or can be lineage specific. For lineage-specific chimerism, cells are sorted based on surface biomarkers followed by DNA analysis on separated cells. Lineage analysis can be done for myeloid cells (CD33 or 14/15), T-cells (CD3), B-cells (CD19), NK cells (CD56), RBC (CD71), and stem cells (CD34; can only be done on BM specimen). Longitudinal analysis of lineage-specific chimerism can be useful to predict disease relapse, graft failure, or successful transplant in cases of immunodeficiency where occasionally only deficient cell lines engraft.

Myeloablative conditioning regimens usually result in high-level chimerism ($>$95%), which is desirable in patients with leukemia, because lower levels ($<$95%) can be associated with a higher risk of relapse. In patients with nonmalignant diseases, sustained chimerism levels greater than 50% are considered curative. Mixed chimerism, however, in patients with immune dysregulation disorders can result in inferior outcomes because of the risk of autoimmunity post-alloHCT, which arises from the residual host immune system.

Frequency of chimerism analysis is highly variable and depends on the patient, center, and physician. Patients with nonmalignant diseases tend to have more frequent analysis because of high risk of graft failure. Patients with leukemia should have chimerism analysis on days 30, 100, 180, and 365 post-alloHCT, at minimum.

12. How is immunomodulation used post-alloHCT?

Patients at high risk for relapse of leukemia should be closely monitored. In some cases, initiating treatment targeted at the disease-initiating mutation may result in a cure. Such interventions include dasatinib for BCR-ABL and some BCR-ABL-like mutations and sorafenib/gilteritinib for FLT3-ITD mutations. When leukemia cells do not have targetable mutations, tapering or withdrawal of immune suppression or infusion of donor lymphocytes may result in immune activation and molecular remission. This approach, however, can result in a significant increase in the incidence of GVHD.

13. Describe the risk of relapse and potential management strategies after alloHCT.

Relapses are the most common cause of treatment failure after alloHCT. Higher risk of relapse has been associated with reduced intensity-conditioning regimens, inadequate disease control before transplant, T-cell depletion, and incomplete T-cell chimerism. Several studies have demonstrated that grades I to II aGVHD and chronic GVHD are associated with decreased risk of relapse because of graft versus leukemia effect.

Management of relapse post-alloHCT depends on the clinical condition of the patient, disease control after relapse, and parental and patient desire to continue treatment. Treatment options for post-alloHCT relapse include chimeric antigen receptor (CAR)-T cells for ALL and acute myeloid leukemia (experimental) or second alloHCT if the patient has disease control, good performance status, and minimal comorbidities. The use of the same donor for a second alloHCT is a subject of debate. Theoretically, a different donor should be used if feasible.

BIBLIOGRAPHY

1. Satwani P, Cooper N, Rao K, Veys P, Amrolia P. Reduced intensity conditioning and allogeneic stem cell transplantation in childhood malignant and nonmalignant diseases. *Bone Marrow Transplant.* 2008;41(2):173–182.
2. Sharma A, Li Y, Huang S, et al. Outcomes of pediatric patients who relapse after first HCT for acute leukemia or MDS. *Bone Marrow Transpl.* 2021;56:1866–1875.
3. Forman SJ, Negrin RS, Antin JH, Appelbaum FR (eds). *Thomas' Hematopoietic Cell Transplantation: Stem Cell Transplantation.* 5th ed. Wiley and Sons, 2015.
4. Martinez-Cibrian N, Zeiser R, Perez-Simon JA. Graft-versus-host disease prophylaxis: pathophysiology-based review on current approaches and future directions. *Blood Rev.* 2021;48:100792.
5. Zeiser R. Advances in understanding the pathogenesis of graft-versus-host disease. *Br J Haematol.* 2019;187(5):563–572.

AUTOLOGOUS HEMATOPOIETIC STEM CELL TRANSPLANTATION FOR CHILDREN AND YOUNG ADULTS

James H. Garvin, Jr

Autologous hematopoietic stem cell transplant (auto HSCT) uses patient-derived stem cells to facilitate recovery from myeloablative high-dose chemotherapy for cancer. The concept is that higher doses of certain agents, particularly alkylators, will be 3 to 15 times more potent than conventional doses and will be useful as consolidation therapy after initial cytoreduction, provided nonhematologic toxicity remains acceptable. Use of intensive chemotherapy may also permit deferral or avoidance of radiotherapy in young children.

1. What are hematopoietic stem cells?

Stem cells are self-renewing blood cell progenitors present in the bone marrow that also circulate at low levels in the peripheral blood. Egress of stem cells from marrow to peripheral blood can be enhanced by administration of hematopoietic growth factors ("mobilization") to facilitate collection ("harvesting") for infusion after myeloablative chemotherapy.

2. What pediatric cancers are treated by auto HSCT?

Current pediatric indications for auto HSCT are newly diagnosed high-risk neuroblastoma and infant medulloblastoma, recurrent germ cell tumors, and recurrent lymphoma (Hodgkin lymphoma and non-Hodgkin lymphoma). Neuroblastoma is most frequent, accounting for 43% of the 3076 pediatric autotransplants reported to the Center for International Blood and Marrow Transplant Research (CIBMTR) between 2008 and 2014 (Khandelwal, 2017). Other pediatric applications of auto HSCT have included relapsed Ewing sarcoma (ES), retinoblastoma, and brain tumors other than medulloblastoma.

3. What are some newer applications of auto HSCT?

Auto HSCT has been used to support recovery from myeloablative or lymphoablative chemotherapy in refractory autoimmune disorders such as juvenile idiopathic arthritis and in pediatric multiple sclerosis after failure of standard therapy.

Another type of auto HSCT involves the genetic modification of patient stem cells for correction or amelioration of certain inherited disorders, referred to as "ex vivo gene therapy." Examples include adenosine deaminase deficiency, X-linked cerebral adrenoleukodystrophy, metachromatic leukodystrophy, and hemoglobinopathies (thalassemia and sickle cell anemia). A growing number of pediatric diseases can be successfully cured by hematopoietic stem cell-based gene therapy (Staal, 2019).

A related procedure is a collection of autologous mononuclear cells by leukapheresis for production of chimeric antigen receptor (CAR) T-cells, modified to express a transgene encoding a tumor-specific CAR, then infusing the manufactured CAR T-cells to treat the cancer. CAR T-cell therapy is approved for relapsed or refractory childhood acute lymphocytic leukemia and may be used as definitive therapy or as a bridge to allogeneic HSCT. Investigational applications of CAR T-cell therapy in pediatrics include lymphoma, acute myeloid leukemia (AML), solid tumors, and central nervous system (CNS) tumors.

4. What are the patient selection criteria for auto HSCT?

Auto HSCT may be considered in high-risk solid tumor malignancies that are chemotherapy-sensitive but not routinely curable with standard chemotherapy regimens, in conjunction with surgery and radiotherapy. In neuroblastoma, auto HSCT will typically follow induction chemotherapy and surgery and precede local irradiation. Auto HSCT is offered to infants with chemotherapy-sensitive brain tumors such as medulloblastoma as a strategy to delay or defer craniospinal irradiation. Auto HSCT is second-line treatment for Hodgkin or non-Hodgkin lymphoma relapsing after initial therapy. Auto HSCT may also be considered in refractory or relapsed solid tumors that remain chemo-sensitive, such as germ cell tumors. Patients should have minimal disease and good performance status at the time of auto HSCT.

For children with relapsed leukemia and other bone marrow cancers, auto HSCT would be limited by the presence of residual disease, and allogeneic HSCT is preferred. Auto HSCT has been pursued in adult AML, where higher treatment failure is offset by lower transplant-related mortality compared with allogeneic HSCT, resulting in comparable overall survival (OS). Auto HSCT has been studied in pediatric AML, but allogeneic HSCT is preferred because OS is superior. For children with relapsed ALL, depending on disease status, and in the absence of randomized trials, referral for CAR T-cell therapy may be weighed against options of novel chemotherapy or allogeneic transplant.

5. When and how are stem cells collected?
Minimum stem cell doses required for engraftment are approximately 2 million viable CD34 positive (CD34+) cells per kg of patient weight per transplant. Peripheral blood stem cells (PBSCs) are collected during recovery from initial conventional-dose chemotherapy, by increasing the dose of filgrastim at early count rise and monitoring circulating CD34+ levels. Leukapheresis is initiated when the peripheral blood CD34+ count reaches 20 million per liter. PBSCs are isolated by continuous flow cell separator in one or more daily sessions. A double lumen pheresis-grade catheter is required, placed in advance or at the time of leukapheresis. Small children may require priming of the pheresis machine with irradiated packed red cells to avoid hypovolemia. Harvest yields can be improved by the addition of plerixafor, a CXCL4 antagonist, to colony-stimulating factors, particularly in heavily pretreated patients. In situations of inadequate PBSC yield, resorting to bone marrow harvest may be considered. After collection, the stem cells are cryopreserved in dimethyl sulfoxide (DMSO).

6. Is tumor cell purging helpful?
Tumor cell contamination of the stem cell graft is a potential problem in neuroblastoma or ES because of marrow involvement at diagnosis. Contaminating tumor cells may increase the risk of relapse post high-dose chemotherapy and auto HSCT. Tumor contamination is less likely with PBSC collection after chemotherapy, compared with bone marrow harvest, and can be addressed by immunomagnetic CD34+ positive selection. Nevertheless, a randomized trial of immunomagnetic purging of PBSC for auto HSCT in high-risk neuroblastoma showed no improvement in outcome and concluded nonpurged PBSCs are acceptable (Kreissman, 2013). This result could be because of incomplete purging, and if so, more effective methods might show a benefit to purging.

7. What about sequential tandem auto HSCT?
Initial experience with auto HSCT was based on single transplant, including the demonstration that auto HSCT improved event-free survival (EFS) in high-risk neuroblastoma (Berthold, 2005) and could delay radiation in young children with newly diagnosed malignant brain tumors (Mason, 1998). The possibility of tandem auto HSCT was introduced for infant brain tumors (Cohen, 2015), and a current trial is comparing outcomes for single versus triple-tandem auto HSCT consolidation. Tandem auto HSCT was also tested in neuroblastoma, including double- and triple-tandem transplant. A randomized trial of sequential double transplant for neuroblastoma showed superior 3-year EFS compared with single auto HSCT (61% vs. 48%), although the randomization rate was low (Park, 2019). Single auto HSCT remains standard for relapsed lymphoma and most solid tumors other than neuroblastoma. Auto HSCT is generally an inpatient procedure, but outpatient auto HSCT for selected children with CNS tumors has been shown to be safe and effective; most patients still require hospital admission at the time of fever/neutropenia.

8. What preparative regimens are used in auto HSCT?
Chemotherapy agents applicable to auto HSCT are chosen based on linear-log dose-toxicity for tumor cells and tolerable organ toxicity despite profound myelosuppression. The regimens chosen for high-dose chemotherapy should have known activity against the particular cancer and will have been shown to give superior outcome compared with continued conventional chemotherapy. For brain tumors, the regimen should include agents capable of CNS penetration, such as thiotepa. Initial experience in pediatric auto HSCT for solid tumors was with high-dose melphalan, then with the combination of carboplatin, etoposide, and melphalan (CEM), and subsequently busulfan-melphalan. Tandem auto HSCT could increase response rates, using repeated cycles of the same regimen (such as carboplatin/thiotepa in CNS tumors) or different regimens given sequentially (such as cyclophosphamide/thiotepa followed by dose-reduced CEM in high-risk neuroblastoma). Total body irradiation (TBI) was used in some early protocols for solid tumors, including ES. In neuroblastoma, (131) I-metaiodobenzylguanidine (MIBG) has single agent activity and has been added to the CEM regimen.

9. What happens after the preparative regimen?
After completion of high-dose chemotherapy, the stem cell product is thawed and infused into the peripheral blood of the recipient using a central venous catheter. Transient complications may include fluid overload, hypertension, and DMSO-related nausea. Filgrastim is initiated after PBSC infusion, and over the next 2 to 4 weeks the PBSC differentiate into progenitors capable of restoring normal peripheral blood counts. The time of neutrophil engraftment after single auto HSCT for high-risk neuroblastoma was 12 days with CEM conditioning and 16 days with busulfan/melphalan conditioning.

10. What are current outcomes for pediatric HSCT?

For newly diagnosed high-risk neuroblastoma, high-dose chemotherapy with auto HSCT improves outcomes over conventional chemotherapy alone, and in a Children's Oncology Group (COG) study, 3-year EFS with double-tandem auto HSCT exceeded 60% (Park, 2019). For young children with metastatic medulloblastoma treated with intensive chemotherapy and single auto HSCT on the Head Start 2 protocol, 3-year EFS was 49%, and radiation was avoided in the majority of survivors younger than 5 years of age (Chi, 2004). A COG study of auto HSCT in relapsed/refractory lymphoma patients with complete response to reinduction chemotherapy resulted in 3-year EFS of 66% (65% in Hodgkin lymphoma and 70% in non-Hodgkin lymphoma; Harris, 2011).

In metastatic or relapsed ES, multimodality treatment including auto HSCT with a TBI-melphalan based regimen was associated with 45% EFS at 6 years, but a prospective analysis of ES patients presenting to a single institution with bone or bone marrow metastases found no improvement in survival with auto HSCT incorporating TBI. High-dose chemotherapy with auto HSCT was not beneficial in recurrent Wilms tumor but continues to be used in protocols for refractory or relapsed germ cell tumors and advanced retinoblastoma.

11. What are some acute complications and late effects of HSCT?

Emesis and stomatitis are anticipated because of the intensity of chemotherapy. The associated decreased oral intake may necessitate parenteral nutrition. Antiemetic prophylaxis with fosaprepitant and a 5-HT3-receptor antagonist is recommended. Palifermin (keratinocyte growth factor) may ameliorate stomatitis. Infection is also anticipated, based on the degree and duration of neutropenia. Pulmonary and gastrointestinal infections predominate. Patients generally receive prophylaxis for herpes simplex virus, *Pneumocystis jirovecii*, and fungal infection. Occasional side effects include hepatic sinusoidal obstruction syndrome, thrombotic microangiopathy, diffuse alveolar hemorrhage, and idiopathic pneumonia syndrome. Overall mortality can approach 5%.

Late effects were reported in a cohort of high-risk neuroblastoma patients with median follow-up of 13.9 years after triple-tandem auto HSCT (Armstrong, 2018). Overall survival was 41%. The most frequent sequela was hearing loss, seen in 17 of 19 patients. The majority of late effects were endocrine-related, including growth failure, hypothyroidism, and hypogonadism. Patients also developed secondary neoplasms and skeletal deformities.

BIBLIOGRAPHY

1. Armstrong AE, Danner-Koptik K, Golden S, et al. Late effects in pediatric high-risk neuroblastoma survivors after intensive induction chemotherapy followed by myeloablative consolidation chemotherapy and triple autologous stem cell transplants. *J Pediatr Hematol/ Oncol.* 2018;40:31–35.
2. Berthold F, Boos J, Burdach S, et al. Myeloablative megatherapy with autologous stem-cell rescue versus oral maintenance chemotherapy as consolidation treatment in patients with high-risk neuroblastoma: a randomised controlled trial. *Lancet Oncol.* 2005;6:649–658.
3. Chi SN, Gardner SL, Levy AS, et al. Feasibility and response to induction chemotherapy intensified with high-dose methotrexate for young children with newly diagnosed high-risk disseminated medulloblastoma. *J Clin Oncol.* 2004;22:4881–4887.
4. Cohen BR, Geyer JR, Miller DC, et al. Pilot study of intensive chemotherapy with peripheral hematopoietic cell support for children less than 3 years of age with malignant brain tumors, the CCG-99703 phase I/II study. A report from the Children's Oncology Group. *Pediatr Neurol.* 2015;53:31–46.
5. Harris RE, Termuhlen AM, Smith LM, et al. Autologous peripheral blood stem cell transplantation in children with refractory or relapsed lymphoma: results of Children's Oncology Group Study A5962. *Biol Blood Marrow Transplantation.* 2011;17:249–258.
6. Khandelwal P, Millard HR, Thiel E, et al. Hematopoietic stem cell transplantation activity in pediatric cancer between 2008 and 2014 in the United States: a Center for International Blood and Marrow Transplant Research report. *Bill Blood Marrow Transplant.* 2017;23:1342–1349.
7. Kreissman SG, Seeger RC, Matthay KK, et al. Purged versus non-purged peripheral blood stem-cell transplantation for high-risk neuroblastoma (COG A3973): a randomized phase 3 trial. *Lancet Oncol.* 2013;14:999–1008.
8. Mason WP, Grovas A, Halpern S, et al. Intensive chemotherapy and bone marrow rescue for young children with newly-diagnosed malignant brain tumors. *J Clin Oncol.* 1998;16:210–221.
9. Park JR, Kreissman SG, London WE, et al. Effect of tandem autologous stem cell transplant vs single transplant on event-free survival in patients with high-risk neuroblastoma. A randomized clinical trial. *JAMA.* 2019;322:746–755.
10. Staal FJT, Aiuti A, Cavazzana M. Autologous stem-cell-based gene therapy for inherited disorders: state of the art and perspectives. *Front Pediatr.* 2019;7:443.

CHAPTER 47

CAR-T CELLS: EXPANDING THE UNIVERSE OF IMMUNOTHERAPY IN CHILDREN WITH MALIGNANT DISEASES

Regina Myers, MD, MS and Prakash Satwani, MD

1. **What are chimeric antigen receptor–T cells?**
   Chimeric antigen receptor (CAR)-T cells are a powerful form of adoptive cell therapy. In their native state, T cells do not express antigens targeted to bind to malignant cells. In CAR-T therapy, T cells are harvested from a patient and then genetically engineered using a viral vector (most commonly a lentiviral or retroviral vector) to produce proteins on their surface that can directly bind to the malignant cells. Binding of CAR-T cells with malignant cells leads to activation and proliferation of CAR-T cells, which results in the killing of malignant cells.

2. **Which antigens can be targeted by CAR-T cells in pediatric malignancies?**
   Several potential antigens have been studied in pediatric malignancies. For B-cell acute lymphoblastic leukemia (B-ALL), CD19 and CD22 have been studied; for T-cell acute lymphoblastic leukemia, it has been CD7 and C5; for acute myelogenous leukemia, CD33 and CD123; for non-Hodgkin lymphoma, CD19; and for neuroblastoma, GD2. The most well-studied CAR to date targets CD19.

3. **Describe the history of CAR-T cell development.**
   In the early 1990s, immunologists Zelig Eshhar and Gideon Gross developed the first CAR-T cells. The original construct for the first Food and Drug Administration (FDA)–approved product, however, tisagenlecleucel (Kymriah), was developed by Dario Campana at St. Jude and then significantly modified by Carl June at University of Pennsylvania for clinical application in patients. The product was then tested in phase I trials of adult and pediatric patients at the University of Pennsylvania and Children's Hospital of Philadelphia (CHOP), respectively. The first pediatric patient treated with CD19 CAR was Emily Whitehead at CHOP, who had relapsed/refractory B-ALL. She achieved remission after the therapy and remains in remission with evidence of circulating CAR-T cells over 9 years later. The technology developed at University of Pennsylvania was later transferred to Novartis, who conducted a global registration trial (the ELIANA trial) of tisagenlecleucel. On August 30, 2017, the FDA approved tisagenlecleucel, which was marketed as Kymriah.

4. **What are the indications for tisagenlecleucel administration in pediatric patients?**
   The FDA-approved label for tisagenlecleucel includes children and young adults who are up to 25 years of age and have B-ALL that is either (1) refractory or (2) in second or greater relapse. The precise definition of refractory ALL is not clearly defined by the FDA.

5. **What are the steps for manufacturing CAR-T cells?**
   Once a patient is deemed eligible for CAR-T cells, the medical team has to take several steps for collection, manufacture, and infusion of CAR-T cells.
   Step 1: Cell collection
   A. Insurance approval: The medical team has to prepare a letter of medical necessity for insurance authorization. The current cost of tisagenlecleucel is $475,000; medical centers must follow FDA-approved indications to infuse tisagenlecleucel; otherwise, they risk not receiving reimbursement.
   B. Washout period: Medications that could affect T-cell function should be discontinued for a period of time before collection. The specific washout period is dependent on the specific medication (e.g., 7 days for intrathecal methotrexate vs. 2–4 weeks for PEG-asparaginase).
   C. Cell counts: It is recommended that patients have an absolute lymphocyte count (ALC) of over 500/ μL and a CD3 of more than 150 to 200/μL to yield the best T-cell collection. It is preferred that patients do not have a substantial number of circulating blasts, but the exact cutoff is not firmly established.
   D. Apheresis process: The majority of children will require placement of an apheresis catheter. The apheresis procedure usually takes 3 to 4 hours because 3 to 5 blood volumes have to circulate through the machine.
   E. After apheresis, the optimal total nucleated cell count needed for successful CAR-T manufacturing is 1×10^9 cells/kg. To manufacture tisagenlecleucel, the cells are frozen and then shipped to Novartis.

Step 2: Manufacturing

A. Cell culture: Cryopreserved cells are thawed at Novartis' facility and put in the cell culture medium. Cells are genetically modified during cell culture process, which takes approximately 2 weeks. Before release, the product undergoes viability and cytokine level testing. Products that meet FDA-release criteria are cryopreserved and shipped back to the home center. Products that are outside of FDA-specification (generally because of viability < 80%) can be administered under an expanded access protocol.

B. Manufacturing failure: Up to 7% of products will fail to manufacture. The causes of manufacturing failure are not fully described. We speculate that it could be related to past chemotherapy exposures, such as doxorubicin, cyclophosphamide, and clofarabine, which can alter the energy metabolism of T cells, rendering them with poor proliferative capacity.

6. What are the steps for bridging chemotherapy and lymphodepletion before CAR-T cell infusion?

Bridging Chemotherapy: The time from leukapheresis to CAR-T infusion is generally 4 to 6 weeks. During that period, most patients will require chemotherapy to decrease or maintain their leukemia burden. It is generally recommended to give the least toxic chemotherapy that will allow for disease control. In addition, it is important to consider avoiding certain agents. For example, inotuzumab ozogamicin is generally not preferred during the bridging period because it can lead to prolonged B-cell aplasia and concerns have been raised about the effectiveness of CD19 CAR in the absence of any CD19$^+$ antigen load.

Lymphodepletion chemotherapy: The goal of lymphodepletion is to provide an in-vivo environment that will result in the expansion, function, and persistence of CAR-T cells. The preferred regimen includes cyclophosphamide (500 mg/m^2 × 2 days) and fludarabine (30mg/m^2 × 4 days). It is hypothesized that these agents result in the depletion of T cells, B cells, and natural killer (NK) cells and the eradication of immunosuppressive T-regulatory cells and cytokines. CAR-T cells can be infused 2 to 14 days after finishing lymphodepletion.

7. What are the steps for infusion of CAR-T cells?

A. Disease assessment: Some centers perform a bone marrow aspiration/biopsy before lymphodepletion; others perform the assessment after lymphodepletion but before CAR infusion.

B. Infection and organ function: Patients should not have any active infections before CAR-T infusion. This includes documenting a negative influenza test during influenza season. The presence of active infection can result in more severe side effects such as severe cytokine release syndrome. Patients should also have adequate organ function before infusion.

C. Setting for infusion: CAR-T cells can be infused in the inpatient or outpatient setting. If performed outpatient, it is important that the patient stays within close proximity of the treating center.

D. Infusion: A single dose of tisagenlecleucel generally ranges from 0.2 to 5.0 × 10^6 CAR-T cells/kg for patients up to 50 kg and 0.1 to 2.5 × 10^8 CAR-T cells for patients over 50 kg. Typically, the actual volume of CAR-T cells is small (<50 mL); thus the infusion can be completed in a few minutes. Infusion-associated reactions are rare, but premedication with acetaminophen and diphenhydramine is advised (corticosteroids need to be avoided).

8. What are the primary toxicities associated with CAR-T cells?

The major unique toxicities of CAR-T cells include cytokine release syndrome (CRS) and immune effector cell-associated neurotoxicity syndrome (ICANS). Other common toxicities include cytopenias, infection, hypogammaglobulinemia, and other organ toxicity.

9. What is the pathophysiology and clinical course of CRS?

The activation and proliferation of CAR-T cells results in the release of various inflammatory cytokines. One of the key cytokines driving toxicity is interleukin-6 (IL-6), which is predominantly released by the macrophages. The first clinical sign of CRS is fever, which generally starts within 1 to 10 days after CAR infusion. Patients with high bone marrow disease burden often have early-onset CRS, with fevers starting within 3 days of infusion. Fevers typically start as low grade but can rapidly become high grade and persistent. In some patients, the CRS can progress to include hypotension and hypoxia. The cornerstone of severe CRS management is administration of tocilizumab, an IL-6 receptor antibody, that has led to rapid reversal of CRS in many cases. Other supportive care measures are also essential. Management of CRS-induced hypotension is slightly different than septic shock. It is recommended that if hypotension persists after 1 to 2 fluid boluses, vasoactive medications be initiated right away. CRS can cause severe capillary leak, and thus administration of excessive fluids can lead to pulmonary edema. Hypoxia management includes supportive care that may include supplement oxygen by nasal cannula, noninvasive positive ventilation, or, in severe cases, mechanical ventilation. In some patients, severe CRS has clinical signs, symptoms, and biochemical features similar to secondary hemophagocytic lymphohistiocytosis. Severe CRS can lead to multiorgan failure and death in a small number of patients. The reported incidence of severe CRS has ranged from 8% to 43% but appears to be declining in recent years because of treatment of patients earlier in their disease course with lower bone marrow leukemic burden.

10. **For patients with severe, refractory CRS, are there other pharmacologic interventions beyond tocilizumab and supportive care?**
   For severe CRS that does not improve with tocilizumab and other supportive care measures, administration of corticosteroids is indicated. There have been concerns raised about the negative impact of corticosteroids on CAR-T cell expansion and persistence. Nevertheless, there are data suggesting that this impact is not substantial, especially in severe CRS after CD19 CAR products. For CRS refractory to both tocilizumab and corticosteroids, other anticytokine therapies have been used, including siltuximab (direct anti-IL-6 antibody), anakinra (IL-1 receptor antagonist), and emapalumab (monoclonal antibody to interferon gamma).

11. **How is CRS graded?**
   There have been several grading systems for CRS described and used. In 2018, however, the American Society of Transplant and Cellular Therapy (ASTCT) developed consensus criteria that have subsequently been widely adopted. This scale grades CRS from grades 1 to 5 and includes a combination of the presence of fever, degree of hypotension, and degree of hypoxia.

12. **Can CRS be prevented?**
   Bone marrow leukemic burden is the primary risk factor associated with the development of severe CRS. The initial CD19 CAR trials demonstrated a 50% risk of severe CRS in patients with more than 40% bone marrow blasts at the time of CAR infusion. Thus it is important, when feasible, to aim to lower the disease burden before infusion. In addition, several recent studies have reported earlier intervention with tocilizumab and/or corticosteroids to mitigate the risk of severe CRS. The results of these studies suggested that earlier intervention at the time of mild CRS may decrease the risk of progression to severe CRS without compromising antitumor efficacy or safety.

13. **What is the incidence, clinical presentation, and management of ICANS?**
   Approximately 20% of patients develop ICANS after CD19 CAR. The median time of onset is 10 days after CAR infusion. The spectrum of symptoms can be highly variable. The most common findings are delirium with impairment of cognition and attention. An expressive or global aphasia can also be seen. Less commonly, seizures can be seen in 3% to 4% of pediatric patients. The most severe and devastating presentation of ICANS is cerebral edema, which can be fatal. Management of ICANS is generally supportive, and ICANS is fully reversible in most cases without specific intervention. In severe ICANS, systemic corticosteroids can be used.

14. **What are other common CAR-associated toxicities?**
   Other potential toxicities include infection, cytopenias, and hypogammaglobulinemia. All patients with fever after CAR-T cell infusion should receive empiric coverage for bloodstream bacterial infections. The choice and duration of antibiotics should be based on institutional guidelines. Although fever is most commonly because of CRS, patients are also at high risk for developing infections because of immunosuppression, presence of an indwelling central venous catheter, and, often, neutropenia. Grade 3 to 4 pancytopenia is seen in many patients in the initial postinfusion period, which can occur as a result of CRS-related inflammation, lymphodepleting chemotherapy, and leukemia. Some patients also experience persistent cytopenias beyond the first month after infusion, which can last many years. The exact incidence and pathophysiology of persistent cytopenias have not yet been well described. In addition, CD19 CAR leads to expected B-cell aplasia, resulting in hypogammaglobulinemia. The hypogammaglobulinemia can persist for many years, especially in patients with ongoing circulating CAR-T cells. Patients should receive immunoglobulin replacement via intravenous or subcutaneous infusion throughout the period of B-cell aplasia, or for immunoglobulin G (IgG) levels less than 400 to 500 mg/dL in patients with B-cell recovery.

15. **How many patients achieve remission with CD19 CAR?**
   Approximately 28 days after infusion, a disease evaluation is performed, including a bone marrow aspirate/biopsy, cerebrospinal fluid analysis, and peripheral blood flow cytometry for CD19. Across different CD19 CAR constructs, including commercial tisagenlecleucel, very high complete remission rates (70%–97%) have been reported at the day 28 timepoint. In addition, the vast majority of patients have been minimal residual disease (MRD)–negative by multiparameter flow cytometry and had B-cell aplasia, indicative of circulating CAR-T cells.

16. **What is the risk of relapse after CD19 CAR?**
   Although remission rates are very high across different CD19 CAR trials and constructs, more than 25% to 50% of patients experience a subsequent relapse in the first 12 to 24 months after infusion. In the global registration trial of tisagenlecleucel, for example, among patients who achieved complete remission, the 24-month relapse-free survival rate was 62%.

17. **What are the mechanisms of relapse after CD19 CAR?**
   There are two overarching mechanisms that lead to relapse after CD19 CAR: (1) loss of CAR-T cell persistence allowing for relapse of residual leukemic cells and (2) escape from CAR-T cell killing through target antigen downregulation or escape. Relapse because of limited CAR-T cell persistence is generally CD19-positive, whereas relapse because of escape from CAR-T cell killing is generally CD19-negative. There is also another specific type of CD19-negative relapse that has been reported after CD19 CAR: lineage switch. Most reports of lineage switch involve patients with *KMT2A*-rearranged B-ALL, a cytogenetic lesion common in infant leukemia, and result in a change from lymphoblastic to myeloid leukemia.

18. **What are the risk factors for relapse after CD19 CAR?**
There are a number of potential factors that may be associated with relapse risk including pre-CAR infusion disease burden, prior therapy received, and duration of CAR-T cell persistence. Several recent studies have identified that high bone marrow disease burden (defined as >5% or >40% depending on the study) is the strongest predictor of relapse after CAR. In addition, prior leukemia-directed therapies may affect relapse risk. A few recent studies have shown worse outcomes in patients with prior blinatumomab exposure. As previously noted, short CAR-T cell persistence also contributes to relapse risk.

19. **For patients who relapse after CAR, are second infusions (or reinfusions) possible?**
Yes, second infusions of CD19 CAR may be possible if the leukemic cells continue to demonstrate surface expression of CD19 antigen after relapse. Many patients have surplus doses of CAR products manufactured at the same time as initial manufacture, which can be stored for future use. A recent study of adult patients with B-ALL, chronic lymphocytic leukemia, or non-Hodgkin lymphoma reported a 20% complete response rate after CD19 CAR reinfusion. There are current clinical trials, including one led by Novartis, testing reinfusions of CD19 CARs in pediatric patients with B-ALL.

20. **What is the role of allogeneic hematopoietic cell transplant after CD19 CAR?**
The role of consolidative allogeneic hematopoietic cell transplant (alloHCT) after achieving MRD negative complete remission after CD19 CAR needs further prospective study. No clinical trials have randomly allocated patients to alloHCT versus no alloHCT, and practice varies by product and by center. Several centers recommend alloHCT for all patients who have not had a prior alloHCT before CD19 CAR. Many centers recommend alloHCT for patients who have short CAR persistence, often defined as B-cell recovery within 6 months after CAR infusion. Other centers have used detection of new MRD-level disease by next-generational sequencing (without MRD detected by flow cytometry) as an indication for alloHCT.

21. **What are the new and future developments in CAR-T for pediatric B-ALL?**
Many new and future developments within CAR-T for B-ALL are focused on strategies to prevent or treat relapse after CD19 CAR. To prevent or treat CD19-positive relapsed disease, approaches being tested include treatment with humanized CD19 CAR products, treatment with immune-checkpoint inhibitors in combination with CAR, and administration of T-cell antigen-presenting cells (T-APCs) after CAR. To prevent or treat CD19-negative relapses, other antigen-targeted CARs (e.g., CD22 CAR) and multiantigen CARs (e.g., CD19/CD22 CAR) are now being tested in early-phase clinical trials. In addition, allogeneic CARs are being developed and tested in patients who are unable to generate autologous products. Further efforts are devoted to new CAR manufacturing platforms that have the potential to manufacture products much faster than the current 2 to 4 week timeframe.

22. **What are the new and future developments in CAR-T beyond B-ALL.**
The landscape of CAR-T for children and young adults is now extending well beyond B-ALL. Several products are currently being tested in early-phase clinical trials, including CD33 and CD123 CARs for acute myeloid leukemia. And many more additional products are in various stages of preclinical development, including CARs for T-cell ALL and CARs for a multitude of solid and brain tumors.

BIBLIOGRAPHY

1. Boettcher M, Joechner A, Li Z, Yang SF, Schlegel P. Development of CAR T cell therapy in children-a comprehensive overview. *J Clin Med.* 2022;11(8):2158.
2. Lee DW, Santomasso BD, Locke FL, et al. ASTCT consensus grading for cytokine release syndrome and neurologic toxicity associated with immune effector cells. *Biol Blood Marrow Transplant.* 2019;25(4):625–638.
3. Maude SL, Laetsch TW, Buechner J, et al. Tisagenlecleucel in children and young adults with B-cell lymphoblastic leukemia. *N Engl J Med.* 2018;378(5):439–448.
4. Maus MV, Alexander S, Bishop MR, et al. Society for immunotherapy of cancer (SITC) clinical practice guideline on immune effector cell-related adverse events. *J Immunother Cancer.* 2020;8(2):e001511.
5. Myers RM, Li Y, Barz Leahy A, et al. Humanized CD19-targeted chimeric antigen receptor (CAR) T cells in CAR-naive and CAR-exposed children and young adults with relapsed or refractory acute lymphoblastic leukemia. *J Clin Oncol.* 2021;39(27):3044–3055.
6. Pulsipher MA, Han X, Maude SL, et al. Next-generation sequencing of minimal residual disease for predicting relapse after tisagenlecleucel in children and young adults with acute lymphoblastic leukemia. *Blood Cancer Discov.* 2022;3(1):66–81.
7. Schultz LM, Baggott C, Prabhu S, et al. Disease burden affects outcomes in pediatric and young adult B-Cell lymphoblastic leukemia after commercial tisagenlecleucel: a pediatric real-world chimeric antigen receptor consortium report. *J Clin Oncol.* 2022;40(9):945–955.

CHAPTER 48

GENE THERAPY FOR HEMOGLOBINOPATHIES AND OTHER DISEASES

Laurie Davis, MD, PhD and Monica Bhatia, MD

Hemoglobinopathies are genetically inherited conditions that originate from the lack or malfunction of components that comprise the hemoglobin (Hb) protein. Sickle cell disease (SCD) and thalassemia are the most common forms of these conditions. SCD is caused by a well-defined point mutation in the β-globin gene and therefore is an optimal target for hematopoietic stem cell (HSC) gene-addition/editing therapy. Similarly, β-thalassemias are caused by point mutations or, more rarely, deletions in the β-globin gene on chromosome 11, leading to reduced (β^+) or absent (β^0) synthesis of the β-chains of Hb. In HSC gene-addition therapy, a therapeutic β-globin gene is integrated into patient HSCs via lentiviral transduction, resulting in long-term phenotypic correction. State-of-the-art gene-editing technology has made it possible to repair the β-globin mutation in patient HSCs or target genetic loci associated with reactivation of endogenous γ-globin expression.

1. **How does gene therapy work?**
   Gene therapy is a therapeutic approach that aims to add, delete, or correct genetic material to treat a disease. Modifying genetic material changes how a protein, or group of proteins, is produced by the cell. In other words, gene therapy aims to give the cell a new set of instructions to change either the amount or type of protein that is produced. By changing the instructions for the production of protein, gene therapy treats the disease at the genetic level.

2. **What is the difference between gene addition and gene editing?**
   Overall, there are two types of gene therapy being studied: gene addition and gene editing. Gene addition treats diseases at the genetic level by adding genetic material to a person's cells to compensate for a missing or faulty gene. Gene editing treats diseases at the genetic level by directly modifying a patient's DNA through a number of different techniques. These techniques are gene inactivation/disruption (also called gene silencing, knockdown, or knockout) and gene correction/insertion.

3. **How does gene addition work?**
   Gene addition therapy is a common gene technique being explored for single-gene diseases—disorders where a mutation occurs in one or both sets of a patient's genes. This gene therapy technique usually involves the insertion of functional (or healthy) copies of a gene (otherwise known as a transgene) into a person's cells by way of a viral vector. Vectors deliver the functional gene to the patient's cells, either *in vivo* or *ex vivo*. Once inside the cell, the transgene provides the cell with instructions that lead to the production of functional proteins. With gene addition therapy, the mutated gene does not need to be replaced or removed. This provides the cell with the instructions that lead to the production of functional genes, while not needing to replace or remove the mutated gene.

4. **What viral vectors have been used in gene therapy?**
   In early trials, a γ-retroviral vector was used to transduce hematopoietic stem cells (HSCs); however, this vector proved to be inadequate for the use of hemoglobinopathies. This was because of its inability to insert target genetic material into nondividing cells such as quiescent HSCs, as well as space limitations within the vector, the relatively large size of the β-globin gene, and that insertion requires promoters. Lentiviral vectors based on the human immunodeficiency virus type 1 (HIV-1) have led to significant advancements in safety and efficacy in genetic delivery into cellular genomes. These vectors have a greater capacity for larger gene sequences and beneficial modifications such as self-inactivation that decrease the risks of insertional oncogenesis. In vivo gene therapy is in the early stages of development using adenoviral vectors, which can be directly injected into the patient's blood.

5. **How does gene editing work?**
   Gene editing involves the creation of targeted breaks in the DNA, with or without instructions to repair them, through a number of different techniques. There are two primary techniques in gene editing: disruption/inactivation and correction/insertion.
   - "Disrupting" or "inactivating" genetic material that is responsible for the genetic disease: This can be achieved by turning off genes that cause disease or disrupting a separate gene that will compensate for the disease-causing gene
   - "Correcting" genetic material by creating a break in the gene and providing a corrective template or "inserting" new genetic material for the cell to use to repair the mutated gene.

6. What is CRISPR?

CRISPR is an acronym for the Clustered Regularly Interspaced Short Palindromic Repeats system found in bacteria and is a specific gene-editing technology.

There are two parts to the CRISPR system: The first is the Cas enzyme itself, and the second is the guide ribonucleic acid (RNA), the tool used to locate the targeted genetic material. Cas proteins (most commonly, Cas9) are a specific class of enzymes that break the target DNA sequence. These proteins work with the guide RNA, which is engineered with a specific sequence that tells the Cas protein where to break the DNA. Once the DNA is cut, this break can be used to repair the broken gene with or without instructions on how to do so.

7. What are the advantages of gene therapy over allogeneic hematopoietic cell transplantation in patients with hemoglobinopathies?

Gene therapy uses autologous (one's own cells), genetically modified HSCs as an alternative to allogenic hematopoietic stem cell transplantation (HSCT) for treating hemoglobinopathies. It circumvents the need for a matched donor and thus avoids the risk of graft versus host disease and graft rejection after HSCT. Furthermore, the conditioning regimen required for the engraftment of genetically modified cells, because of their autologous origin, does not include immunosuppressive drugs.

8. Have other disorders used gene therapy techniques as a curative option?

Gene therapy has successfully treated several primary immunodeficiencies (PIDs) including adenosine deaminase (ADA) severe combined immunodeficiency (SCID), X-linked SCID, Artemis SCID, Wiskott-Aldrich syndrome, X-linked chronic granulomatous disease, and leukocyte adhesion deficiency-I. In all, gene therapy for PIDs has progressed over the recent decades to be equal or better than allogeneic HSCT in terms of efficacy and safety.

9. What has been the experience of gene therapy in immunodeficiencies?

Initial studies of gene therapy for PIDs in the 1990s to 2000s used integrating murine gamma-retroviral vectors. Although these studies showed clinical efficacy in many cases, especially with the administration of marrow cytoreductive conditioning before cell reinfusion, these vectors caused genotoxicity and development of leukoproliferative disorders in several patients. More recent studies have used lentiviral vectors in which the enhancer elements of the long terminal repeats self-inactivate during reverse transcription ("SIN" vectors). These SIN vectors have excellent safety profiles and have not been reported to cause any clinically significant genotoxicity.

10. What are the current inclusion criteria for the use of gene therapy in patients with hemoglobinopathies?

In patients with SCD, current trials include those with severe symptoms such as acute chest syndrome, multiple pain crises, recurrent priapism, and/or splenomegaly. β-thalassemia patients have been required to have severe phenotypes causing transfusion dependence to be eligible for these gene therapy trials.

11. How is gene therapy performed?

Gene-modifying therapy for hemoglobinopathies is currently being offered in the United States only through clinical trials. The process is lengthy and is similar regardless of whether the approach is a gene addition or gene editing one. It is divided into four stages:

A. Stage 1 – Screening: Patients are screened to determine whether they are eligible candidates for the clinical trial. This includes a detailed history and physical examination as well as blood tests and organ function testing. If all criteria are met based on these assessments, the patient proceeds to Stage 2.

B. Stage 2 – Stem Cell Collection and Manufacturing: Patients are then admitted to the hospital to undergo peripheral blood stem cell collection. Stem cells will be released from the bone marrow using a medication called plerixafor and collected through an intravenous (IV) line. Each collection cycle is 3 days, and some patients may require more than one cycle to obtain sufficient numbers of stem cells. These stem cells will then be collected and sent to a central lab where they will be modified depending on the approach (gene addition vs. gene editing).

C. Stage 3 – Preparative Chemotherapy and Infusion: Once the cells have been modified, they are returned back to the patient's treating center. The patient is then admitted to undergo myeloablative chemotherapy. This creates space in the bone marrow allowing the cells to proliferate. Engraftment of these cells usually takes approximately 3 to 4 weeks, during which time the patient will be hospitalized.

D. Stage 4 – Follow-Up: Upon discharge, the patient is followed monthly for the first 6 months and then every 3 months for the first 2 years for lab work and physical assessments. After the first 2 years, the patient is then transitioned to a long-term follow-up study for an additional 13 years.

12. What is the landscape of current gene therapy trials?

Gene addition for β-thalassemia: Betibeglogene autotemcel (Beti-cel) ex vivo gene therapy integrates functional copies of a modified form of the β-globin gene (β^{A-T87Q}-globin gene) into a patient's own HSCs. The efficacy and safety of this treatment has been studied in 5 clinical trials: two phase I/II trials (HGB-204 and HGB-205), two phase III trials (NorthStar-2 (HGB-207) and North-Star 3 (HGB-212)), and one long-term follow-up study. A total of 63 patients with transfusion-dependent β-thalassemia (TDT) from the phase I/II and phase III trials have received an infusion of beti-cel. All patients had successful neutrophil and platelet engraftment, which occurred after a median of 26 days (range 13–39) and 46 days (range 13–94), respectively. In the phase III trials, the primary endpoint was transfusion independence (TI), which was defined as a weighted average hemoglobin of at least 9 g/dL without any packed red blood cell transfusions for a continuous period of at least 12 months. Of evaluable patients, 32 patients (89%) have achieved TI. Additionally, over a median follow-up of 42 months (range 23–87 months) across the phase I/II and phase III trials, no patients who have achieved TI have lost TI. There have been no deaths, and the serious adverse events reported have all been attributed to the myeloablative conditioning.

Gene addition for SCD: Lovotibeglogene autotemcel (lovo-cel) gene therapy is an investigational one-time treatment being studied for SCD that is designed to add functional copies of a modified form of the β-globin gene (β^{A-T87Q}-globin gene) into a patient's own HSCs. Once patients have the β^{A-T87Q}-globin gene, their red blood cells (RBCs) can produce antisickling hemoglobin (HbA^{T87Q}) that decreases the proportion of HbS, with the goal of reducing sickled RBCs, hemolysis, and other complications. Lovo-cel has been studied in four clinical trials: two phase I/II trials (HGB-205 and HBG-206), one phase III trial (HGB-210), and one long-term follow-up study. As of February 2021, a total of 49 patients have been treated with lovo-cel, with up to 6 years of patient follow-up, in the HGB-205 (n = 3), HGB-206 (n = 44), and HGB-210 (n = 2) clinical studies. The HGB-206 total includes Group A (n = 7), B (n = 2), and C (n = 35), representing progressive adaptations to the manufacturing and treatment processes. In the Group C cohort of the phase I/II HGB-206 study, no severe vaso-occlusive events (VOEs) were reported with up to 24 months of follow-up in patients with a history of at least four severe VOEs and at least 6 months of follow-up.

13. **What are the potential risks of gene therapy?**
Ex vivo gene therapy carries a risk of secondary malignancy and infertility as engraftment of genetically modified HSCs primarily depends on the use of a myeloablative (typically busulfan based) conditioning regimen. Although newer lentiviral viral vectors have improved safety profiles, there is the potential for insertional mutagenesis/oncogenesis. This can result in the insertion of viral promoters upstream of a pro-oncogene or within a regulatory gene, resulting in aberrant expression of cell cycle regulatory proteins, which can lead to cellular dysfunction, myelodysplasia, or the development of malignancy such as leukemia or lymphoma.

14. **Have there been reports of insertional oncogenesis in patients undergoing gene therapy?**
Although insertional oncogenesis has been identified as a potential risk with transgene therapy, there have been no reports of insertional oncogenesis and no malignancies in the TDT trials for beti-cel. Nevertheless, cases of myelodysplastic syndrome (MDS) and acute myeloid leukemia (AML) have been reported in clinical trials using a lentiviral vector. In patients with SCD who have received lovo-cel, one case of MDS and one case of AML were reported; the MDS was revised to transfusion-dependent anemia, and the European Medicines Agency judged that the viral vector was unlikely to be the cause of either case. Nevertheless, three cases of MDS have also been reported with elivaldogene autotemcel, used to treat adrenoleukodystrophy (ALD), with at least one case deeming the lentiviral vector to be the cause.

15. **What are the results of gene-editing trials in hemoglobinopathies?**
In January 2021, the first report of successful clinical utilization of ex vivo CRISPR-Cas9 gene editing of autologous stem cells designed to reduce erythrocyte specific BCL11A expression was reported in adult patients with SCD or β-thalassemia. Currently, the CLIMB THAL-111 and CLIMB SCD-121 trials, for patients with TDT and SCD, respectively, have completed enrollment with patients in various stages of follow-up. In these studies, patients are infused with CTX001, autologous CRISPR-Cas9-edited CD34+ hematopoietic stem and progenitor cells (HSPCs) that were genetically edited to reactivate the production of fetal hemoglobin by downregulating the production of BCL11a expression.

16. **What are the potential barriers to using gene therapy?**
Major barriers to gene therapy include cost of therapy, treatment-related toxicities, and psychosocial issues inherent to hemoglobinopathy patient populations. Although hospitalization, conditioning, and cell harvesting costs alone can represent a significant financial burden, the genetic alteration of the harvested stem cells can continue to elevate the total cost of therapy. The initial therapy offered for SCD and thalassemia patients has been estimated to be $1.8 million per patient, which has been justified because of the significant potential of accumulated cost caused by the need for chronic therapies over the lifetime of these patients. The use of busulfan in the required preparatory conditioning regimen represents a risk for future infertility and secondary malignancies. Alternative reduced intensity conditioning using alternative regimens and in vivo viral gene therapy vectors are under investigation in attempts to mitigate this toxicity. Because of neurologic sequelae of hemoglobinopathies, psychosocial factors can become a barrier to gene therapy. After transitioning to adult providers, patients can have decreased cognitive abilities because of their underlying vascular damage, which can limit access to health care and overutilization of emergency room services. Often this mode of healthcare access for pain crises can be complicated by opioid stigmatization and lack of continuity of care with specialists, which further exacerbates this health care disparity. Lastly, gene therapy is currently only being offered on clinical trials at select centers with a narrow inclusion criterion, making this an unrealistic option for many patients with TDT and SCD.

BIBLIOGRAPHY

1. A Study Evaluating the Efficacy and Safety of LentiGlobin BB305 Drug Product in Beta-Thalassemia Major and Sickle Cell Disease. https://ClinicalTrials.gov/show/NCT02151526.
2. Arnold SD, Brazauskas R, He N, et al. Clinical risks and healthcare utilization of hematopoietic cell transplantation for sickle cell disease in the USA using merged databases. *Haematologica*. 2017;102(11):1823–1832.
3. Cavazzana M, Antoniani C, Miccio A. Gene therapy for β-Hemoglobinopathies. *Mol Ther*. 2017;25(5):1142–1154.
4. Demirci S, Uchida N, Tisdale JF. Gene therapy for sickle cell disease: an update. *Cytotherapy*. 2018;20(7):899–910.
5. Frangoul H, Altshuler D, Cappellini MD, et al. CRISPR-Cas9 gene editing for sickle cell disease and β-thalassemia. *N Engl J Med*. 2021;384(3):252–260.
6. Gene Transfer for Sickle Cell Disease. https://ClinicalTrials.gov/show/NCT03282656.
7. Harrison C. First gene therapy for beta-thalassemia approved. *Nat Biotechnol*. 2019;37(10):1102–1103.
8. High KA, Roncarolo MG. Gene therapy. *N Engl J Med*. 2019;381(5):455–464.
9. Hulbert ML, Shenoy S. Hematopoietic stem cell transplantation for sickle cell disease: progress and challenges. *Pediatr Blood Cancer*. 2018;65(9), e27263.
10. Ikawa Y, Miccio A, Magrin E, Kwiatkowski JL, Rivella S, Cavazzana M. Gene therapy of hemoglobinopathies: progress and future challenges. *Hum Mol Genet*. 2019;28(R1):R24–R30.
11. Johnson FL, Look AT, Gockerman J, Ruggiero MR, Dalla-Pozza L, Billings 3rd FT. Bone-marrow transplantation in a patient with sickle-cell anemia. *N Engl J Med*. 1984;311(12):780–783.
12. Morrison C. $1-million price tag set for Glybera gene therapy. *Nat Biotechnol*. 2015;33(3):217–218.
13. Olowoyeye A, Okwundu CI. Gene therapy for sickle cell disease. *Cochrane Database Syst Rev*. 2018;11(11):CD007652.
14. Rachmilewitz EA, Giardina PJ. How I treat thalassemia. *Blood*. 2011;118(13):3479 3488.
15. Rai P, Malik P. Gene therapy for hemoglobin disorders - a mini-review. *J Rare Dis Res Treat*. 2016;1(2):25–31.
16. Ribeil JA, Hacein-Bey-Abina S, Payen E, et al. Gene therapy in a patient with sickle cell disease. *N Engl J Med*. 2017;376(9):848–855.
17. Safety and Efficacy of Gene Therapy of the Sickle Cell Disease by Transplantation of an Autologous CD34 + Enriched Cell Fraction That Contains CD34 + Cells Transduced ex Vivo With the GLOBE1 Lentiviral Vector Expressing the βAS3 Globin Gene in Patients With Sickle Cell Disease (DREPAGLOBE). https://ClinicalTrials.gov/show/NCT03964792.
18. Stem Cell Gene Therapy for Sickle Cell Disease. https://ClinicalTrials.gov/show/NCT02247843.
19. Thompson AA, Walters MC, Kwiatkowski J, et al. Gene therapy in patients with transfusion-dependent β-thalassemia. *N Engl J Med*. 2018;378(16):1479–1493.

CHAPTER 49

HEMATOPOIETIC CELL TRANSPLANTATION FOR MALIGNANT DISORDERS

Larisa Broglie, MD, MS

1. **How do the goals of autologous transplantation and allogeneic transplantation differ?**

   Hematopoietic cell transplantation (HCT) is the act of restoring hematopoiesis by infusing hematopoietic stem cells. The cells that are infused can be from another person (allogeneic) or previously collected cells from the recipient (autologous). The goals and expectations between allogeneic and autologous transplantation differ.

   Autologous transplantation is most used for children with chemotherapy-sensitive malignancies, such as solid tumors or relapsed lymphomas. During these transplants, higher doses of chemotherapy are used and significant myelosuppression occurs as a result. An infusion of autologous hematopoietic stem cells overcomes this myelosuppression and allows for earlier bone marrow recovery, reducing potential infectious complications. For this reason, autologous transplantation can also be referred to as high-dose chemotherapy with autologous stem cell rescue. Incorporation of tandem autologous HCT to consolidation therapy improved event-free survival (EFS) for patients with high-risk neuroblastoma from 30% to 61% at 3 years. Similarly, patients with relapsed Hodgkin lymphoma show an increased EFS from 34% to 55% with the use of autologous HCT in treatment for relapsed disease.

   Conversely, allogeneic transplantation seeks to restore a defective bone marrow by replacing it with that from a healthy donor. In the case of hematologic malignancies, the bone marrow has produced a clonal population of leukemic blasts that have evaded detection by the patient's own immune system. During allogeneic transplant, high doses of chemotherapy or radiation are given to eliminate any remaining malignant cells. Then, donor hematopoietic stem cells are infused, which will then reconstitute the bone marrow and become the dominant hematopoietic and immune cells in the body. The healthy immune system can then surveil for any recurrence of malignant cells and effectively eliminate them; this is known as graft versus leukemia (GVL). In this way, allogeneic transplantation was one of the first immunotherapies that was developed.

2. **What are the indications for allogeneic transplant in patients with acute lymphoblastic leukemia?**

   Most patients with acute lymphoblastic leukemia (ALL) do not require allogeneic transplant. Patients with high risk for relapse, however, are considered for allogeneic transplant. Patients who are unable to achieve a morphologic remission (<5% bone marrow blasts) after induction chemotherapy or who have persistent minimal residual disease (MRD) should be referred for consideration of allogeneic transplant in first complete remission.

   For patients that relapse after therapy, early relapses are at higher risk of subsequent relapses and death and should be considered for allogeneic transplant in second remission. Patients who relapse less than 18 months from initial diagnosis were noted to have an extremely poor outcome with only 21% overall survival (OS) with chemotherapy alone. It was found that allogeneic transplant showed a significant survival benefit for patients with a bone marrow relapse within 36 months from initial diagnosis. The probability of relapse was lower with use of allogeneic transplant—43% probability of relapse with HCT using a total body irradiation (TBI)–based regimen with matched sibling transplant compared with 69% probability of relapse with chemotherapy alone. This corresponded to a leukemia-free survival (LFS) of 23% with chemotherapy alone and 41% with a TBI-containing transplant. Use of unrelated donor transplant also showed improved EFS; patients who received an unrelated donor transplant had an EFS of 44% compared with no survival (0%) for patients with high-risk disease who received chemotherapy alone. Since the integration of allogeneic HCT (AlloHCT) for these patients with high-risk disease, and improvement in supportive care strategies, survival outcomes have continued to improve over time.

   Lastly, patients who suffer a third relapse with ALL should be considered for allogeneic transplant if able to achieve remission.

3. **What is the standard of care conditioning regimen for patients with ALL?**

   The standard of care allogeneic transplant approach for patients with ALL uses a TBI–based conditioning regimen. Patients who were treated with non-TBI containing conditioning chemotherapy were found to have higher relapse rates. In a study published in 2000, LFS was 50% with TBI-cyclophosphamide regimes compared with 35% using a chemotherapy-based approach (busulfan-cyclophosphamide). A recent randomized trial from Europe confirmed these results with an EFS of 86% for patients receiving TBI-based conditioning compared with 58% in those receiving chemotherapy-based conditioning.

4. **In patients with acute myeloid leukemia, what side effects should be considered in patients who have received gemtuzumab ozogamicin?**
Gemtuzumab ozogamicin is an anti-CD33 monoclonal antibody that is conjugated to calicheamicin. It has efficacy against CD33+ acute myeloid leukemia (AML) and is incorporated into upfront treatment; however, treatment carries a risk of veno-occlusive disease of the liver (VOD) in patients who subsequently receive myeloablative allogeneic transplantation. In one study, 64% of patients that received gemtuzumab experienced VOD with transplant compared with 8% of patients who did not receive gemtuzumab.

5. **Which patients with AML require consideration of allogeneic transplantation?**
Survival among children with AML remains suboptimal. Nevertheless, incremental progress in survival after AlloHCT has occurred over the last 3 decades. Relapsed AML is the most common indication for AlloHCT. In the current era, 40% of newly diagnosed AML pediatric patients receive AlloHCT because of a high risk of relapse. After AlloHCT, the 5-year AML-free survival in the current era is approximately 60%. Mortality because of transplant-related toxicities and relapse of AML after AlloHCT are the main causes of treatment failure.

6. **What is the effect of minimal residual disease before allogeneic transplant?**
Among leukemia patients undergoing AlloHCT, the MRD is one of the most important prognostic indicators of relapse after AlloHCT. MRD is measured by flow cytometry (ALL and AML) and next-generation sequencing (NGS) for ALL. The sensitivity of leukemia detection in flow cytometry is 1 leukemia cell among 10,000 normal cells and NGS is 1 leukemia cell among 1 million normal cells. Within reasonable limits, every effort should be made to achieve MRD negative status by flow cytometry before AlloHCT because positive MRD increases the risk of relapse by 30% to 40%.

7. **What is the association between graft versus host disease and relapse?**
After allogeneic transplant, a patient becomes a mixed chimera; hematopoietic cells are from a donor, but the remainder of the body remains recipient in origin. The donor T cells can recognize the recipient as foreign and attack; this is known as graft versus host disease (GVHD). GVHD suggests that the donor immune system recognizes differences in the recipient, which includes surveillance for any recurrence of malignancy. Therefore GVHD can act as a surrogate for GVL which, in turn, is associated with less relapse.

The GVL effect was first demonstrated when it was noted that relapse rates were highest in patients receiving allogeneic transplants from identical twins (41% probability of relapse) and where T cells were removed from the hematopoietic cell graft (34%) and lowest when patients were noted to have acute or chronic GVHD (17% and 20%, respectively).

BIBLIOGRAPHY
1. Corbacioglu S, Carreras E, Ansari M, et al. Diagnosis and severity criteria for sinusoidal obstruction syndrome/veno-occlusive disease in pediatric patients: a new classification from the European society for blood and marrow transplantation. *Bone Marrow Transplant.* 2018;53(2):138–145.
2. Davies SM, Ramsay NK, Klein JP, et al. Comparison of preparative regiments in transplants for children with acute lymphoblastic leukemia. *J Clin Oncol.* 2000;18(2):340–347.
3. Horowitz MM, Gale RP, Sondel PM, et al. Graft-versus-leukemia reactions after bone marrow transplantation. *Blood.* 1990;75(3):555–562.
4. Jodele SJ, Dandoy CE, Myers K, et al. High-dose carboplatin/etoposide/melphalan increases risk of thrombotic microangiopathy and organ injury after autologous stem cell transplantation in pediatric patients with neuroblastoma. *Bone Marrow Transplant.* 2018;53(10):1311–1318.
5. Matthay KK, Villablanca JG, Seeger RC, et al. Treatment of high-risk neuroblastoma with intensive chemotherapy, radiotherapy, autologous bone marrow transplantation, and 13-cis-retinoic acid. Children's Cancer Group. *N Engl J Med.* 1999;341(16):1165–1173.
6. Peters C, Dalle JH, Locatelli F, et al. Total body irradiation or chemotherapy conditioning in childhood ALL: a multinational, randomized, noninferiority phase III study. *J Clin Oncol.* 2021;39(4):295–307.
7. Peters C, Schrappe M, von Stackelberg A, et al. Stem-cell transplantation in children with acute lymphoblastic leukemia: a prospective international multicenter trial comparing sibling donors with matched unrelated donors-The ALL-SCT-BFM-2003 trial. *J Clin Oncol.* 2015;33:1265–1274.
8. Schmitz N, Pfistner B, Sextro M, et al. Aggressive conventional chemotherapy compared with high-dose chemotherapy with autologous haemopoietic stem-cell transplantation for relapsed chemosensitive Hodgkin's disease: a randomised trial. *Lancet.* 2002;359(9323):2065–2071.
9. Wadleigh M, Richardson PG, Zahrieh D, et al. Prior gemtuzumab ozogamicin exposure significantly increases the risk of veno-occlusive disease in patients who undergo myeloablative allogeneic stem cell transplantation. *Blood.* 2003;102(5):1578–1582.

CHAPTER 50

STEM CELL TRANSPLANTATION FOR CHILDREN WITH NONMALIGNANT DISORDERS

Jennifer Krajewski, MD and Monica Bhatia, MD

The concept of stem cell transplant was first performed in 1956 in a patient with leukemia; however, this was quickly applied to nonmalignant disorders only a decade later in a patient with severe combined immunodeficiency. In patients with nonmalignant conditions, the goal is to replace a missing gene or enzyme in the hematopoietic/immune systems or to replete a bone marrow that is not functioning. Historically, conditioning regimens have been myeloablative, mimicking those used in malignant conditions, but myeloablative conditioning regimens are associated with numerous short- and long-term complications such as acute and chronic graft versus host disease (GVHD), infections, infertility, and organ damage. Full-donor chimerism levels are usually associated with success in the malignant setting, but in the nonmalignant setting, mixed-donor chimerism levels can be curative. Lowering the intensity of conditioning regimens has been used in an attempt to decrease complications, but this can also be associated with higher rates of graft failure and rejection. When approaching transplantation for nonmalignant disorders, careful consideration must be made regarding conditioning regimens. The goal is to decrease toxicity but at the same time provide enough ablation for cure.

1. **What special considerations should be accounted for when performing a bone marrow transplant in a patient with Fanconi anemia?**
   Fanconi anemia (FA) is an inherited DNA repair disorder with heterogeneous clinical manifestations, including congenital anomalies, progressive cytopenias to frank bone marrow (BM) failure, and both hematologic and solid malignancies. FA patients are particularly sensitive to chemotherapy and radiation therapy, as first demonstrated by Gluckman et al. This study reported the dismal outcomes for 5 FA patients undergoing human leukocyte antigen (HLA)–matched sibling donor (MSD) BM transplant (BMT) with "standard dose" cyclophosphamide (CY). All 5 patients experienced severe acute GVHD, leading to death in 4. The current goal of conditioning regimens for FA patients is to eliminate radiation and minimize the use of CY by including fludarabine and busulfan as alternatives. In terms of graft source, BM from an HLA-MSD is the graft of choice when it is available; however, sibling cord blood units can also be used as a source, and the first successful cord blood transplant occurred in a patient with FA. For FA patients without an HLA-MSD, an HLA-matched unrelated donor (MUD) is the second best option, and for those without an HLA-matched unrelated marrow donor, there is no clear next best choice.

2. **What complications related to FA still need to be monitored even after BMT?**
   Compared with the general population, FA patients have a markedly higher risk of malignancy, particularly squamous cell carcinomas of the aeroesophageal and/or anogenital tracts, in addition to myelodysplastic syndromes (MDS) and acute myeloid leukemia (AML). In contrast to the general population, the peak hazard for solid tumors increases in a linear manner after the age of 10 years, increasing by over 10% per year after the age of 40. Because of this increased risk of epithelioid tumor risk, all patients should undergo frequent evaluations of the aeroesophageal tract (biannual dental evaluations and annual direct endoscopic laryngoscopy) and anogenital tracts (annual Pap smears and evaluations). Patients should additionally be encouraged to reduce risk by avoiding environmental exposures such as alcohol, tobacco products, and ultraviolet radiation.

3. **What are the indications to proceed to BMT in a patient with Kostmann syndrome?**
   Kostmann syndrome is an inherited hematological disorder with severe neutropenia with an absolute neutrophil count (ANC) less than 0.2×10^9/L and early onset of severe bacterial infections. BMT is the only curative option for Kostmann syndrome, but the successful reduction in infections with the use of GCSF has improved the overall long-term survival in those unable to receive a transplant. Nevertheless, these patients have a higher risk of transforming events, such as MDS or leukemia. Patients who do not respond to GCSF or who need very high doses of GCSF (15–20 micrograms/kg/day) to see a response should be considered for MSD or MUD BMT. In addition, patients who have BM dysplasias or cytogenetic abnormalities, including an isolated GCSFr mutation, should be considered for BMT.

4. **How do you diagnose a patient with acquired severe aplastic anemia?**
   Acquired severe aplastic anemia (SAA) is regarded as the result of an immune-mediated destruction of hematopoietic cells. It is defined as pancytopenia with a hypocellular BM in the absence of an abnormal infiltrate or marrow fibrosis. The diagnosis of acquired SAA is based on the exclusion of other disorders that can cause pancytopenia and on the well-known Camitta criteria. To diagnose SAA, there must be two of the following: hemoglobin concentration less than 100 g/L, platelet

count less than 50×10^9/L, neutrophil count less than 1.5×10^9/L. The modified Camitta criteria is used to assess severity. A BM biopsy is mandatory and will confirm an empty marrow; it should also exclude MDS, leukemia, or marrow metastasis from solid tumors. Cytogenetics and/or fluorescence in situ hybridization (FISH) analysis should also be sent to determine any chromosomal abnormalities.

5. **What is the treatment for a newly diagnosed patient with SAA?**
For newly diagnosed patients with SAA, the standard of care in those with an MSD is BMT. Event-free survival (EFS) rates in pediatric patients with an MSD are estimated in various studies to be between 85 and 100%. For those without a **sibling donor,** immunosuppressive therapy (IST) is given consisting of equine antithymocyte globulin (ATG) and cyclosporine, with hematological recovery in 50% to 70% of patients and excellent long-term survival among responders. For those who do not respond, alternate donor transplants are recommended. Additionally, some are considering alternate donor transplants as upfront therapy in those without sibling donors if they have a well-matched donor. Dufour et al. recently reported on the outcome of 29 children with acquired SAA treated with unrelated grafts as first-line treatment. The 2-year overall survival (OS) and EFS were 96% and 92%, respectively. These results appeared equal to a historical matched group of HLA identical sibling BMT and superior to patients receiving either an MSD or MUD transplant after failure of IST. In addition, results using haplo-identical related donors have been promising in patients who fail IST, with a recent study showing a 100% OS at 21 months post-BMT with minimal GVHD,[6] and trials are ongoing evaluating the use of haplo-identical related BMT as upfront therapy.

6. **What post-BMT complications are SAA patients more at risk for?**
In the 1970s, long-term survival after allogeneic marrow transplantation was only 45%, thought to be because of high rates of graft rejection and higher rates of severe acute GVHD. The problem of graft rejection was predicted from preclinical studies and attributed to sensitization of patients to minor non-HLA antigen disparities with their respective donors through prior blood transfusions. Nevertheless, the risk for graft rejection can be minimized by using leukocyte-poor blood products, by irradiating blood products before transfusion, and by introducing a conditioning regimen that includes ATG. After these changes were adopted clinically, graft rejection rates declined to 4%.
The incidence of GVHD has decreased through strategies such as the use of combination GVHD prophylaxis and the use of post-transplant cyclophosphamide in haplo-identical BMT.

7. **When is the best time to transplant a patient with severe combined immunodeficiency?**
Early transplantation before 3.5 months is associated with better overall survival. With early transplantation and aggressive monitoring and treatment of infections, survival rates may be as high as 97%. The Primary Immune Deficiency Treatment Consortium (PIDTC) recently performed a retrospective analysis of the largest cohort of severe combined immunodeficiency (SCID) patients in North America published to date. In this study, the likelihood of having an active infection at the time of transplant was significantly higher (52%) for patients transplanted at older than 3.5 months of age compared with those transplanted at younger than 3.5 months of age. Early diagnosis is crucial, as is the inclusion of SCID on the newborn screen to allow for earlier detection of patients with this disorder.

8. **Under what circumstances can you perform BMT for a patient with SCID without using pretransplant conditioning?**
Transplants done with MSDs, MUDs, and haplo-identical maternal donors in which there is maternal chimerism in the recipient all engraft readily without conditioning, although the likelihood of reconstituting B-cell immunity decreases with each kind of donor as HLA mismatch increases. SCID type also influences the decision regarding conditioning because some types are much more likely than others to recover B-cell function without conditioning. An advantage of using conditioning, particularly in uninfected patients, is the increased chance of achieving donor myeloid chimerism and being off immunoglobulin replacement therapy in patients surviving beyond 2 years after HSCT.
Adenosine deaminase deficiency (ADA) is a rare inherited disorder that leads to SCID. Unlike other SCID forms, two other options are available for treatment of ADA-SCID: enzyme replacement therapy (ERT) with pegylated bovine ADA, and autologous haematopoietic stem cell gene therapy (GT). MSD transplants represent a successful treatment option with high survival rates and excellent immune recovery. Unfortunately, mismatched parental donor transplants have a poor survival outcome and should be avoided unless other treatments are unavailable. ERT and GT both show excellent survival, and therefore the choice between ERT, MUD transplant, or GT is difficult and dependent on several factors, including accessibility to the different modalities, response of patients to long-term ERT, and the attitudes of physicians and parents to the short- and potential long-term risks associated with different treatments.

9. **Chronic granulomatous disease is associated with what late complications if the patients do not undergo BMT early in life?**
Chronic granulomatous disease (CGD) is a genetic disease. In CGD, mutations in any one of five different genes can cause a defect in an enzyme called phagocyte NADPH oxidase. Certain white blood cells use this enzyme to produce hydrogen peroxide, which these cells need to kill certain bacteria and fungi. There is a genetic form (X-linked recessive) of CGD that primarily affects males. The remaining cases of CGD are inherited as autosomal recessive traits, which can affect both males and females. Treatment of CGD consists of continuous antibiotic therapy to help prevent infections. BMTs have proven to be successful in some affected individuals with CGD. The orphan drug, Actimmune (interferon gamma-1b), has been approved by the Food and Drug Administration (FDA) for the treatment of CGD.

A recent French study found many complications in adult patients with CGD who have not undergone a transplant, including growth failure, chronic dyspnea, chronic digestive complications, and poor educational achievement (only half of the patients were attending high school at the age of 16 years). Another study focused on the pulmonary manifestations of adult patients with CGD, and only 25% of them had normal pulmonary function testing results, with 58% and 17% found to have a restrictive or obstructive physiology, respectively.

10. **When should a patient with Wiskott Aldrich syndrome undergo BMT, and what is the preferred type of BMT?**
Wiskott Aldrich syndrome (WAS) is primary immunodeficiency disease resulting in recurrent infections, eczema, and microthrombocytopenia. The clinical symptoms are caused by loss of function mutations in the *WAS* gene. Expressed only in hematopoietic cells, *WAS* encodes the WAS protein (WASp), a key actin cytoskeletal regulator that coordinates assembly of actin filaments in response to cell signalling events. Defects in WASp function have been shown to impair cellular processes in myeloid and lymphoid lineage cells.

In its classical form, significant combined immune deficiency, autoimmune complications, and risk of hematological malignancy necessitate early correction with stem cell transplantation or GT. The presence of autoimmunity, particularly autoimmune hemolytic anemia or thrombocytopenia, is associated with a twofold to threefold risk of poor prognosis. In addition, the absence of WASp expression correlated best with measures of infection, particularly opportunistic infection; bacterial infection was four times more likely in WASp-negative patients compared with WASp-positive patients, whereas fungal and *Pneumocystis* infection was only seen in WASp-negative patients. Because of this, WASp-negative patients should be strongly considered for early BMT.

HLA-identical sibling donor transplantation remains the treatment of choice for WAS. Nevertheless, alternative donors should be considered, especially for patients with risk factors. One retrospective analysis found that in a multivariate analysis on all BMTs done for WAS, transplant era significantly impacted OS and the extent of HLA mismatch did not significantly affect the incidence of acute GVHD, chronic GVHD, or survival.

11. **What are the curative therapy options for patients with hemoglobinopathies?**
BMT is the only curative option for both sickle cell disease (SCD) and β-thalassemia. Initially, this option was limited to those with MSDs; however, clinical trials are being conducted to investigate the use of unrelated and mismatched related donors, including haplo-identical donors. In addition, gene therapy is also being investigated as a curative option for both thalassemia and SCD. Many trials are underway to investigate how to best offer these curative therapies to as many hemoglobinopathy patients as possible.

12. **What is the preferred donor for patients with SCD?**
MSD is the preferred source, with most recent trials demonstrating an OS and disease-free survival rate of over 95% for patients undergoing this type of BMT. Unfortunately, only about 15% of SCD patients will have a matched sibling who does not also have SCD, so alternative donor options are greatly needed. Of note, a matched sibling who has sickle cell trait is an acceptable donor.

13. **What sickle cell complications warrant considering curative therapy?**
Any pediatric SCD patient with severe symptoms such as history of stroke, recurrent vaso-occlusive crises, recurrent acute chest syndromes, or evidence of pulmonary hypertension should be considered for curative therapy. As the OS rate has increased because of a decrease in transplant-related morbidity and mortality, adult patients up to the age of 45 are now being considered as well. For patients who are fortunate to have MSDs, further trials are investigating if patients with mild symptoms can be safely cured. Eventually, the goal is to be able to offer curative therapy to every patient because the life expectancy for SCD patients is significantly shorter than healthy adults even when patients have a mild clinical course in childhood.

14. **What transplant complications are more likely in SCD patients undergoing BMT, and what can be done to decrease their risk?**
Because of the vascular changes induced by SCD, patients are more at risk for neurologic complications such as posterior reversible encephalopathy syndrome, seizures, and hemorrhage during and after BMT. Minimizing thrombocytopenia and hypomagnesemia and preventing hypertension above baseline blood pressure can help decrease these chances. In addition, all SCD patients should receive seizure prophylaxis as long as they are on immunosuppression, especially when using a calcineurin inhibitor.

15. **What evaluations are especially important when evaluating an SCD patient before undergoing curative therapy?**
All SCD patients should undergo a complete organ evaluation (heart, lungs, brain, kidneys, liver, eyes) before BMT to ensure there is not any asymptomatic organ damage from SCD that would make curative therapy too risky. In particular, patients with iron overload (i.e., history of serum ferritin over 1000 or history of chronic transfusions) need to undergo assessment of liver iron and the presence of cirrhosis or fibrosis. Significant fibrosis is typically an exclusion criterion from curative therapy because of the increased risk of having side effects from the chemotherapy and other supportive care medications. Magnetic resonance imaging (MRI) or angiography (MRA) of the brain is especially important to ensure there is no evidence of a silent recent stroke because curative therapy would need to be delayed to ensure conditioning does not cause progression of the acute stroke.

16. **What pretransplant findings make BMT riskier for a patient with thalassemia?**
    Patients over the age of 7 and patients with hepatomegaly greater than 5 cm have historically been at higher risk for post-transplant complications. The Pesaro group developed a prognostic scheme to predict transplant outcomes in patients younger than 17 years of age in the 1980s. This prognostic scheme included three variables all related to iron burden: lifetime quality of chelation received before transplantation, hepatomegaly (defined as more than 2 cm below the costal margin), and presence of liver fibrosis pretransplant as determined by hepatic biopsy examination. These variables stratified patients into three groups: Class I patients in whom there were none of the adverse risk factors, Class II in whom one or two adverse risk factors were present, and Class III, who exhibited all three. Outcomes were found to be remarkably different between these three groups; however, this classification was developed when deferoxamine was the only available chelation therapy. Nevertheless, the important and still applicable concept stemming from the Pesaro classification is that constant lifelong control of iron overload, with prevention of iron-related tissue damage, is crucial for successful transplantation. In the last decade, almost all transplant centers have followed this simple classification for predicting the risks and benefits of HSCT in thalassemia patients. Nevertheless, reducing the intensity of conditioning regimens has helped offset this, but the introduction of gene therapy as a curative therapy provides a safe curative option for more patients.

BIBLIOGRAPHY

1. Bacigalupo A. How I treat acquired aplastic anemia. *Blood.* 2017;129(11):1428–1436.
2. Bhatia M, Sheth S. Hematopoietic stem cell transplantation in sickle cell disease: patient selection and special considerations. *J Blood Med.* 2015;6:229–238.
3. Bhatia M, Walters MC. Hematopoietic cell transplantation for thalassemia and sickle cell disease: past, present and future. *Bone Marrow Transplant.* 2008;41(2):109–117.
4. Burroughs LM, Woolfrey AE, Storer BE, et al. Success of allogeneic marrow transplantation for children with severe aplastic anaemia. *Br J Haematol.* 2012;158(1):120–128.
5. Camitta BM, Nathan DG. Anemia in adolescence. 2. Hemoglobinopathies and other causes. *Postgrad Med.* 1975;57(2):151–155.
6. Clay J, Kulasekararaj AG, Potter V, et al. Nonmyeloablative peripheral blood haploidentical stem cell transplantation for refractory severe aplastic anemia. *Biol Blood Marrow Transplant.* 2014;20(11):1711–1716.
7. Dufour C, Veys P, Carraro E, et al. Similar outcome of upfront-unrelated and matched sibling stem cell transplantation in idiopathic paediatric aplastic anaemia. A study on behalf of the UK Paediatric BMT Working Party, Paediatric Diseases Working Party and Severe Aplastic Anaemia Working Party of EBMT. *Br J Haematol.* 2015;171(4):585–594.
8. Dunogué B, Pilmis B, Mahlaoui N, et al. Chronic granulomatous disease in patients reaching adulthood: a nationwide study in France. *Clin Infect Dis.* 2017;64(6):767–775.
9. Dupuis-Girod S, Medioni J, Haddad E, et al. Autoimmunity in Wiskott-Aldrich syndrome: risk factors, clinical features, and outcome in a single-center cohort of 55 patients. *Pediatrics.* 2003;111(5 Pt 1):e622–e627.
10. Ebens CL, MacMillan ML, Wagner JE. Hematopoietic cell transplantation in Fanconi anemia: current evidence, challenges and recommendations. *Expert Rev Hematol.* 2017;10(1):81–97.
11. Fioredda F, Calvillo M, Bonanomi S, et al. Congenital and acquired neutropenias consensus guidelines on therapy and follow-up in childhood from the Neutropenia Committee of the Marrow Failure Syndrome Group of the AIEOP (Associazione Italiana Emato-Oncologia Pediatrica). *Am J Hematol.* 2012;87(2):238–243.
12. Gallo S, Woolfrey AE, Burroughs LM, et al. Marrow grafts from HLA-identical siblings for severe aplastic anemia: does limiting the number of transplanted marrow cells reduce the risk of chronic GvHD? *Bone Marrow Transplant.* 2016;51(12):1573–1578.
13. Gaspar HB, Aiuti A, Porta F, Candotti F, Hershfield MS, Notarangelo LD. How I treat ADA deficiency. *Blood.* 2009;114(17):3524–3532.
14. Georges GE, Doney K, Storb R. Severe aplastic anemia: allogeneic bone marrow transplantation as first-line treatment. *Blood Adv.* 2018;2(15):2020–2028.
15. Gluckman E, Devergié A, Bourdeau-Esperou H, et al. Transplantation of umbilical cord blood in Fanconi's anemia. *Nouv Rev Fr Hematol.* 1990;32(6):423–425.
16. Imai K, Morio T, Zhu Y, et al. Clinical course of patients with WASP gene mutations. *Blood.* 2004;103(2):456–464.
17. Locatelli F, Bruno B, Zecca M, et al. Cyclosporin A and short-term methotrexate versus cyclosporin A as graft versus host disease prophylaxis in patients with severe aplastic anemia given allogeneic bone marrow transplantation from an HLA-identical sibling: results of a GITMO/EBMT randomized trial. *Blood.* 2000;96(5):1690–1697.
18. Lucarelli G, Galimberti M, Polchi P, et al. Marrow transplantation in patients with thalassemia responsive to iron chelation therapy. *N Engl J Med.* 1993;329(12):840–844.
19. Pai SY, Logan BR, Griffith LM, et al. Transplantation outcomes for severe combined immunodeficiency, 2000-2009. *N Engl J Med.* 2014;371(5):434–446.
20. Railey MD, Lokhnygina Y, Buckley RH. Long-term clinical outcome of patients with severe combined immunodeficiency who received related donor bone marrow transplants without pretransplant chemotherapy or post-transplant GVHD prophylaxis. *J Pediatr.* 2009;155(6):834–840.e831.
21. Salvator H, Mahlaoui N, Catherinot E, et al. Pulmonary manifestations in adult patients with chronic granulomatous disease. *Eur Resp J.* 2015;45(6):1613–1623.
22. Shin CR, Kim MO, Li D, et al. Outcomes following hematopoietic cell transplantation for Wiskott-Aldrich syndrome. *Bone Marrow Transplant.* 2012;47(11):1428–1435.
23. Srivastava A, Shaji RV. Cure for thalassemia major - from allogeneic hematopoietic stem cell transplantation to gene therapy. *Haematologica.* 2017;102(2):214–223.

24. Storb R, Etzioni R, Anasetti C, et al. Cyclophosphamide combined with antithymocyte globulin in preparation for allogeneic marrow transplants in patients with aplastic anemia. *Blood.* 1994;84(3):941–949.
25. Storb R, Floersheim GL, Weiden PL, et al. Effect of prior blood transfusions on marrow grafts: abrogation of sensitization by procarbazine and antithymocyte serum. *J Immunol.* 1974;112(4):1508–1516.
26. Wahlstrom JT, Dvorak CC, Cowan MJ. Hematopoietic stem cell transplantation for severe combined immunodeficiency. *Curr Pediatr Rep.* 2015;3(1):1–10.

CHAPTER 51

COMPLICATIONS ASSOCIATED WITH ALLOGENEIC HEMATOPOIETIC CELL TRANSPLANTATION IN CHILDREN

Charlotte Alme, MD and Prakash Satwani, MD

1. **Why is it important to understand complications after allogeneic hematopoietic cell transplantation?**
   Allogeneic hematopoietic cell transplantation (AlloHCT) is a lengthy and complex process. The majority of the patients sustain complications after AlloHCT. These complications can have a significant impact on survival, quality of life, cost, and healthcare utilization. Hence, it is crucial to understand the landscape of complications after alloHCT.

2. **How do we classify complications after AlloHCT?**
   Complications after alloHCT can be divided into early complications (0–100 days), intermediate complications (101–180 days), late complications (6–24 months), and very late complications (>24 months).
   A. **Early complications** are predominantly related to:
      a. Conditioning regimens (i.e., mucositis, infections, kidney, liver, and lung injury) Immunological responses (i.e., engraftment syndrome, acute graft-versus-host disease [aGVHD], idiopathic pneumonia syndrome, and graft rejection) and/or
      b. Polypharmacy (i.e., posterior reversible encephalopathy syndrome from calcineurin inhibitors, renal insufficiency because of antibiotics and calcineurin inhibitors, liver injury because of antibiotics, total parenteral nutrition, myelosuppression because of mycophenolate mofetil and antiviral medications).
   B. **Intermediate complications** are usually because of the presence of aGVHD and chronic GVHD (cGVHD) and because of the immunosuppressive therapies used to control these complications. This often predisposes patients to bacterial, viral, and fungal infections.
   C. **Late complications** often are a byproduct of cGVHD therapy. The backbone of cGVHD therapy includes steroids, which can predispose patients to osteopenia and avascular necrosis of the bones, short stature, chronic hypertension, and adrenal suppression.
   D. **Very late complications** are not infrequent and many of those complications are related to conditioning regimens, including alkylating agents and total body irradiation. These complications include gonadal failure resulting in early menopause, infertility, growth retardation, thyroid dysfunction, cataracts, and second malignancies.

3. **What are the most common infections after transplant and their time course?**
   After alloHCT, children are at risk for several opportunistic infections. The majority of the infections among transplant patients are derived from the host gastrointestinal (GI) tract, skin, and/or respiratory system. Because of a weakened host innate immune system, gut dysbiosis, central lines, and other catheters, patients are at risk for bacterial, fungal, and viral infections. Additionally, once discharged after alloHCT, patients are not only at risk of opportunistic infections but also community-acquired infections such as, but not limited to, influenza, respiratory syncytial virus, and parainfluenza. Patterns of infection are time dependent as summarized in Figure 51.1.

4. **What are the most significant viral infections after-AlloHCT?**
   Viral infection in alloHCT recipients are associated with significant morbidity and mortality because of the direct cytopathic effect of viruses and the myriad of side effects related to antiviral medications. Viral infection can be further described as viral reactivation or disease. Viral reactivation is defined as detection of virus on polymerase chain reaction (PCR) testing of blood, and viral disease is defined as direct organ injury from the cytopathic effects of a virus. Fortunately, in the current era because of weekly PCR-based surveillance, the majority of the viral infections are detected in the viremia phase and preemptive treatment may prevent progression to viral disease.
   The most common viral infections diagnosed in alloHCT recipients are cytomegalovirus (CMV), Epstein-Barr virus (EBV), adenovirus, bladder kidney virus (BKV), and human herpesvirus-6 (HHV-6). Risk factors associated with viral reactivation are past history of viral infection in donor and/or recipients, delayed immune reconstitution because of in-vivo or ex-vivo T-cell depletion, stem cell transplant (SCT) using cord blood units, GVHD, and/or treatment of GVHD. From a viral infection perspective, the optimal donor is the one who has similar serostatus to the recipient;

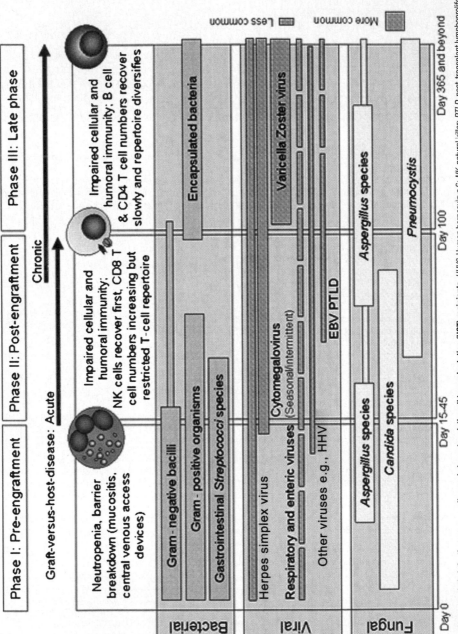

Figure 1.1 Phases of opportunistic infections among allogeneic hematopoietic cell transplantation (HCT) recipients. *HHV6*, Human herpesvirus 6; *NK*, natural killer; *PTLD*, post-transplant lymphoproliferative disease. (From Mackall C, Fry T, Gress R, et al. Background to hematopoietic cell transplantation, including post transplant immune recovery. *Bone Marrow Transplant.* 2009;44(8):457–462.)

a mismatch in serostatus can lead to a higher incidence of viral infection and often necessitates the need for prolonged antiviral therapy.

There are two types of management strategies:

A. Prophylactic: Patients at risk for CMV reactivation receive ganciclovir/valganciclovir or letermovir prophylaxis; however, patients must have frequent CMV PCR performed.

B. Preemptive: Patients at risk undergo weekly PCR testing for common viral infections, and patient receives antiviral therapy once PCR becomes positive.

The most common viral infections are described in more detail, as follows:

A. **EBV, including post-transplant lymphoproliferative disease (PTLD):** EBV, either as reactivation or primary infection, can cause potentially fatal EBV-PTLD, as well as hepatitis, colitis, nephritis, and pneumonia. Compared with solid organ transplant, EBV PTLD after alloHCT occurs early, usually within the first 6 months. Most of the cases are detected early because the majority of centers perform weekly quantitative EBV PCR for 3 to 6 months after alloHCT. EBV PTLD should be suspected in PCR-positive patients with unexplained fever, lymphadenopathy, hepatosplenomegaly, tonsillar hypertrophy, night sweats, weight loss, and cytopenia. These symptoms tend to progress very rapidly.

    a. **Diagnosis:** Preferably, patients should undergo a positron emission tomography (PET)–computed tomography (CT) scan and a lymph node/tissue biopsy. Nevertheless, some patients may be too ill (hemodynamic instability) to undergo these procedures, and in those instances, treatment can be started based on EBV PCR positivity and symptomatology. Once the patient is clinically stable, a lymph node biopsy should be attempted.

    b. **Treatment:** Reduce immunosuppression first if possible. If no response is seen, administer rituximab, 375 mg/m^2 intravenously (IV) once weekly for up to max four doses in total; a response rate of up to 80% is seen with rituximab. Other therapies include donor-derived or third-party EBV-specific cytotoxic T cells (EBV-CTLs), which have demonstrated significant efficacy in clinical trials. For patients who are unresponsive to rituximab and CTLs, chemotherapy regimens similar to non-Hodgkin lymphoma have been used; however, effectiveness is questionable.

B. **CMV:** CMV is the most common opportunistic infection after alloHCT. The risk of reactivation is 40% to 50% in CMV-positive recipients. Patients at risk for CMV reactivation (if recipient and/or donor is CMV immunoglobulin G [IgG] positive) should have weekly CMV-qPCR and receive prophylactic letermovir for 100 days after alloHCT (currently Food and Drug Administration [FDA] approved for patients >18 years of age). CMV can cause multiorgan disease, pneumonia, gastroenteritis, and retinitis.

    a. **Treatment:** IV ganciclovir or oral (PO) valganciclovir, foscarnet, and cidofovir are effective, but all have significant side effects (myelotoxicity and nephrotoxicity). Patients who do not have an optimal response or are unable to tolerate anti-CMV medications can receive CMV-CTLs infusions from their alloHCT donor if they are CMV antibody positive or from a third-party bank. CMV-CTLs have been demonstrated to be safe and effective but not always readily available and may take time to manufacture.

C. **Adenovirus:** Adenovirus is one of the most challenging viral infections because it can cause serious end-organ damage and its treatment is very toxic and not very successful. Adenovirus can cause pneumonia, colitis, hepatitis, keratoconjunctivitis, hemorrhagic cystitis, encephalitis, and myocarditis, with many patients having multiorgan involvement. Adenovirus is much more common in children than adults because children shed this virus for months to years. It can be detected in the stool and nasopharyngeal aspirates up to 2 weeks before a positive blood qPCR.

    a. **Diagnosis/Monitoring:** After alloHCT, it is crucial to perform weekly monitoring by blood qPCR. Early detection and treatment is critical because adenovirus tends to replicate rapidly.

    b. **Treatment:** IV Cidofovir 5 mg/kg/week. Cidofovir administration can cause significant nephrotoxicity, and patients must receive hyperhydration and probenecid to help avoid this complication. The large amounts of fluid can also be problematic in those with impaired kidney or cardiac function. Probenecid protects renal tubules and increases plasma cidofovir concentration. Adenovirus-specific CTLs could be beneficial in patients not responding to cidofovir. However, adenovirus-specific CTLs are available at only a few centers in the United States.

D. **HHV-6:** The clinical presentation and management of HHV-6 in pediatric alloHCT is controversial. The incidence of HHV-6 viremia/infection is close to 20%, and the majority of infections occur early after alloHCT. Routine surveillance of HHV-6 is complicated by the fact that HHV-6 could be genomically inserted in donor myeloid cells, which could be challenging to differentiate from primary infection. HHV-6 should be suspected in a patient with unexplained fever, in cases of delayed engraftment/graft failure, and in patients with encephalopathy. In terms of management of HHV-6, the consensus is that only limbic encephalitis should be treated with foscarnet. Patients may develop nephrotoxicity with foscarnet, and in those cases, ganciclovir is another potential treatment option.[2]

E. **Bladder kidney virus (BKV):** BKV is a ubiquitous human polyomavirus with an affinity for uroepithelium. BKV can cause hemorrhagic cystitis in up to 20% of alloHCT recipients, resulting in microscopic hematuria (grade 1 hematuria) to macroscopic hematuria (grade 2) to macroscopic hematuria with blood clots (grade 3), potentially causing postrenal failure because of urinary obstruction (grade 4). This virus and its treatment can potentially lead to both acute and chronic renal injury. The treatment of BK hemorrhagic cystitis is symptomatic and includes increased hydration to prevent blood clot formation in the bladder, and intermittent or permanent urinary catheterization if the patient has clot formation. Continuous bladder irrigation is challenging but an effective modality to prevent clot formation. Supportive and adjuvant therapies include spasmolytics such as ditropan and analgesics such as pyridium. Antiviral treatment with IV cidofovir is controversial; some centers use IV cidofovir

(1 mg/kg) once a week without probenecid. In refractory cases, intravesicular cidofovir can be considered. Some centers have used BKV-specific CTLs to control BKV-induced hemorrhagic cystitis.

5. **What is acute graft-versus-host disease, and how does it affect the outcomes of transplant?**
   Acute GVHD occurs when donor T cells recognize recipient antigens as foreign. There are three steps involved in the pathophysiology of aGVHD: (1) T cells are presented with host antigen by host antigen–presenting cells; (2) donor T cell is activated because of the host antigen presentation; and (3) target organ injury is activated by the T cells/cytokine (skin, GI tract, and liver).

   The single most important risk factor associated with the occurrence of aGVHD is the degree of human leukocyte antigen (HLA) mismatch between recipient and donor. Historically, the incidence of aGVHD (grades II–IV) is in the range of 20% after HLA-matched sibling, 40% after 10/10 HLA-matched unrelated donor, and 60% after a mismatched unrelated donor alloHCT. Nevertheless, advances in graft processing (stem cell enrichment with T-cell depletion, αβ-T cell depletion and post-transplant cyclophosphamide) has resulted in lower rates (in the range of 20%–40%) of aGVHD in haplo-identical ($\geq$5/10 HLA match) and HLA mismatched unrelated alloHCT. In vivo T cell-depletion using serotherapy with antithymocyte globulin (ATG) or alemtuzumab is a common practice when unrelated donors are used (matched or mismatched). Serotherapy increases the risk of relapse and viral infections but decreases the risk of both acute and chronic GVHD. As previously described, ex-vivo T-cell-depletion is becoming popular, and more and more centers are becoming proficient with this technology. The advantage of ex-vivo depletion over in-vivo depletion is the precision of the number of T cells that can be infused, whereas the extent of T-cell depletion in-vivo with serotherapy is unpredictable.

   A. **Prophylaxis:** The standard of care for aGVHD prophylaxis is a calcineurin inhibitor (tacrolimus or cyclosporine) plus methotrexate. In patients without evidence of GVHD, tapering of tacrolimus/cyclosporine typically starts around 3 months in patients with malignant disease and at 6 months in those with nonmalignant diseases.

   B. **Staging and grading of aGVHD:** Because aGVHD involves multiple organs, each organ is staged individually and stages are merged to assess the grade. The treatment decision and prognostication of outcomes is evaluated by aGVHD grading. Among patients with leukemia, grades I/II aGVHD are associated with improved disease-free survival, potentially because of the graft-versus-leukemia effect. Nevertheless, grades III and IV aGVHD are considered severe and are associated with poor outcomes because of the risk of severe/life-threatening opportunistic infection resulting from the intense immunosuppression needed to control aGVHD. Hence, escalation of anti-infection prophylaxis is crucial to prevent opportunistic infections.

Stage	Skin (maculopapular rash)	Liver (bilirubin in mg/dL [μmol/liter])	Gastrointestinal (GI) (stool volume/day)
1	>25% of body surface area (BSA)	2–3 (34–50)	280–555mL/m^2
2	25%–50% of BSA	>3–6 (51–102)	556–833mL/m^2
3	>50% of BSA	>6–15 (103–255)	>833mL/m^2
4	Generalized erythroderma, bullae, desquamation	>15 (˃255)	Severe abdominal pain with/without ileus or grossly bloody stools
Grade			
1	1–2	0	0
2	3 or	1 or	1
3	2–3	2–3 or	2–4
4	4	4	

Glucksberg staging/grading.[9]

   C. **Treatment:** Among patients with grades II to IV aGVHD, the standard of care is to start with steroids (prednisolone/methylprednisolone 2 mg/kg/day) with tapering as soon as possible to the lowest effective dose. Additionally, dose of prophylactic GVHD medications such as cyclosporine A or tacrolimus are generally increased to higher serum concentrations until a response to treatment is observed and steroids are tapered. Approximately one-third of pediatric patients have a suboptimal response to steroids. Recently the FDA approved ruxolitinib (an inhibitor of the JAK1 and JAK2 protein kinases) for the treatment of steroid refractory aGVHD in patients older than 12 years of age. Other therapies that have been used in the management of steroid refractory aGVHD include mesenchymal stromal cells, etanercept, infliximab, basiliximab, mycophenolate mofetil (MMF), sirolimus, ATG, and extracorporeal photopheresis (ECP). Among patients with grade I skin aGVHD, topical immunosuppressive treatments with steroids and tacrolimus creams have been used, and among those patients with aGVHD of the gut, oral budesonide can be helpful.

6. **What is chronic GVHD?**
   Chronic GVHD is less common among children (20%–40%) than adults (<60%). CGVHD can have a significant impact on quality of life. The biggest risk factor for the development of cGVHD is previous aGVHD and peripheral blood SCT. It is caused by an impaired immune tolerance between both alloreactive and autoreactive donor-derived T and B cells, resulting in chronic inflammation and scarring. The overall survival in those with mild cGVHD in malignant conditions is better than for patients without cGVHD because of less relapse.

A. Symptoms usually start between 3 months and 2 years after SCT and can include the following:
   a. Sclerotic or nonsclerotic skin changes
   b. Itchy, dry (sicca) eyes often preceded by light sensitivity
   c. Dry oral mucosa if salivary glands are involved. Lichenoid ulcerations, gingivitis, dental abnormalities
   d. Genital lesions with vulvovaginitis, balanitis, phimosis
   e. Joints and fascia: Can cause reduced range-of-motion, myositis, and pain
   f. Liver involvement resembles cholestasis and may necessitate a liver biopsy
   g. GI tract: dysphagia (esophagus), nausea, vomiting, diarrhea, and malabsorption
   h. Pulmonary GVHD presents with progressive shortness of breath and poor exercise tolerance.
   i. Cytopenias
B. **Treatment:** The mainstay of therapy includes steroids with or without a calcineurin inhibitor (CNI; e.g., cyclosporine/tacrolimus or sirolimus). Mild cGVHD can be treated with topical steroids and/or tacrolimus cream or low-dose prednisolone. Moderate to severe cGVHD requires treatment with oral steroids with CNI. Recently the FDA approved 3 new drugs for cGVHD that is unresponsive to first-line therapy: ibrutinib (protein kinase inhibitor), ruxolitinib (mentioned previously), and belumosudil (serine/threonine kinase inhibitor). cGVHD tends to be slow in terms of response and may require weeks to months to respond. It is crucial that patients receive antimicrobial prophylaxis for the prevention of infections.

7. **What is transplant-associated thrombotic microangiopathy?**
Transplant-associated thrombotic microangiopathy (TA-TMA) is underdiagnosed but a serious complication after alloHCT. Signs, symptoms, and laboratory parameters associated with TA-TMA are often challenging to decipher. The reported incidence of TA-TMA is around 10% to 30% and usually occurs early (1–2 months) after alloHCT. High-dose chemotherapy/radiation therapy, aGVHD, infections, and calcineurin inhibitors have been associated with TA-TMA. These risk factors potentially cause vascular endothelial injury, resulting in the activation of the complement cascade, which ultimately results in microthrombi formation.

   TA-TMA should be suspected if a patient requires two antihypertensive medications to control blood pressure, and has elevated lactate dehydrogenase (LDH), and thrombocytopenia. Usually TA-TMA is associated with renal insufficiency/proteinuria, direct antiglobulin negative hemolytic anemia, low haptoglobin, severe GI bleeding, pain, vomiting, diarrhea, pleural/pericardial effusions, pulmonary hypertension, and neurological disease (seizures).
A. **Diagnosis:** The definitive diagnosis is with a renal biopsy demonstrating microangiopathy. Nevertheless, because of thrombocytopenia or other morbidities, a renal biopsy may not be feasible. One of the promising biomarkers associated with TMA is elevated soluble C5b9 (membrane attack complex or terminal complement complex) levels. Soluble C5b9 as a biomarker is very sensitive and useful in guiding the administration of eculizumab therapy. Nevertheless, this test is limited by the slow turnaround of the results.
B. **Treatment:** Terminal complement blockade with eculizumab for those with proteinuria and/or elevated SC5b9. Patients with very high levels of SC5b9 may require higher doses or more frequent doses to control the microangiopathy with the goal to continue eculizumab until hematologic parameters normalize. Patients receiving eculizumab are at high risk for infectious complications and must receive meningococcal prophylaxis before beginning treatment as well as during treatment and for a while after completing treatment with eculizumab.

8. **What is graft rejection/failure, and how do you treat it?**
Graft failure is a devastating complication after alloHCT, with an incidence of approximately 10%.[13,14] In cases of neutropenic graft failure, patients are at risk for severe life-threatening infections. Nonneutropenic graft failures are usually associated with autologous hematopoietic recovery and have a better prognosis compared with neutropenic graft failures.

   Risk factors associated with graft failure are reduced intensity conditioning, the use of unrelated cord blood grafts, the use of bone marrow (BM) rather than peripheral blood stem cells (PBSC), development of donor HLA–specific antibodies among alloHCT recipients, a lower dose of infused CD34 cells (more often seen in cord blood and BM grafts), HLA-mismatch, ABO mismatch, and T-cell depletion. Treatment includes re-transplanting the patient, as soon as possible if neutropenic graft failure. It is important to try to figure out why there was an initial graft failure so that treatment for re-transplant can be modified so this does not happen again with the following transplant. This could include using a new donor, increasing the intensity of conditioning regimen, or using PBSCs rather than BM.

9. **What is veno-occlusive disease of the liver or sinusoidal obstructive syndrome?**
Veno-occlusive disease of the liver (VOD) or sinusoidal obstructive syndrome (SOS)[15,16] is characterized by damage to sinusoidal endothelial cells in the liver. Endothelial injury results in two major changes: (1) leakage of vascular contents in the space of Disse, resulting in increased pressure on hepatocytes and compression of bile canaliculi, which diminishes bile flow to major bile ducts that ultimately results in hyperbilirubinemia, and (2) endothelial damage, resulting in formation of thrombi in the sinusoids, which ultimately results in portal hypertension.

   Refractory thrombocytopenia could be an early clue, but the major clinical features of SOS are painful hepatomegaly, ascites, weight gain, and bilirubin greater than 2 mg/dL. Reversal of portal vein blood flow on ultrasound is pathognomonic of SOS/VOD but is a late finding and is associated with severe VOD. In children with VOD, 20% to 30% may not have elevated bilirubin (anicteric SOS/VOD).

   The incidence of VOD/SOS in children undergoing alloHCT is 10% to 20%. Risk factors associated with occurrence of VOD/SOS are use of inotuzumab and gemtuzumab before alloHCT, high busulfan levels, total body irradiation, young age, certain diseases (thalassemia, osteopetrosis, hemophagocytic lymphohistiocytosis [HLH], and neuroblastoma), previous liver disease (bilirubin >1.5 mg/dL), and second transplants. Established Seattle or Baltimore criteria are useful in establishing diagnosis but have low sensitivity and could delay diagnosis and treatment. Recent guidelines published by Cairo et al. are more practical and prognostic.

The use of ursodeoxycholic acid as prophylaxis in alloHCT patients has resulted in decreased liver injury. Nevertheless, the impact of ursodeoxycholic acid on the incidence of VOD is not clear. The key to successful management of VOD/SOS is a high index of suspicion and early intervention with defibrotide, maintenance of euvolemia with cautious use of diuretics, and placement of pleural/ascites drain if the patient becomes significantly volume overloaded.

10. **Discuss some noninfectious pulmonary complications and treatment.**
   Noninfectious pulmonary complications[17] are very challenging to diagnose and often associated with high mortality. The majority of these complications are diagnoses of exclusion and probably multifactorial in origin. To establish a diagnosis, infections must be ruled out. To exclude infectious causes, a number of tests may be needed, including blood samples for antigens associated with infectious organisms (i.e., aspergillus galactomannan), blood and sputum cultures, nasopharyngeal swabs for viral respiratory pathogens, and chest x-ray (CXR)/computerized tomography (CT). For those with suspected pulmonary infections, there may also be a need for bronchoscopy with bronchoalveolar lavage (BAL) and/or lung biopsy.
   A. Idiopathic pneumonia syndrome (IPS) is an immune-mediated, diffuse alveolar injury without underlying renal, cardiac, or infectious cause. The incidence of IPS is less than 10%. Patients typically present with fever, nonproductive cough, dyspnea, tachypnea, hypoxemia, and rales around 3 to 4 weeks from alloHCT. CXR demonstrates new multilobar infiltrates. In true cases of IPS, a BAL is negative for infections. IPS is probably related to activation of donor T cells or cytokines released by T cells and macrophages. The treatment include steroids, tumor necrosis factor (TNF) α-inhibitor (etanercept), or cytokine-inhibition with anti-interleukin (IL)-6 (tocilizumab). The mortality is 60% to 80% and approaches 95% if the patient requires mechanical ventilation.
   B. Diffuse alveolar hemorrhage (DAH) is a result of damage to the alveolar capillary basement membrane. It is usually seen in the first month after alloHCT, presenting with dyspnea, dry cough, hypoxemia, and, on rare occasions, hemoptysis. Exact etiology of DAH is unknown. Nevertheless, immune dysregulation, infections, and conditioning regimen have been implicated in the causation of DAH. Treatment is mainly supportive but also includes high-dose steroids. Unfortunately, DAH can be rapidly progressive, and results in very high mortality.

11. **What are some late effects from total body irradiation?**
   Usually, total body irradiation (TBI) is given as 2 Gray fractionated doses, to a total of 12 Gray. Fractionation is associated with less toxicity and better antileukemia effect. TBI is usually not offered to children younger than 4 years because of neurological toxicity. TBI is predominantly used as a part of conditioning regimens in patients with acute lymphoblastic leukemia (ALL). It is occasionally used for acute myelogenous leukemia (AML) and, rarely, for nonmalignant diseases (low dose [2–4 Gray]) to improve engraftment.
   One of the major concerns in children is growth failure because of damage to the epiphyseal growth plates from TBI. The final adult height among TBI recipients can be shorter that those not receiving TBI by a few inches. TBI can also result in other endocrine abnormalities, including growth hormone deficiency, thyroid hormone disturbances, and delayed puberty. Gonadal failure and infertility are also common.
   Organ-specific damage because of TBI includes:
   A. Heart: Late, progressive cardiotoxicity, especially if combined with anthracyclines or cyclophosphamide. This can result in cardiomyopathy, arrhythmias, and sudden death.
   B. Eyes: Posterior, subcapsular cataracts, usually 1 to 3 years after TBI.
   C. Brain/neuropsychological effects: Spectrum of deficits, including specific learning disabilities, attention deficit, and memory impairment. Younger children are more severely affected, and girls more than boys. There is also an increased risk in those with previous cranial irradiation.
   D. Oral cavity: Impaired growth of permanent teeth, tooth or root shortening, agenesis, decay, decreased saliva, disrupted enamel formation, and hypoplasia of the mandible and maxilla.

BIBLIOGRAPHY

1. Al Hamed R, Bazarbachi AH, Mohty M. Epstein-Barr virus-related post-transplant lymphoproliferative disease (EBV-PTLD) in the setting of allogeneic stem cell transplantation: a comprehensive review from pathogenesis to forthcoming treatment modalities. *Bone Marrow Transplant.* 2020;55(1):25–39.
2. Balduzzi A, Dalle JH, Jahnukainen K, et al. Fertility preservation issues in pediatric hematopoietic stem cell transplantation: practical approaches from the consensus of the Pediatric Diseases Working Party of the EBMT and the International BFM Study Group. *Bone Marrow Transplant.* 2017;52(10):1406–1415.
3. Cahn JY, Klein JP, Lee SJ, et al. Prospective evaluation of 2 acute graft-versus-host (GVHD) grading systems: a joint Société Française de Greffe de Moëlle et Thérapie Cellulaire (SFGM-TC), Dana Farber Cancer Institute (DFCI), and International Bone Marrow Transplant Registry (IBMTR) prospective study. *Blood.* 2005;106(4):1495–1500.
4. Cairo MS, Cooke KR, Lazarus HM, et al. Modified diagnostic criteria, grading classification and newly elucidated pathophysiology of hepatic SOS/VOD after haematopoietic cell transplantation. *Br J Haematol.* 2020;190(6):822–836.
5. Corbacioglu S, Carreras E, Ansari M, et al. Diagnosis and severity criteria for sinusoidal obstruction syndrome/veno-occlusive disease in pediatric patients: a new classification from the European society for blood and marrow transplantation. *Bone Marrow Transplant.* 2018;53(2):138–145.

6. Dulery R, Salleron J, Dewilde A, et al. Early human herpesvirus type 6 reactivation after allogeneic stem cell transplantation: a large-scale clinical study. *Biol Blood Marrow Transplant.* 2012;18(7):1080–1089.

7. Dvorak CC, Higham C, Shimano KA. Transplant-associated thrombotic microangiopathy in pediatric hematopoietic cell transplant recipients: a practical approach to diagnosis and management. *Front Pediatr.* 2019;7:133.

8. Einsele H, Ljungman P, Boeckh M. How I treat CMV reactivation after allogeneic hematopoietic stem cell transplantation. *Blood.* 2020;135(19):1619–1629.

9. Gatza E, Reddy P, Choi SW. Prevention and treatment of acute graft-versus-host disease in children, adolescents, and young adults. *Biol Blood Marrow Transplant.* 2020;26(5):e101–e112.

10. Haider S, Durairajan N, Soubani AO. Noninfectious pulmonary complications of haematopoietic stem cell transplantation. *Eur Respir Rev.* 2020;29(156).

11. Jodele S, Laskin BL, Dandoy CE, et al. A new paradigm: diagnosis and management of HSCT-associated thrombotic microangiopathy as multi-system endothelial injury. *Blood Rev.* 2015;29(3):191-204.

12. Kruizinga MD, van Tol MJD, Bekker V, et al. Risk factors, treatment, and immune dysregulation in autoimmune cytopenia after allogeneic hematopoietic stem cell transplantation in pediatric patients. *Biol Blood Marrow Transplant.* 2018;24(4):772–778.

13. Lindemans CA, Leen AM, Boelens JJ. How I treat adenovirus in hematopoietic stem cell transplant recipients. *Blood.* 2010;116 (25):5476–5485.

14. Ozdemir ZN, Civriz Bozdağ S. Graft failure after allogeneic hematopoietic stem cell transplantation. *Transfus Apher Sci.* 2018;57 (2):163–167.

15. Ruderfer D, Wu M, Wang T, et al. BK virus epidemiology, risk factors, and clinical outcomes: an analysis of hematopoietic stem cell transplant patients at Texas Children's Hospital. *J Pediatric Infect Dis Soc.* 2021;10(4):492–501.

16. Sarantopoulos S, Cardones AR, Sullivan KM. How I treat refractory chronic graft-versus-host disease. *Blood.* 2019;133(11):1191 1200.

17. Tomblyn M, Chiller T, Einsele H, et al. Guidelines for preventing infectious complications among hematopoietic cell transplantation recipients: a global perspective. *Biol Blood Marrow Transplant.* 2009;15(10):1143–1238.

18. Wolff DLA. Chronic Graft-Versus-Host Disease. In: Carreras E, Dufour C, Mohty M, Kröger N (eds). *The EBMT Handbook.* Springer Open, 2019:331–345.

INDEX

Note: Page numbers followed by *f* indicate figures, *t* indicate tables, and *b* indicate boxes.